The Musculoskeletal System

Commissioning Editor: Timothy Horne
Development Editor: Lulu Stader
Project Manager: Janaki Srinivasan Kumar
Designer/Design Direction: Charles Gray
Illustration Manager: Gillian Richards

SYSTEMS OF THE BODY

The Musculoskeletal System

BASIC SCIENCE AND CLINICAL CONDITIONS

SECOND EDITION

Philip Sambrook OAM MBBS
MD LLB FRACP
Florance & Cope Professor of Rheumatology
Institute of Bone & Joint Research
University of Sydney
Royal North Shore Hospital
St Leonards, Sydney, Australia

Thomas Taylor DPHIL(Oxon)
FRACS FRCS FRCS(Ed)
Emeritus Professor
Department of Orthopaedics and Traumatic Surgery
University of Sydney
Royal North Shore Hospital
St Leonards, Sydney, Australia

Leslie Schrieber MD, FRACP
Associate Professor
Department of Rheumatology
University of Sydney
Royal North Shore Hospital
St Leonards, Sydney, Australia

Andrew M. Ellis OAM MBBS
FRACS(Orth) FAOrthA
Visiting Medical Officer Orthopaedics
and Traumatic Surgery
Royal North Shore Hospital
St Leonards, Sydney, Australia
LTCOL Royal Australian Army Medical Corps.

Illustrations by Ethan Danielson

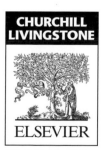

CHURCHILL
LIVINGSTONE

ELSEVIER

EDINBURGH LONDON NEW YORK OXFORD PHILADELPHIA ST LOUIS SYDNEY TORONTO 2010

CHURCHILL
LIVINGSTONE
ELSEVIER

First Edition © 2001 Elsevier Limited.
Second Edition © 2010 Elsevier Limited. All rights reserved.

ISBN: 978-0-7020-3377-3

British Library Cataloguing in Publication Data
A catalogue record for this book is available from the British Library

Library of Congress Cataloging in Publication Data
A catalog record for this book is available from the Library of Congress

Notice
Knowledge and best practice in this field are constantly changing. As new research and experience broaden our knowledge, changes in practice, treatment and drug therapy may become necessary or appropriate. Readers are advised to check the most current information provided (i) on procedures featured or (ii) by the manufacturer of each product to be administered, to verify the recommended dose or formula, the method and duration of administration, and contraindications. It is the responsibility of the practitioner, relying on their own experience and knowledge of the patient, to make diagnoses, to determine dosages and the best treatment for each individual patient, and to take all appropriate safety precautions. To the fullest extent of the law, neither the Publisher nor the Editors assume any liability for any injury and/or damage to persons or property arising out of or related to any use of the material contained in this book.

The Publisher

 ELSEVIER your source for books, journals and multimedia in the health sciences

www.elsevierhealth.com

Printed in China

Working together to grow
libraries in developing countries

www.elsevier.com | www.bookaid.org | www.sabre.org

ELSEVIER **BOOK AID International** Sabre Foundation

The Publisher's policy is to use **paper manufactured from sustainable forests**

Chapter 1 Rheumatoid arthritis and the hand
Leslie Schrieber MD FRACP
Associate Professor, Department of Rheumatology, Sydney Medical School, Royal North Shore Hospital, St Leonards, Sydney, Australia

Chapter 2 Soft tissue rheumatic disease involving the shoulder and elbow
David H. Sonnabend MB BS MD BSc(Med) FRACS FAOrthA
Professor, Department of Orthopaedics and Traumatic Surgery, Sydney Medical School, Royal North Shore Hospital, Sydney, Australia

Chapter 3 Nerve compression syndromes
Michael Tonkin MB BS MD FRCS(EdOrth) FRACS
Professor of Hand Surgery, Sydney Medical School, Royal North Shore Hospital, Sydney, Australia

Chapter 4 Back pain
Les Barnsley BMed(Hons) GradDipEpi PhD FRACP FAFRM(RACP)
Associate Professor, Department of Medicine, Sydney Medical School, Head of Department of Rheumatology, Concord Hospital, Sydney, Australia

Chapter 5 Bone structure and function in normal and disease states
Philip Sambrook OAM MB BS MD LLB FRACP
Florance & Cope Professor of Rheumatology, Institute of Bone & Joint Research, Sydney Medical School, Royal North Shore Hospital, St Leonards, Sydney, Australia

Chapter 6 Articular cartilage in health and disease
Christopher B. Little BSc MSc BVMS PhD Diplomate ACVS
Associate Professor, Raymond Purves Bone and Joint Research Laboratories, Kolling Institute of Medical Research, Institute of Bone and Joint Research, Sydney Medical School, Royal North Shore Hospital, St Leonards, Sydney, Australia

and

Lyn March MB BS MSc PhD FRACP FAFPHM
Associate Professor, Department of Medicine, Sydney Medical School, and Director of Rheumatology, Westmead Hospital, Sydney, Australia

Chapter 7 Crystal arthropathies and the ankle
Neil McGill MB BS BSc(Med) FRACP
Visiting Rheumatologist, Royal Prince Alfred Hospital, Sydney, Australia

Chapter 8 Disorders of skeletal muscle
Rodger Laurent MD MMedEd, FRACP
Senior Staff Rheumatologist, University of Sydney, Royal North Shore Hospital, St Leonards, Sydney, Australia

Chapter 9 Autoimmunity and the musculoskeletal system
Nicholas Manolios MD PhD FRACP FRCPA
Associate Professor, Department of Medicine, University of Sydney, and Director of Rheumatology, Westmead Hospital, Sydney, Australia

Chapter 10 Trauma and the musculoskeletal system
Andrew M. Ellis OAM MBBS FRACS(Orth) FAOrthA
Visiting Medical Officer, Orthopaedics and Traumatic Surgery, Royal North Shore Hospital, St Leonards, Sydney, Australia
LTCOL Royal Australian Army Medical Corps.

and

Thomas Taylor DPhil(Oxon) FRACS FRCS FRCS(Ed)
Emeritus Professor, Department of Orthopaedics and Traumatic Surgery, Sydney Medical School, Royal North Shore Hospital, St Leonards, Sydney, Australia

Chapter 11 Infection and the musculoskeletal system
Sydney Nade DSc MD MB BS BSc(Med) FRCS FRACS MRCP(UK) FAOrthA
Clinical Professor, Discipline of Surgery, Sydney Medical School, Sydney, Australia

ACKNOWLEDGEMENTS

This project has been made possible mainly as a result of the teaching staff in the Departments of Medicine and Surgery at the University of Sydney. We also wish to thank the leadership of Timothy Horne, Lulu Stader and Janaki Srinivasan and their wonderful team of illustrators to whom we are indebted.

This book is aimed primarily at medical students. In the past, many medical courses have been structured to teach, progressively, anatomy, physiology, pathology, pharmacology and, finally, clinical medicine. In line with new curricula of many medical schools, the aim of this book is to integrate basic with clinical science, using a problem-based learning approach. The first edition was a great success with much positive feedback and we have kept that model in the second edition, while updating the book to reflect the many new advances in the field. However, the self-assessment material now appears on the book's website.

Since musculoskeletal disorders account for about 20% of all visits to primary care physicians, it is essential that medical students have a good working knowledge and understanding of the relevant basic and clinical sciences to allow them to diagnose and treat such disorders. We believe that the ideal approach is problem-based learning and each chapter is devoted to a specific musculoskeletal pathology, illustrated by an appropriate case or cases. The book has been developed for that purpose. It is not

a comprehensive textbook of rheumatology or orthopaedics, however many primary care physicians will find it useful to revise and update their knowledge about specific diseases.

In each chapter, a major rheumatic disease is introduced by a clinical case. This is followed by the relevant basic science in an integrated fashion so that the anatomy, biochemistry and physiology necessary to understand that disease are explained. Each of the chapters is written by a different experienced clinician; however, the approach to each follows a similar format that makes it easy for the reader to understand.

We are proud of the second edition of this book and confident that it represents a novel and practical guide to the teaching of musculoskeletal disorders in most medical schools. We anticipate that this will translate to better management of musculoskeletal conditions by primary care physicians.

CONTENTS

CONTENTS

RHEUMATOID ARTHRITIS AND THE HAND

Leslie Schrieber

Chapter objectives

After studying this chapter you should be able to:

1. Explain the structure and function of synovial joints.

2. Understand the relevant anatomy of the hand and wrist joints.

3. Discuss the basic function of the immune system.

4. Understand the aetiopathogenesis of rheumatoid arthritis.

5. Describe the pathological changes that occur in inflammatory arthritis.

6. Recognize the common clinical presentations and features of rheumatoid arthritis and their pathophysiological basis.

7. Develop an approach to the differential diagnosis of inflammatory arthritis.

8. Describe extra-articular manifestations of rheumatoid arthritis and explain their pathophysiological basis.

9. Understand the principles that govern the team approach to the management of rheumatoid arthritis.

10. Describe the clinical pharmacology and use of non-steroidal anti-inflammatory drugs, corticosteroids, disease-modifying anti-rheumatic drugs and biological therapies in the treatment of rheumatoid arthritis.

11. Discuss the place of orthopaedic surgery in the treatment of rheumatoid arthritis.

12. Appreciate the long-term prognosis of rheumatoid arthritis.

Introduction

Synovial joints, the most mobile type of joints in the body, are susceptible to inflammatory injury leading to arthritis. The synovium is a common target of a variety of insults including direct microbial infection, crystal deposition and autoimmune attack, e.g. in rheumatoid arthritis (RA). This chapter will review normal synovial joint structure and function, the processes that lead to inflammatory arthritis, an approach to differential diagnosis, and the principles of treatment of RA. The topic and discussion will be illustrated by a patient with inflammatory arthritis found to have RA. It is the commonest chronic inflammatory rheumatic disease, affecting 1–2% of the population. RA not only produces extensive morbidity, but also is associated with a reduction in life expectancy.

Essential anatomy and physiology

Synovial joint anatomy

There are three types of joints in the body: synarthroses, amphiarthroses and diarthroses (synovial joints). Synarthroses are joints that have an interlocking suture line between adjacent bones (e.g. skull bones)—this provides a very strong bond. The synarthrosis grows during maturation of the developing brain and is eventually replaced by bony union between the adjacent bones. Amphiarthroses are joints that have fibrocartilage between adjacent bones—this allows for flexibility. They are found in the rib cage, the sacroiliac joint and between vertebral bodies—the intervertebral discs.

Case 1.1   Rheumatoid arthritis: 1

Case history

Mrs Gale is a 43-year-old woman who, together with her husband, runs a domestic cleaning company. She presents with a 9-month history of painful hands and wrists. Her symptoms started with occasional early-morning stiffness and swelling in her right knee, followed shortly afterwards by similar symptoms in her hands and wrists. Mrs Gale says she is no longer able to help her husband in the cleaning business. The pain is getting worse. Physical examination reveals symmetrical soft-tissue swelling in all of the proximal interphalangeal and metacarpophalangeal joints of both hands and wrists. Her right knee joint is swollen and has an effusion. The metatarsophalangeal joints are tender to palpation.

A provisional diagnosis of an inflammatory arthritis, probably rheumatoid arthritis, is made. Interpretation of this presentation requires knowledge of synovial joint structure in general and the hands in particular as well as knowledge of the immune system in health and disease.

Synovial, or diarthrodial joints, are the commonest type of joint and are the most mobile. They possess a synovial membrane, have a cavity that contains synovial fluid, and are subclassified into ball and socket (e.g. hip), hinge (e.g. interphalangeal) and saddle (e.g. first carpometacarpal) types. These joints (Fig. 1.1) allow the cartilaginous surfaces of the joint ends to move efficiently and smoothly, with low frictional resistance. Different designs allow for different movements, including flexion (bending), extension (straightening), abduction (movement away

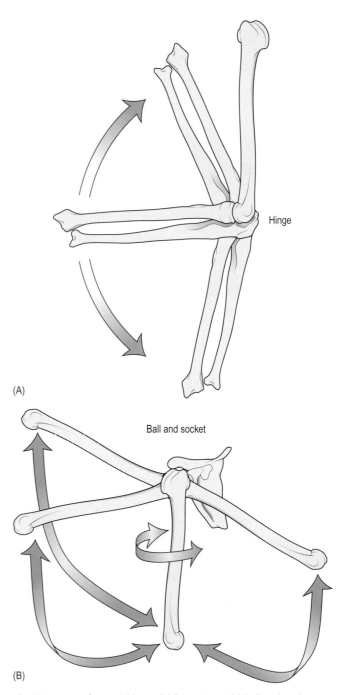

Hinge

(A)

Ball and socket

(B)

Fig. 1.1 Types of synovial joint: (A) hinge joint; (B) ball and socket joint.

from midline), adduction (movement towards midline), and rotation. They are more susceptible to inflammatory injury than are other types of joints.

Synovial joints are surrounded by a capsule that defines the boundary between articular and periarticular structures (Fig. 1.2). Reinforcing the capsule are ligaments and muscular tendons, which act across the joint. The joint capsule, ligaments and tendons are composed principally of type 1 collagen fibres—type 1 collagen is the major fibrous protein of connective tissue.

The synovium has a lining layer that consists of special cells called synoviocytes and is normally one to three cells thick. There is no basement membrane separating the synoviocyte layer from the subintima (Fig. 1.3). There are at least two different types of synoviocyte cell: type A and type B. Type A are of bone marrow-derived macrophage (phagocyte or 'hungry cell') lineage and type B are fibroblast-like mesenchymal (connective tissue) cells. Other cell types in this layer include dendritic cells—antigen-processing cells involved in generating an immune response. The synoviocytes lie in a stroma composed of collagen fibrils and proteoglycans (a diverse group of glycosylated proteins that are abundant in the extracellular matrix of connective tissues), which is continuous with the subintima. The latter may be fibrous, fatty or areolar (contain loose connective tissue). It contains a dense network of fenestrated capillaries (small blood vessels) that facilitate the exchange of molecules between the circulation and the synovium. The vessels are derived from branches of the arterial plexus that supplies the joint capsule and juxta-articular bone. There is also a lymphatic supply—a vascular system involved in removing large molecules from the synovium. The latter is innervated and pain sensitive, particularly during inflammation.

Synovial joint physiology

Normal synovial joints are highly effective in allowing low-friction movement between articulating surfaces. Articular cartilage is elastic, fluid-filled and supported by a relatively impervious layer of calcified cartilage and bone. Load-induced compression of cartilage forces interstitial fluid to flow laterally within the tissue through adjacent cartilage. This assists in protecting the cartilage against mechanical injury.

Synovial fluid (Fig. 1.4) is present in small quantities in normal synovial joints. It is a clear, relatively acellular,

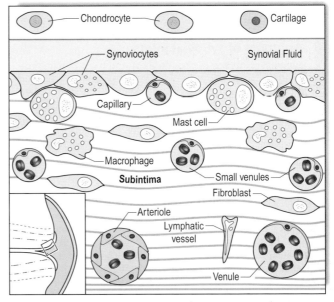

Fig. 1.3 Histology of a normal synovial joint.

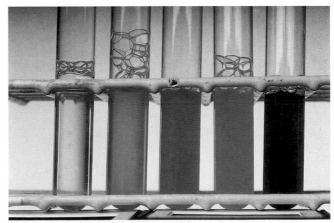

Fig. 1.4 Synovial fluid—macroscopic appearance, from left to right: normal or osteoarthritis; inflammatory (e.g. rheumatoid arthritis); gout; septic; and haemarthrosis (blood).

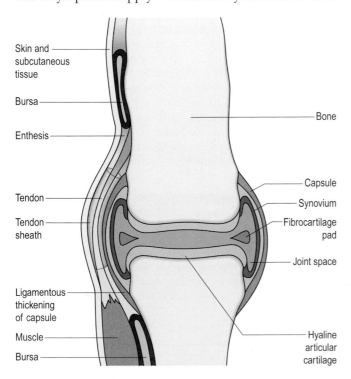

Fig. 1.2 Structure of a synovial joint.

RHEUMATOID ARTHRITIS AND THE HAND

viscous fluid that covers the surface of synovium and cartilage. Synovial fluid is an ultrafiltrate of blood to which hyaluronic acid is added. Hyaluronic acid is secreted by synoviocytes and is the molecule responsible for synovial fluid viscosity, acting as a lubricant for synovial–cartilage interaction. Synovial fluid represents an important site for exchange of nutrients and metabolic by-products between plasma and the surrounding synovial membrane. The synovial cavity can be used to advantage as a site in which therapeutic agents are introduced, e.g. intra-articular corticosteroids to treat inflamed synovium, as well as for diagnostic aspiration.

Normal synovial fluid contains only small quantities of low molecular weight proteins compared with plasma. The barrier to the entry of proteins probably resides within the synovial microvascular endothelium (cells that line the synovial microcirculation).

Interesting facts

Anatomy of synovial joints

Synovial joints are the commonest and most mobile type of joint in the body. They possess a synovial membrane and have a cavity that contains synovial fluid. They are subclassified into ball and socket (e.g. hip), hinge (e.g. interphalangeal) and saddle (e.g. first carpometacarpal) types.

Interesting facts

Synovial fluid

Synovial fluid, present in small quantities in normal synovial joints, is a clear, relatively acellular, viscous fluid that covers the surface of synovium and cartilage. It is an ultrafiltrate of blood to which hyaluronic acid is added. Hyaluronic acid is secreted by synoviocytes and is the molecule responsible for synovial fluid viscosity, acting as a lubricant for synovial–cartilage interaction.

Anatomy of the hand and wrist joints

Joints and synovial membranes

The proximal and distal interphalangeal joints are true hinge joints whose movements are restricted to flexion and extension. Each joint has a thin dorsal (upper surface) capsular ligament strengthened by expansion of the extensor tendon, a dense palmar (under surface) ligament, and collateral ligaments on either side of the joint. The metacarpophalangeal joints are also considered hinge joints and their ligaments resemble those of the interphalangeal joints. When the fingers are flexed, the heads of the metacarpal bones form the rounded prominences of the knuckles, with the joint space lying about 1 cm distal (peripheral) to the apices of the knuckles. Figure 1.5 shows the relationship of the dorsal and lateral aspects of the joint space, synovial membrane and the articular capsule to adjacent structures.

The wrist or radiocarpal joint is formed proximally by the distal end of the radius and the articular disc, and distally by a row of carpal bones, the scaphoid, lunate, pisiform and triquetrum (Fig. 1.5A). The articular disc joins the radius to the ulnar and separates the distal end of the ulnar from the wrist joint proper. The wrist joint is surrounded by a capsule and supported by ligaments.

The distal radioulnar joint is adjacent to but not normally part of the wrist joint, since the articular disc divides these joints into separate cavities (Fig. 1.5A). The midcarpal joint is formed by the junction of the proximal and distal rows of the carpal bones. Limited flexion, extension and some rotation occur in the midcarpal joint. Pronation and supination occur primarily at the proximal and distal radioulnar articulations.

Tendons

The long flexor tendons of the muscles of the forearm are enclosed in a common flexor tendon sheath that begins proximal to the wrist crease and extends to the midpalm (Fig. 1.6). Part of the common flexor tendon sheath lies in the carpal tunnel and is bounded anteriorly by the flexor retinaculum (a ligament that lies on the volar surface of the wrist). Thickening of the synovial membrane of the flexor tendons because of synovitis can cause carpal tunnel syndrome (see Ch. 3).

The extensor tendons of the forearm pass through fibro-osseous tunnels on the dorsum of the wrist. These tunnels, which are lined with a synovial sheath, are bounded superficially by the extensor retinaculum and on the deep surface by the carpal bones and ligaments. A depression over the dorsolateral aspect of the wrist when the thumb is extended and abducted is called the anatomical snuffbox. It is formed by the tendons of abductor pollicis longus and extensor pollicis brevis muscles and is limited proximally by the radial styloid process. Tenderness in this region can be due to stenosing tenosynovitis of these tendons (a condition called de Quervain's tenosynovitis). In this condition, placing the thumb in the palm of the hand, flexing the fingers over the thumb and adducting the wrist will usually produce severe pain (Finkelstein's manoeuvre).

Essential immunology

The immune system has developed principally as a means to help the host combat microbial infection. The human body uses a number of mechanisms to achieve this objective, some innate and non-specific, others involving exquisitely precise targeted processes.

Innate mechanisms

Innate defence mechanisms include the protective effects of intact skin and mucosa in combating microbes. Normal skin acts as an impermeable barrier to most infectious agents. Mucus secreted by the membranes lining the inner surfaces of the body (e.g. nasal and bronchial mucosa) acts as a protective barrier that prevents bacteria adhering to epithelial cells.

A variety of white blood cells, including polymorphonuclear neutrophils (PMNs) and macrophages, can act as important lines of defence against microbial attack. These cells, derived from bone marrow precursors, are capable of eliminating microbes following their phagocytosis (uptake). The cells are rich in digestive enzymes that aid in elimination of these microbes. PMNs are short-lived cells, whereas macrophages may remain in connective tissues for prolonged periods. PMNs are principally involved in host defence against pus-forming bacteria, while macrophages are better at combating intracellular microbes, including certain bacteria, viruses and protozoa. No prior exposure to the microorganism is necessary for these leukocytes to act.

Another innate line of defence against microbes is the complement system. This comprises over 20 proteins. The complement system is able to respond rapidly to a trigger stimulus, resulting in activation of a sequential cascade in which one reaction is the enzymatic catalyst of the next (Fig. 1.7). The most important complement component is C3, which facilitates the uptake and removal of microbes by enhancing their adherence to the surface of phagocytic cells. Biologically active fragments of C3–C3a, and C5a are able to attract PMNs (called chemotaxis) as well as activating these cells. Activated complement components later in this sequence, C6, 7, 8 and 9, form a complex—the membrane attack complex—on the surface of target cells and this is able to punch holes in the cell membrane, resulting in target cell lysis.

There are a variety of other humoral defence mechanisms mediated by soluble factors that assist in containing microbial infection. These include acute phase proteins such as C-reactive protein, alpha-1-antiprotease and alpha-2-macroglobulin and the interferons. The latter are a family of broad-spectrum antiviral agents that are synthesized by cells when infected by viruses. They limit the spread of virus to other cells.

Humans as well as many lower-order animals have developed more selective mechanisms to combat infection, involving humoral or antibody and cellular systems.

Antibodies

Antibodies are remarkable proteins produced by bone-marrow derived B lymphocytes, which are able to differentiate into plasma cells. Antibodies are adaptor molecules that are capable of binding to phagocytic cells, activating complement and binding to microbes. Each antibody has a unique recognition site for a particular microbe—the Fab end of the molecule, which binds microbes (Fig. 1.8). Molecules in the microorganism that evoke and react with antibodies are called antigens. The Fc end of the antibody molecule contains domains capable of binding and activating the first component of complement

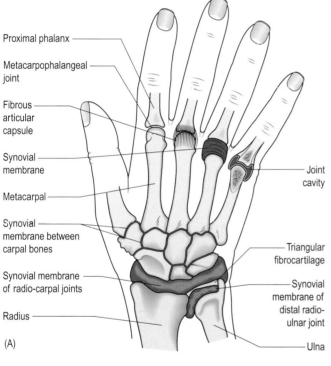

Proximal phalanx
Metacarpophalangeal joint
Fibrous articular capsule
Synovial membrane
Metacarpal
Synovial membrane between carpal bones
Synovial membrane of radio-carpal joints
Radius
(A)
Joint cavity
Triangular fibrocartilage
Synovial membrane of distal radio-ulnar joint
Ulna

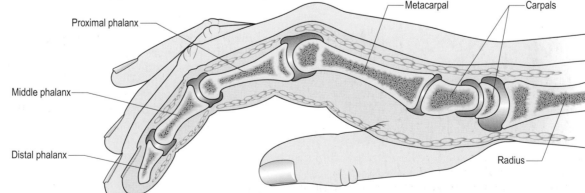

Metacarpal
Carpals
Proximal phalanx
Middle phalanx
Distal phalanx
Radius
(B)

Fig. 1.5 Relationship of the synovial membranes of the wrist and metacarpal joints to adjacent bones: (A) dorsal view; (B) sagittal view showing in addition proximal and distal interphalangeal joints.

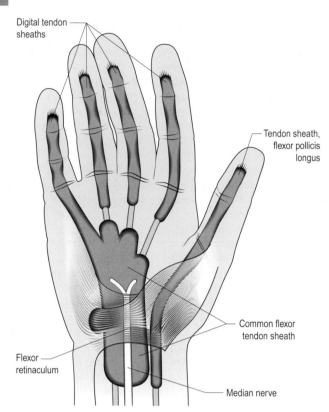

Fig. 1.6 Palmar view of the hand showing distribution of the synovial sheaths and flexor tendons.

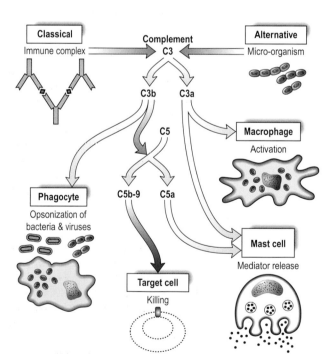

Fig. 1.7 The complement system: the classical complement pathway is activated by immune complexes of antibodies and antigens, while the alternative pathway is promoted by the lipopolysaccharide component of the cell wall of bacteria. Both result in conversion of C3 to C3b, which activates the terminal lytic complement sequence.

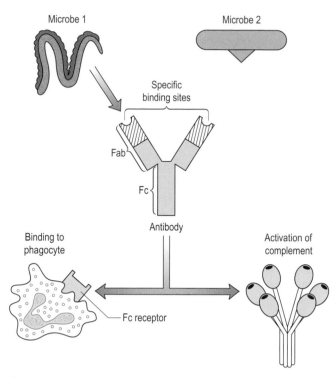

Fig. 1.8 The structure of an immunoglobulin: the antibody is an adaptable molecule able to bind specifically to microbial antigen 1, but not antigen 2 via its Fab end. The Fc end is able to activate complement and to bind to the Fc receptor on host phagocytic cells.

as well as binding to phagocyte Fc receptors. There are five antibody subtypes, classified by variations in the structure of the Fab region: IgG, IgM, IgA, IgD and IgE.

There is an enormous variety of B lymphocytes, each programmed to synthesize a single antibody specificity. These antibodies are expressed on the lymphocyte cell surface and act as a receptor for antigens. This process is highly selective; for example, antibodies that recognize tetanus toxoid antigen do not recognize influenza virus, and vice versa. On exposure to antigen, B lymphocytes with the corresponding cell surface antibody specificity, bind to the cell and deliver activation signals. This leads to their differentiation into plasma cells and synthesis and secretion of specific antibodies. The activated B lymphocytes also undergo proliferation, resulting in expansion of the number of clones capable of producing the same antibody. Antibody production in response to antigenic challenge is referred to as an acquired immune response.

Even after the elimination of a microbial antigen trigger, some B lymphocytes remain and have a 'memory' of this exposure. On subsequent challenge with the same antigen, the body responds by synthesizing antibody faster and in greater quantities than on the first exposure. This is the secondary immune response.

The ability to recognize a particular antigen and distinguish it from a different antigen is related to the ability to distinguish between self-antigen and non-self (i.e. foreign) antigens. There is an active process by which self-antigen fails to induce an immune response, known as tolerance.

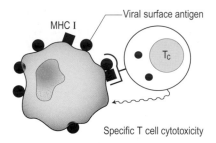

Fig. 1.9 Cytotoxic T cells are able to recognize viral surface antigen in association with MHC class 1 molecules and subsequently lyse the target cell.

In some circumstances, tolerance is broken and the individual produces self-directed antibodies known as autoantibodies. These may give rise to autoimmune diseases. Another autoimmune disease, systemic lupus erythematosus, is discussed in Chapter 9.

Cell-mediated immunity

Many microbes live inside host cells out of the reach of antibodies. Viruses can live inside host cells, such as macrophages, where they replicate. Thus a different form of immune defence, known as cell-mediated immunity, is required to combat intracellular infection. This involves T or thymus-derived lymphocytes. T cells only recognize antigen when it is presented on the surface of a host cell. There are T cell receptors present on the cell surface, distinct from antibody receptors, which recognize antigen. A further complexity is that antigen is recognized in association with another cell surface molecule known as the major histocompatibility complex (MHC) expressed on the target cell. The MHC plays an important role in organ transplant rejection.

A macrophage that has been infected with a virus is able to process small antigenic components of the virus and place these on its surface. A subpopulation of T lymphocytes, known as T helper cells, primed to that antigen, recognize and bind to the combination of antigen and class 2 MHC molecules. These T cells also secrete a range of soluble products known as lymphokines. The latter include gamma interferon, which stimulates microbicidal mechanisms in the macrophage that help to kill the intracellular microbe.

There is also another subpopulation of T lymphocytes, known as cytotoxic T cells, which recognize antigen expressed on the surface of target cells in association with MHC class 1 molecules (Fig. 1.9). The cytotoxic T cell comes into direct contact with the target cell and kills it. Just as is true for B cells, T cells selected and activated by binding antigen undergo clonal proliferation and mature to produce T helper and cytotoxic cells and produce memory cells. The latter can be reactivated upon further antigenic challenge.

For maximal T cell responses, second signals are usually required. Two of the co-stimulatory molecules

through which these signals are provided are CD28 and CD40 ligand. Both of these molecules are expressed by synovial T cells in RA. One of the newer biological therapies for RA, Abatacept, specifically targets this interaction.

In summary, a wide range of innate and adaptive immunological mechanisms has evolved to protect the host against microbial infection. In some circumstances the host becomes a target for these responses, resulting in autoimmune disease.

Pathology

Synovitis

To gain a better appreciation of the processes occurring within an inflamed joint, it is necessary to understand synovial pathology. However, in clinical practice a synovial biopsy is not routinely performed as part of the diagnosis of inflammatory arthritis.

In RA, the classical example of an inflammatory arthropathy, the synovium undergoes characteristic histological changes, but these are not disease-specific. Eventually, they may progress to destruction of articular cartilage and result in joint subluxation or ankylosis (bridging of adjacent bones).

In the early stages of RA, the synovium becomes oedematous (contains excess fluid), thickened, hyperplastic (cells multiply excessively) and develops villus-like projections as found in normal small intestine (Fig. 1.10A). The synovial lining layer undergoes cellular proliferation and becomes multilayered. One of the earliest histological changes is injury to the synovial microvasculature, with swelling of endothelial cells, widened interendothelial gaps and luminal occlusion. There is dense synovial cellular infiltration with prominent perivascular T lymphocytes, plasma cells and macrophages, but few neutrophils (Fig. 1.10B). Prominent fibrin deposition is characteristic. Lymphoid nodular aggregates composed principally of CD4 T (helper) cells may be found in the synovial stroma (Fig. 1.10C), but are more likely to develop later in the disease. By contrast, in the synovial fluid there is a predominance of neutrophils. RA often involves periarticular structures including tendon sheaths and bursae.

In the later stages of RA, the inflamed synovium develops a hyperaemic, fibrovascular granulation tissue known as *pannus* (Latin: 'piece of cloth'), which includes new blood vessel formation (angiogenesis). This spreads over and subsequently invades the articular cartilage. The pannus eventually destroys articular cartilage and invades bone, causing juxta-articular erosions and subchondral cysts. These can be seen on plain radiography and at an even earlier stage of disease using magnetic resonance imaging (MRI). It may lead to fibrosing ankylosis and loss of joint mobility. Joint instability and subluxation (partial dislocation) may arise from damage to the joint capsule, ligaments and tendons, as the inflammatory process extends. This may subsequently heal with fibrosis and

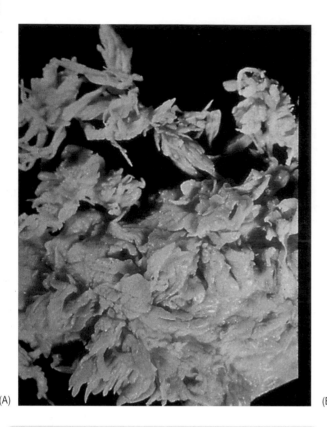

(A)

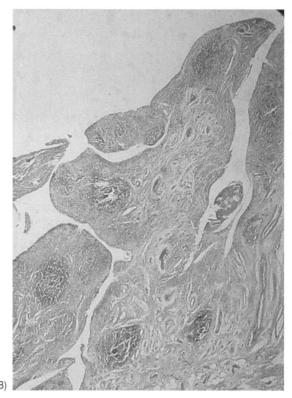

(B)

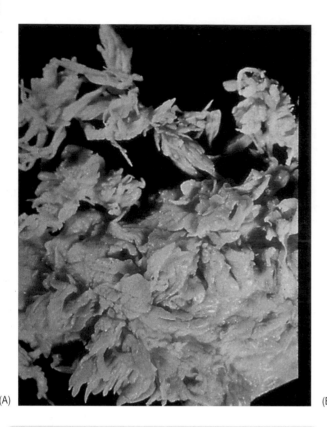

(C)

Fig. 1.10 Histopathology of a joint with rheumatoid arthritis.
(A) Early disease: low-power micrograph of inflamed synovium.
(B) Lymphoid nodular aggregates in synovial stroma (C) Diagram of
the histopathology of a rheumatoid joint.

lead to fixed deformities. The destruction of cartilage predisposes to secondary osteoarthritis.

Although RA predominantly involves synovial joints, it is a systemic disease and may affect many tissues and organs including skin, blood vessels, heart, lungs, muscles and eyes. The most characteristic extra-articular feature is the rheumatoid nodule, found in 25% of patients, typically in subcutaneous tissues over pressure areas. Rheumatoid nodules have a characteristic microscopic appearance, consisting of three distinct layers—a central zone of fibrinoid necrosis (pink-staining dead material) surrounded by palisading (fence-like) phagocytes arranged radially, and granulation tissue with inflammatory cells.

The synovium in the seronegative spondyloarthropathies may be difficult to distinguish microscopically from RA. Typically there is inflammation both in the synovium and bony entheses (the site of ligamentous and capsular insertion into bone)—enthesitis. The synovium does not usually develop extensive pannus formation and consequently, there is less invasion of bone and articular cartilage compared with RA. The enthesis becomes infiltrated by a non-specific granulation tissue. In severe forms of the disease, enthesopathy is followed by calcification and ossification, particularly in the spine and capsules of peripheral joints.

Differential diagnosis of inflammation of the synovium

Synovial joints are susceptible to inflammatory injury, probably because of their rich network of fenestrated

Box 1.1 Common causes of inflammatory arthritis

Microbial

- *Staphylococcus aureus*
- *Neisseria gonorrhoeae*
- Lyme disease (*Borrelia burgdorferi*)
- Hepatitis B virus
- Epstein–Barr virus
- Ross River fever virus

Crystal

- Sodium urate
- Calcium pyrophosphate dihydrate

Seronegative spondyloarthropathies

- Ankylosing spondylitis
- Psoriatic arthritis
- Arthritis associated with chronic bowel inflammation—ulcerative colitis and Crohn's disease
- Reactive arthritis

Autoimmune

- Rheumatoid arthritis
- Systemic lupus erythematosus

Other

- Polymyalgia rheumatica

capillaries. The synovium has only a limited number of ways in which it can respond to injury.

The synovium may be the target of a large number of insults including microbes, e.g. *Staphylococcus aureus* leading to septic arthritis; crystals, e.g. sodium urate leading to gouty arthritis; or autoimmune attack, e.g. RA in which the trigger is unknown (Box 1.1).

Determining the aetiological basis for synovitis may be difficult. Tender soft-tissue swelling and fluid (effusion) of synovial joints (as seen with Mrs Gale) indicates that the joint is inflamed, i.e. synovitis. Information on the following may enable a more precise diagnosis to be made:

- the pattern and distribution of joint involvement (symmetrical versus asymmetrical)

- the number of joints involved—one (monoarthritis), a few (<6—oligoarthritis) or multiple (>6—polyarthritis)

- the duration of inflammation (days, weeks or months)

- the type of trigger; and

- the presence of extra-articular features, e.g. fever, rashes.

The sudden onset of painful swelling of one joint—monoarthritis—raises the possibility of infection.

Microorganisms may lodge in the joint from a direct penetrating injury or, more commonly, by haematogenous (blood-borne) spread from a distant site during bacteraemia. Clinical pointers include fever and constitutional symptoms—sweating, rigors (shivers), malaise. However, these symptoms are not specific for infection and may occur in patients with RA. A cutaneous source of infection may give a clue, e.g. a boil or carbuncle. In the case of sexually active young women, *Neisseria gonorrhoeae* infection needs to be considered. This subject is covered in more detail in Chapter 11.

Sudden onset of monoarthritis, particularly in the big toe, in an older male raises the suspicion of crystal-induced arthritis due to sodium urate deposition. Uric acid, the end product of purine metabolism, may precipitate out of its usually soluble state, deposit in the synovium and produce acute inflammation. An acute attack is typically triggered by agents (alcohol and certain drugs) that raise serum uric acid levels and precipitate sodium urate crystal deposition. Clinically it presents with the sudden onset of exquisite pain in a joint—frequently the first metatarsophalangeal joint. The patient exhibits the classic signs of inflammation—local heat, erythema (redness), tenderness, swelling and loss of function. Another type of crystal that commonly produces monoarthritis is calcium pyrophosphate dihydrate. This usually affects middle-aged females and involves the knee joint. Crystal arthritis is covered in greater depth in Chapter 7.

Involvement of one or a limited number of joints in an asymmetric distribution raises the possibility of seronegative (i.e. rheumatoid factor negative) spondyloarthritis. The spondyloarthropathies, as the name implies, often have spinal involvement and include ankylosing spondylitis, psoriatic arthritis, colitic arthritis and reactive arthritis. These conditions typically manifest as an asymmetric arthritis involving one or several joints, including the spine and/or sacroiliac joints. There are often associated features that give clues to the diagnosis, e.g. presence of psoriasis (a red, scaly skin rash) or a history of inflammatory bowel disease (e.g. episodes of bloody diarrhoea). A recent episode of non-specific urethritis or bowel infection with *Salmonella* or *Shigella* microorganisms should raise the possibility of reactive arthritis. Patients may give a history of eye inflammation (e.g. iritis—inflammation of the iris) resulting in episodes of painful red eyes, or inflammation of ligamentous or tendinous insertions into bone (enthesitis) resulting in painful heels, for example. Patients with seronegative spondyloarthropathies frequently have a family history of the condition and there is an association with the white blood cell marker (histocompatibility locus antigen) HLA-B27. The latter is found in over 95% of Caucasian males with ankylosing spondylitis, but in only 6–8% of the normal population. How this genetic marker leads to disease predisposition is poorly understood. Tests for the autoantibody rheumatoid factor are negative—hence the term seronegative.

The pattern of disease onset in RA is quite variable. Although it often presents insidiously with the development of a symmetrical inflammatory arthritis involving multiple joints over weeks to months, a monoarticular onset, especially involving the knee (as in Mrs Gale's case), may antedate the development of symmetrical arthritis. The joints most commonly affected in polyarthritis with RA are the small joints of the hands (proximal interphalangeal and metacarpophalangeal joints), wrists, elbows, feet, knees and ankles. Later in the disease, large joints such as the hip and shoulder may be involved, but not usually at presentation. A family history of RA is often present. The patient usually complains of joint stiffness, especially in the morning, joint swelling and pain. The patient may also have systemic symptoms, such as weight loss and fatigue.

Polymyalgia rheumatica is an inflammatory arthropathy characterized by pain and stiffness, usually of sudden onset, predominantly affecting the limb girdle areas (shoulders and hips). It usually occurs in older subjects, is generally associated with a moderate to markedly elevated erythrocyte sedimentation rate (ESR) and C-reactive protein levels and is rapidly responsive to corticosteroids. It is often associated with giant cell arteritis, especially in the temporal arteries but any artery can be affected. Headache is the most common symptom but visual symptoms suggesting arteritis include transient and permanent visual loss. Biopsies characteristically show infiltrations of macrophages, T cells and multinucleated giant cells, the hallmark of the disease.

Aetiopathogenesis of rheumatoid arthritis

There are a diverse range of aetiologies for inflammatory arthritis—infection, crystal and autoimmune. The first two are discussed in the chapters on bone and joint infection (Ch. 11) and crystal arthritis (Ch. 7), respectively. Here, the aetiopathogenesis of RA is discussed (Fig. 1.11).

Although the cause of RA is unknown, genetic, microbial and immunological factors are thought to play a role in disease susceptibility. RA is one of a group of conditions in which immunogenetic responses are important.

As such, it joins the majority of autoimmune diseases in which genes known to exert influence on the immune response (immune response genes) are involved in disease pathogenesis. However, because the antigen(s) that trigger RA are unknown, the precise details remain elusive.

Major histocompatibility complex (MHC) genes, present on chromosome 6 in man, are important in determining host immune responses to foreign antigens. They play a vital role in organ transplantation and determine whether rejection of a graft occurs. They are also

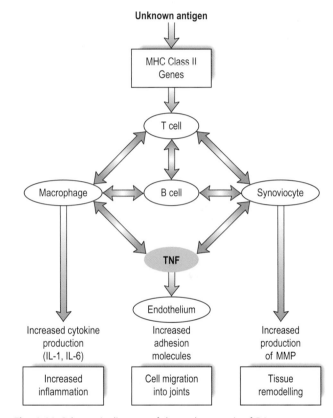

Fig. 1.11 Schematic diagram of the pathogenesis of RA.

Case 1.1 Rheumatoid arthritis: 2

Establishing the diagnosis

It comes to light that Mrs Gale's mother had severe RA and was disabled by her disease. Mrs Gale complains of fatigue, but gives no history of rashes, weight loss or change in bowel habit. The history of polyarthritis of insidious onset, symmetrical pattern of joint involvement, prominent early morning joint stiffness and positive family history of RA suggest a diagnosis of RA. However, to establish the diagnosis, radiological and laboratory investigation are warranted. A number of investigations are usually performed; the focus here is on synovial fluid analysis and joint X-rays.

Synovial fluid analysis

Synovial fluid aspiration, performed at the bedside, using a sterile no-touch technique is often helpful in determining the cause of inflammatory arthritis (Table 1.1). Typically in RA, the fluid is macroscopically (i.e. to the naked eye) cloudy, owing to the increased number of white cells it contains, and of low viscosity because of the biochemical degradation of hyaluronic acid (Fig. 1.4). This contrasts with normal synovial fluid, which is clear, colourless and highly viscous. Other features of the fluid may provide a diagnosis for the inflammatory arthritis, e.g. the presence of needle-shaped birefringent crystals in gout, or bacteria in septic arthritis.

Case 1.1 Rheumatoid arthritis: 2 (continued)

Table 1.1 Synovial fluid analysis in inflammatory arthritis

	Normal	RA	Gout	Septic
Colour	Colourless	Yellow	Yellow	Yellow
Clarity	Clear	Cloudy	Cloudy	Purulent
Viscosity	High	Low	Low	Low
White cell count (/mm³)	<1500	2–50 000	5–50 000	50–500 000
% neutrophils	<5	30–80	50–80	>95
Crystals	No	No	Yes	No
Bacteria	No	No	No	Yes

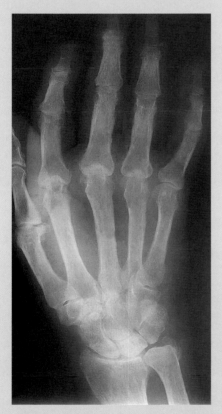

Fig. 1.12 X-ray showing bony erosion of metacarpophalangeal joint and proximal interphalangeal joint.

Joint X-rays

Plain X-rays of the hands and feet often provide useful diagnostic information in patients with inflammatory arthritis. The earliest changes in RA involving the hands are soft-tissue swelling of proximal interphalangeal and metacarpophalangeal joints. This corresponds with synovitis of affected joints. There is periarticular osteoporosis (bone thinning) thought to be secondary to increased blood flow through inflamed joints and local release of cytokines (molecules that are released by activated cells and are involved in signalling to other cells). However, these changes are not specific for RA and simply reflect joint inflammation. The most characteristic feature is the development of bony erosions that start at the periphery of the joint where the synovium reflects off the joint capsule. Erosions correspond with the site of local invasion by inflammatory synovial tissue, known as pannus, which grows into the adjacent bone and cartilage (Fig. 1.12), discussed below.

involved in predisposition to autoimmune diseases such as RA and systemic lupus erythematosus. There is a linkage of certain genes in this complex, known as DR, with susceptibility to RA. The best-described association of RA is with HLA-DR4.

Family studies have found that HLA haplotype sharing (i.e. individuals sharing the same genetic markers) is increased in family members affected by RA. Molecular analysis of the DR alleles (variations at this gene locus) associated with RA suggests that the genetic contribution

of MHC genes to RA is approximately 25%. Other genes thought to play a role in disease susceptibility to RA include immunoglobulin genes, genes controlling glycosylation patterns of immunoglobulin (i.e. the different type and amount of carbohydrate present) and T cell receptor genes. It must be remembered that RA has a complex multifactorial pathogenesis and, while immune response genes are important, environmental factors also play a role.

A microbial aetiology of RA has been postulated for many decades. Microorganisms that have been proposed to play a role include mycoplasma, mycobacteria and a number of viruses, e.g. Epstein–Barr virus. However, there is no convincing evidence for a microbial cause of RA.

That immunological and inflammatory processes play a role in the pathological expression of RA is undisputed. Although RA is a systemic disease, its hallmark is chronic inflammation in the synovium of multiple joints. It is best viewed as being an autoimmune disease, triggered by an unknown antigen. The initiating event of joint damage is thought to be triggering of autoreactive CD4 T helper lymphocytes by antigen(s) presented to these T cells. In early lesions, activated/memory T cells predominate in pericapillary sites beneath the synovial membrane. Accompanying the T cells are neutrophils, mast cells and mononuclear phagocytes that mature to activated macrophages.

In the earliest lesions, there is an increase in vascularity driven by angiogenesis-stimulating factors released from macrophages and fibroblasts. Both vessels and infiltrating cells have enhanced expression of intercellular adhesion molecules, especially intercellular adhesion molecule-1 (ICAM-1). As the lesion progresses, lymphoid cells organize into microenvironments similar to that seen in lymph nodes. Dendritic cells (specialized cells that present antigens to the immune system effectively) are found in these environments and are thought to provide the basis of local antibody production by B cells and ongoing T cell activation. Mature memory T cells promote antibody synthesis with little negative feedback.

Despite the importance of T cell involvement, the most active cells in synovial lesions are macrophages. The macrophage-derived cytokines interleukin (IL) -1, -6 and -8, tumour necrosis factor-alpha (TNF-α), and granulocyte-macrophage colony-stimulating factor (GM-CSF) are found in abundance within the rheumatoid synovium. Interleukins are a group of peptides that signal between cells of the immune system. By contrast, only low levels of T cell-derived cytokines, e.g. IL-2, IL-4 and interferon-gamma, can be detected. TNF-α is thought to be a central cytokine in the perpetuation of the inflammatory response. Indeed, anti-TNF treatment by monoclonal antibodies to TNF-α or TNF receptor blockade has been demonstrated to have a dramatic effect in reducing inflammatory disease activity in RA. Fibroblast-like cells also contribute to the cytokine network, particularly IL-6 and transforming growth factor beta (TGF-β). The latter is a downregulatory cytokine (i.e. it decreases inflammatory activity).

Pro-inflammatory cytokines predominate in rheumatoid synovium. They are responsible for:

- activation of adhesion molecule expression on blood vessels

- synovial recruitment of inflammatory cells (lymphocytes and other leukocytes)

- continuing activation of macrophages, fibroblasts and dendritic cells

- promoting angiogenesis.

Macrophages, neutrophils and fibroblasts produce large quantities of proteolytic enzymes including matrix metalloproteinases (MMPs)—enzymes that require cleavage by other proteases to become active. The matrix metalloproteinases—collagenase, gelatinase and stromelysin—mediate the degradation of joint tissues that accompanies the development of pannus.

Large quantities of antibody are present within the joint, including local production of rheumatoid factors (RF). The latter are autoantibodies of the IgM, IgG and IgA classes characterized by antigenic binding determinants on the constant region of human IgG. IgM RF are found in the serum of 70% of patients with RA and are associated with severe joint disease and extra-articular features, e.g. vasculitis (inflammation of blood vessels). Patients who have IgM RF in their serum are said to be seropositive. RF may participate in some of the clinical phenomena that occur in RA, e.g. vasculitis leading to leg ulcers or nodules. However, they are not specific for RA and may occur in other autoimmune diseases, e.g. Sjögren's syndrome, and occasionally in infectious diseases, e.g. bacterial endocarditis.

Recently, another auto-antibody has been described in the serum of patients with RA, namely anti-citrullinated protein antibodies and are highly specific for that disease. Citrullination is catalysed by peptidyl arginine deaminase. Citrullinated proteins are found in the synovium of patients with RA, but are not unique to that site or to that disease. Diagnostic kits which detect cyclic citrullinated protein antibodies are now challenging RFs as the most valuable test in the diagnosis of RA.

Pathophysiological basis of symptoms and signs of rheumatoid arthritis

Although RA is an autoimmune multisystem disease, its primary clinical manifestation usually relates to the involvement of synovial joints. The clinical features vary in severity between patients, as well as fluctuating over time in individual patients. The initial presentation of the disease is most commonly as a symmetrical inflammatory polyarthritis involving the hands (Fig. 1.13). Why the disease causes symmetrical joint involvement is unknown. The patient experiences pain, stiffness and swelling in the joints, that is characteristically worse in the morning. Joint swelling and pain are due to the presence of active inflammation in the synovium, i.e. synovitis or effusion. Systemic symptoms may be due to the presence of circulating cytokines such as TNF-β.

Joint deformity is not a typical feature of early disease and usually occurs only after the disease has been present for some time. Deformity arises secondary to damage caused by the pannus invading cartilage and bone. Radiological bone erosions may not be present at the time of diagnosis, but usually develop over months, or longer, with ongoing active disease. They reflect invasion of bone by pannus. Typical deformities include ulnar deviation of the digits at the metacarpophalangeal joints

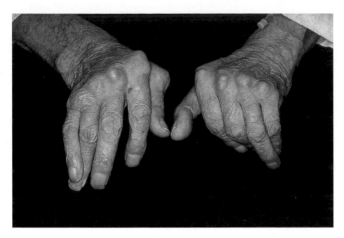

Fig. 1.13 The hands in rheumatoid arthritis.

Rheumatoid arthritis: 3

Case note: Management

Mrs Gale reports that she has noticed the development of small painless nodular lumps over the extensor surfaces of both elbows. Her general practitioner explains that she has RA and that the lumps are rheumatoid nodules. She will need to be treated with a comprehensive management programme. She is referred to the local branch of the Arthritis Foundation for information and is advised to attend their patient education programme. She is recommended to undertake a period of rest and commenced on naproxen 500 mg b.d., a non-steroidal anti-inflammatory drug. She is referred to a rheumatologist for advice about the use of disease-modifying anti-rheumatic drugs.

and swan-neck deformities of the fingers. Ulnar deviation results from the fingers being pulled in the ulnar direction by the natural pull of the forearm muscles in the presence of subluxation (partial dislocation) at the metacarpophalangeal joints. In a swan-neck deformity, the proximal interphalangeal joint is hyperextended and the distal interphalangeal joint flexed.

The temporal pattern of these clinical manifestations varies between patients. About one-third experience prolonged periods of remission. Another third demonstrate fluctuating disease activity characterized by periods of active joint inflammation interspersed with periods of more quiescent disease. The remaining third manifest progressive deforming joint damage with declining functional status over time. Mortality rates are increased in those with the most severe forms of the disease.

Rheumatoid arthritis as a systemic disease

RA may be more accurately termed rheumatoid disease, as it is a multisystem disease (Fig. 1.14), with the major clinical manifestation being polyarthritis. In addition to joint pain, stiffness and swelling, patients with RA often have systemic clinical features that can include fatigue, weight loss, low-grade fever and myalgia (muscle pain). Lymphadenopathy (enlarged lymph glands) is present in about 30% of patients with active disease, usually of axillary, epitrochlear (near the elbow) or inguinal regions, and biopsy shows reactive hyperplasia.

Patients often have a normochromic (normal colour), normocytic (normal-sized red blood cells) anaemia. This occurs commonly in patients with chronic inflammatory or infectious diseases and is due to ineffective bone marrow production of red blood cells. It is known as the anaemia of chronic disease. If the haemoglobin level drops below 10 g/L, other explanations besides RA should be looked for. Thrombocytosis (elevation of platelet count), common in active disease, returns to normal when the arthritis is controlled. The erythrocyte sedimentation

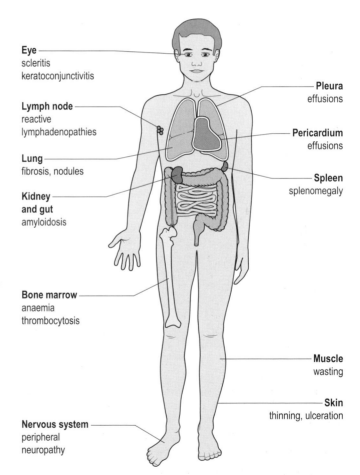

Eye
scleritis
keratoconjunctivitis

Lymph node
reactive
lymphadenopathies

Lung
fibrosis, nodules

**Kidney
and gut**
amyloidosis

Bone marrow
anaemia
thrombocytosis

Nervous system
peripheral
neuropathy

Pleura
effusions

Pericardium
effusions

Spleen
splenomegaly

Muscle
wasting

Skin
thinning, ulceration

Fig. 1.14 The organs commonly involved in rheumatoid arthritis.

rate (ESR) and serum C-reactive protein levels are often elevated and are used as markers of disease activity. The ESR is determined by counting the number of millimetres the red blood cells have settled from the top of the serum in a capillary tube after 60 minutes.

Rheumatoid nodules occur in 25% of patients, most commonly on the extensor surfaces of the forearms, but they can occur at any site where there is pressure (Fig. 1.15). Subcutaneous nodules are usually only removed if they cause discomfort or become ulcerated, and may recur if the arthritis remains active. They are also found in internal organs, e.g. in the lungs, spleen, heart valves, eyes, and other viscera.

Vasculitis may also occur in RA. The most common type is a mild obliterative endarteritis (the vessels are occluded), which produces painless infarcts in the finger-nail beds and paronychia. These lesions frequently appear in crops, heal without tissue damage and, accordingly, do not require specific treatment. Leukocytoclastic vasculitis (inflammation of small blood vessels with 'nuclear dust') in the skin may also occur and manifest as palpable purpura (small raised purple lesions). This type of vasculitis most commonly occurs in the legs and heals without scarring. The most serious type of vasculitis in RA is a necrotizing vasculitis of small to medium-sized arteries and requires aggressive treatment. Its manifestations depend upon the site of involvement but include necrotizing skin lesions and ulcers when dermal vessels are affected, intestinal infarction and mononeuritis multiplex—involvement of multiple discrete peripheral nerves.

RA can also involve the heart, pericarditis (inflammation of the sac that surrounds the heart) being the most common cardiac manifestation. Small, usually asymptomatic, pericardial effusions have been reported in up to 40% of patients with RA. Histology shows a fibrinous pericarditis. Only a very small number of patients have larger pericardial effusions that become symptomatic. A mild myocarditis (inflammation of the heart muscle) can also occur in RA. It is rarely symptomatic and usually associated with a normal electrocardiogram. Valvular abnormalities occasionally occur in RA, most frequently of the aortic valve, and are usually due to fibrous valvular scarring.

The most common respiratory manifestation of RA is pleural involvement, typically manifesting as an asymptomatic pleural effusion. Occasionally, it can produce frank pleurisy (pleuritis). Rheumatoid nodules may also be found in the lung and can be difficult to distinguish from other causes of pulmonary nodules. Pulmonary fibrosis may occur secondary to chronic lymphocytic and monocytic infiltrate in the pulmonary interstitium or rarely as an adverse reaction to treatment with agents such as gold or methotrexate.

There are several types of eye involvement. Scleritis, or inflammation of the sclera, results in a painful, red eye (Fig. 1.16). Scleritis can lead to thinning of the sclera, called scleromalacia, which may rarely perforate the eye—scleromalacia perforans. Episcleritis, or inflammation in the loose connective tissue that lies between the conjunctiva and the sclera, is less likely to be symptomatic or as serious as is scleritis. It usually resolves rapidly with no residual abnormalities.

Several neuropathies can occur as part of RA, including a peripheral neuropathy (glove and stocking pattern of involvement), entrapment neuropathy caused by soft tissue swelling (the commonest example being carpal tunnel syndrome—see Ch. 3) and mononeuritis multiplex.

Treatment of rheumatoid arthritis

The management of patients with RA is very complex. This section is restricted to providing the principles

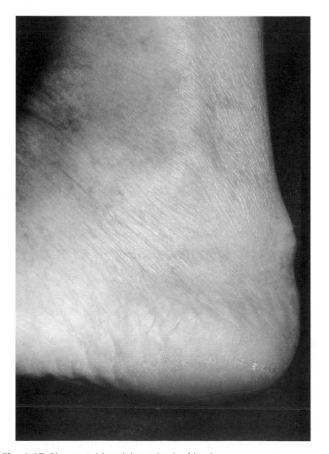

Fig. 1.15 Rheumatoid nodules at back of heel.

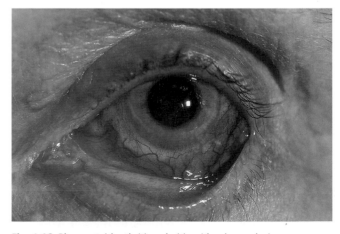

Fig. 1.16 Rheumatoid arthritis: scleritis with scleromalacia.

guiding management. For a more comprehensive coverage of this subject, the reader is directed to textbooks of rheumatology.

Modern approaches involve recognition of the importance of the therapeutic team in the optimal management of patients with RA. The team comprises of a rheumatologist (who usually acts as team leader), family physician, orthopaedic surgeon, allied health members including physiotherapist, occupational therapist, social worker, nurse and patient educator, the patient and his or her immediate family. While not all members of this team are required in the management of every patient, at times each may be called on to contribute his or her expertise.

Rest is therapeutic during periods of active disease. Controlled trials of rest therapy have demonstrated its therapeutic benefit. This does not imply that bed rest is required for all patients. Therapy may simply involve rest periods taken during the day. Exactly how rest reduces inflammation is unknown. Rest has to be balanced with exercise, best supervised by an experienced physiotherapist. Exercises include passive joint movement during periods of active disease, which are used to preserve a full range of joint motion, and active exercises including isometrics to reverse muscle wasting. The latter often develops in muscles adjacent to inflamed joints as a result of disuse.

Patients often experience depressive symptoms, marital disharmony and financial hardship as a result of having a chronic painful debilitating disease. The social worker can help with these aspects of the patient's care. In more advanced cases, the orthopaedic surgeon plays an important role, usually in performing synovectomy for a chronically inflamed joint that has failed to respond to medical therapy or in reconstructive surgery to replace irreversibly damaged joints.

Pharmacological treatment principles (Table 1.2) include providing analgesia, reducing joint inflammation, preventing joint damage and inducing remission.

Analgesics

Analgesics, including paracetamol/acetaminophen, have no anti-inflammatory effects. They can be used every 4–6

Table 1.2 Principles of drug treatment in RA

Drug type	Action
Analgesics	Pain relief
Non-steroidal anti-inflammatory drugs	Reduce inflammation
Corticosteroids	Reduce inflammation
Disease-modifying anti-rheumatic drugs	Induce remission and prevent joint destruction
Biological therapy	Induce remission and prevent joint destruction

hours for pain relief if necessary. They seldom produce side-effects and are well tolerated.

Non-steroidal anti-inflammatory drugs

Non-steroidal anti-inflammatory drugs (NSAIDs), of which aspirin is the historical prototype, inhibit the cyclooxygenase enzymes. NSAIDs act quickly (within hours to a few days) and reduce joint inflammation by inhibiting the production of inflammatory cyclooxygenase products, particularly the prostaglandins—small lipid molecules with potent effects on many steps in the inflammatory process. This provides symptomatic relief, with a reduction in joint pain, stiffness and swelling. They do not, however, prevent the development of joint erosions or damage. Furthermore, their effect rapidly reverses on drug cessation. Nevertheless, they have made an important contribution to the symptomatic treatment of patients with RA.

These drugs, of which there are a large number, are potent anti-inflammatory agents. Commonly used agents include diclofenac, naproxen, ketoprofen, sulindac, piroxicam, indomethacin and ibuprofen. They vary in their plasma half-lives, potency and degree of gastrointestinal toxicity. NSAIDs are usually administered orally, in conjunction with food, sometimes as an enteric-coated formulation to reduce gastrointestinal toxicity. They are occasionally given as a suppository, which also reduces, but does not eliminate, upper gastrointestinal toxicity. Unfortunately, many RA patients do not have the manual dexterity to insert a suppository. A number of NSAIDs are available as gels that can be applied topically to inflamed joints.

As a class of drugs, their use has been limited by adverse effects, particularly upper gastrointestinal toxicity, e.g. gastritis and peptic ulcer formation. In susceptible individuals, NSAIDs are nephrotoxic, by inhibiting prostaglandin-dependent compensatory renal blood flow. Some NSAIDs have characteristic adverse effects, e.g. headaches with indomethacin. By contrast, other NSAIDs have certain advantages, e.g. relative renal sparing with sulindac.

Two classes of cyclooxygenase enzymes have been described: COX-1 and COX-2. COX-1 enzymes are expressed constitutively in gastric mucosa, kidneys and other organs and are not inducible. By contrast, COX-2 enzymes are not usually constitutively expressed in tissues, but can be induced by certain molecules, e.g. cytokines at sites of inflammation. Traditional NSAIDs, as described above, inhibit both COX-1 and COX-2 enzymes (Fig. 1.17). However, selective COX-2 inhibitors have been developed, which have minimal effects on the COX-1 enzyme. These agents provide anti-inflammatory effects with less upper gastrointestinal toxicity. Celecoxib and rofecoxib were the first of this novel class of compounds. However, Rofecoxib was withdrawn because of a higher risk of patients developing myocardial infarction. The cardiovascular safety of Celecoxib and of non-selective NSAIDs remains under a cloud. At time of writing, a definitive statement on their cardiovascular safety cannot be made. It seems wise to minimize or avoid their use in patients at high risk or with a previous history of cardiovascular disease.

> ### Interesting facts
>
> #### NSAIDs and cardiovascular risk
>
> Over the past 30 years, the main toxicity concern of NSAIDs has been the upper gastrointestinal toxicity system. However, since 2000 there has been increasing interest in the cardiovascular risk of NSAIDs, particularly the COX-2 selective inhibitor Rofecoxib (Vioxx). This culminated in its international withdrawal from the market. The cardiovascular risk of NSAIDs, whether COX-2-selective or not remains under a cloud.

Corticosteroids

The corticosteroids (or glucocorticoids) are hormones produced by the adrenal glands. They have potent anti-inflammatory and immunosuppressive properties. Their effect in RA, when used at high doses, is dramatic. Corticosteroid analogues have been produced synthetically by chemical modification of the natural hormone cortisol. This has resulted in a range of compounds with varying potencies and differential toxicities. By far the most commonly used compound is prednisone, which is four to five times as potent as cortisol and has less mineralocorticoid activity, resulting in less fluid retention.

Prednisone is administered orally and acts rapidly to reduce inflammation, resulting in a lessening of joint swelling, pain and stiffness in RA. They bind to cytoplasmic cortisol receptors and are transported into the nucleus where they interfere with RNA processing of protein molecules. Corticosteroids act on a wide variety of target cells including leukocytes. They inhibit leukocyte chemotaxis (directed motion towards a stimulus), preventing circulating polymorphs, monocytes and lymphocytes from reaching sites of inflammation. They reduce vascular permeability and inhibit the production of cytokines and arachidonic acid metabolites, such as prostaglandins and leukotrienes.

Despite clinical efficacy, corticosteroids are toxic if used at high doses for prolonged periods. Corticosteroids

have important effects on bone metabolism resulting in osteoporosis and eventual non-traumatic fractures (discussed in Ch. 5). They interfere with glucose metabolism and are diabetogenic. Corticosteroids cause salt and water retention and may precipitate or exacerbate hypertension. They interfere with ocular lens metabolism resulting in cataract formation. Their immunosuppressive action, while beneficial in reducing inflammation in RA, results in increased susceptibility to a wide range of bacterial and opportunistic infections, e.g. herpes zoster virus and fungal infections.

In general, corticosteroid side-effects are dose- and time-related. In order to limit toxicity, corticosteroids should be used for as short a time and at as low a dose as possible to achieve an anti-inflammatory effect. In recent years, a number of different regimens have been introduced to improve efficacy, while minimizing toxicity. These include the use of intermittent pulses of high-dose corticosteroids, e.g. monthly intravenous methylprednisolone. It has recently been demonstrated that continuous low-dose daily oral prednisone (<7.5 mg/day) retards the development of bony erosions with minimal toxicity.

Another route frequently used to administer corticosteroids is intra-articular injection of depot preparations. This approach aims to deliver a high dose of corticosteroid, which is retained within the joint and reduces local inflammation with limited systemic absorption. This approach is effective in controlling local disease activity.

In patients with life- or major organ-threatening rheumatoid vasculitis, high-dose systemic treatment with

> ### Case 1.1 Rheumatoid arthritis: 4
>
> #### Case note: Corticosteroid treatment
>
> Despite 2 weeks of complete rest and a course of naproxen, Mrs Gale has only partly improved, remains in pain and cannot function effectively. After a telephone call by her general practitioner to a rheumatologist, she is advised to commence oral prednisone 10 mg per day as a morning dose.

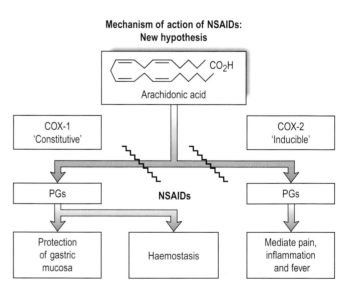

Fig. 1.17 The cyclooxygenase system: arachidonic acid is converted to prostaglandins by the enzyme cyclooxygenase (COX). There are two forms of this enzyme: COX-1 and COX-2. COX-1 produces prostaglandins responsible for maintaining normal stomach, kidney, intestine and platelet function. COX-2 produces prostaglandins found at inflammatory sites. Conventional NSAIDs block both COX-1 and COX-2. COX-2-specific inhibitors block only COX-2; thus they inhibit only those prostaglandins responsible for inflammation.

corticosteroids for prolonged periods is usually required. Drugs to protect against the development of osteoporosis, such as vitamin D and calcium, bisphosphonates, or, in postmenopausal women, hormone replacement therapy are all deserving of consideration (see Ch. 5).

Disease-modifying anti-rheumatic drugs

Disease-modifying anti-rheumatic drugs (DMARDs) are a group of disparate compounds that in general share an important feature—the potential to retard the development of bony erosions in RA. Drugs in this category include gold compounds, sulfasalazine and the antimalarial drug hydroxychloroquine. Immunosuppressive drugs are also sometimes considered in this group. These include the folic acid antagonist methotrexate, the antimetabolite azathioprine, the alkylating agent cyclophosphamide, cyclosporin, which inhibits the production of IL-2 by T lymphocytes, and recently the pyrimidine antagonist leflunomide. Methotrexate is the most widely prescribed drug in this group.

There is no single mechanism by which these agents work. In general, they have a delayed onset of clinical action, measured in weeks to months rather than hours to days as with NSAIDs and corticosteroids. They all have potential toxicity and require careful and regular monitoring. Their initiation should be under the guidance of a rheumatologist. A detailed description of these drugs, their mechanism of action and toxicity profile is beyond the scope of this chapter.

There is a changing view on the way in which anti-rheumatic drugs, especially the DMARDs, are best used in RA. These agents are now introduced at the time of diagnosis rather than waiting for the appearance of radiological erosions, as was formerly done. The radiological and clinical outcome of patients with RA treated with DMARDs early in disease has improved. DMARDs are now being used in combination rather than as single agents, much as oncologists have used combination chemotherapy to treat haematological malignancy.

Case 1.1 Rheumatoid arthritis: 5

Case note: Treatment with a disease-modifying anti-rheumatic drug

Mrs Gale has her first appointment with the rheumatologist. She has had a good symptomatic response to oral prednisone and has markedly reduced joint pain and stiffness. Nevertheless, the rheumatologist recommends that she be commenced on a disease-modifying anti-rheumatic drug. He discusses the various options available and they decide to add enteric-coated sulfasalazine initially at 500 mg per day. She is told about possible adverse drug effects and the need for regular blood counts to monitor for toxicity.

Combinations of drugs with different mechanisms of action and different profiles of toxicity have been chosen. Combinations shown to be superior to single-agent DMARD treatment include: hydroxychloroquine, sulfasalazine plus methotrexate; and cyclosporin plus methotrexate.

Interesting facts

Biological therapy for rheumatoid arthritis

At the time of writing the first edition of *The Musculoskeletal System* in 2000, the clinical role of biological therapy for RA was still unclear. However, that position has changed. There has been a dramatic expansion in both the range of diseases in which it is being applied and the range of agents that are now available. In the rheumatic field this has broadened to include psoriatic arthritis, ankylosing spondylitis as well as RA. Targets have now broadened from those directed against TNF-α to include B cells, co-stimulatory molecules, IL-1 receptor antagonist and IL-6 receptor.

Biological treatments

A new era is emerging with the introduction of biological agents in the treatment of RA. These include monoclonal antibodies directed against B cells (e.g. Mabthera) or co-stimulatory molecules (e.g. Abatacept) and those against inflammatory cytokines, e.g. TNF-α. Another approach is the use of soluble cytokine receptors, e.g. soluble TNF receptors, IL-1 receptor antagonists and IL-6 receptor. This approach is proving to be highly effective in both suppressing joint inflammation and in preventing the development of bony erosions. The main reservations are their high cost and uncertainty about their long-term safety.

In summary, the medical treatment of RA is complex and not for the occasional practitioner. It involves the use of specialized drugs with significant toxicity and requires considerable expertise in their appropriate use.

Surgery for rheumatoid arthritis

A significant number of RA patients require the skills of an orthopaedic surgeon at some stage of their disease. Two types of surgery are commonly used—synovectomy and reconstructive or joint-replacement surgery.

Synovectomy is the surgical removal of synovium from an inflamed joint. It can be performed as an open procedure or by arthroscopy, depending on the joint involved and the skill of the surgeon. The main indication is persistent arthritis in a joint, which fails to settle, despite medical therapy, including repeated intra-articular depot corticosteroid injections. The site most commonly treated is the knee. Less commonly treated are other joints or inflamed tendon sheaths—tenosynovitis requires synovectomy. Results are good with better symptomatic and radiographic outcome for an involved joint, compared with medical therapy, even after 3 years.

Case 1.1 Rheumatoid arthritis: 6

Case note: Response to drug treatment

Some 3 years later, Mrs Gale is managing reasonably well on treatment with prednisone 5 mg per day, sulfasalazine 2 g per day, vitamin D and a calcium supplement. She is able to help with the family business, but has persistent synovitis in her right knee, despite repeated intra-articular depot corticosteroid injections. The latter produce only temporary relief of symptoms. She is referred to an orthopaedic surgeon for consideration of a synovectomy.

Case 1.1 Rheumatoid arthritis: 7

Case note: Response to surgical treatment

Mrs Gale undergoes an arthroscopic synovectomy with a good result. One year later she notices a recurrence of generalized joint pain, stiffness and fatigue. Blood tests indicate that her inflammatory parameters (ESR and C-reactive protein) have worsened. Her rheumatologist advises revision of her anti-rheumatic medications, with the addition of methotrexate.

Reconstructive or joint-replacement surgery is reserved for patients with irreversibly damaged joints and severe articular cartilage loss, who are experiencing pain on using the joint, e.g. when walking short distances, and loss of function. The joints most commonly replaced are: the knee, hip, shoulder and metacarpophalangeal joints of the hands. There are many types of artificial joints with different biomechanical properties. Some require the use of cement to hold the joint prosthesis in place, while uncemented prostheses have been developed more recently. The results of surgery, particularly for knee and hip joint replacement, are excellent with markedly reduced pain and improved joint function. Half-lives for cemented knee and hip prostheses are approximately 8–10 years. Surgical revision is now a common procedure. The main local adverse outcomes of joint replacement surgery are cement loosening and, uncommonly, but very seriously, secondary bacterial infection. It is hoped that the use of uncemented prostheses will eliminate loosening of prostheses and result in longer prostheses half-life.

Other types of surgery are performed less commonly on RA patients, including bony fusion, particularly for unstable wrists, and carpal tunnel release for a median nerve entrapped in the carpal tunnel by persistently inflamed synovium (see Ch. 3).

Prognosis

The natural history of untreated RA is poor. It is associated not only with severe morbidity, but a shortening of life-expectancy by 7–10 years. Patients die as a result of premature cardiovascular disease, infection or extra-articular disease. It has been claimed that the prognosis for untreated RA is similar to that of treated Hodgkin's disease.

DMARDs slow disease progression, both clinically and radiologically, although complete remission off therapy is seldom achieved. It is thought that the earlier introduction of DMARDs and the use of combination therapy or biologicals can substantially improve the long-term prognosis and reduce mortality.

Further reading

Hochberg, M.C., Silman, A.J., Smolen, J.S., Weinblatt, M.E., Weisman, M.H. (Eds.), 2008. Rheumatology, fourth ed. Mosby, Philadelphia.

Moore, K.L., Dalley, A.F., 1999. Clinically Oriented Anatomy, fourth ed. Williams & Wilkins, Baltimore.

SOFT TISSUE RHEUMATIC DISEASE INVOLVING THE SHOULDER AND ELBOW

2

David H. Sonnabend

Chapter objectives

After studying this chapter you should be able to:

1. Understand normal shoulder anatomy and function.

2. Appreciate the pathological processes involved in the most common shoulder diseases.

3. Understand the epidemiology of rotator cuff pathology.

4. Assess the risk factors commonly associated with rotator cuff disease.

5. Understand the general principles of medical and surgical treatment of rotator cuff disease.

6. Understand common soft tissue conditions affecting the elbow.

Introduction

In the musculoskeletal system, disorders of the soft tissues (muscles, tendons, ligaments, fascia, capsules, etc.) are often considered separately from those of the hard tissues (bone and cartilage). Indeed 'soft tissue rheumatism' is a term frequently applied to miscellaneous disorders causing musculoskeletal pain arising from structures outside the joint, such as bursae, tendons, ligaments and muscles. 'Fibromyalgia' is also sometimes included under this heading, but will be considered separately in Chapter 8. Upper limb pain in general, and shoulder pain in particular, is commonly due to disease of these soft tissues. Careful history-taking often provides a provisional diagnosis. Different age groups suffer different pathologies. Physical examination should be both general and directed towards the most likely diagnoses. Specific investigations, some of them expensive, should be used thoughtfully, and not in a shotgun fashion. Multiple modalities of treatment should be considered and may be employed simultaneously. These include rest, physical modalities, such as ice and heat, physiotherapy, specific exercise programmes (including stretching and strengthening), and both non-steroidal anti-inflammatory medication and corticosteroids by injection. Surgery is sometimes the definitive treatment, and in appropriate cases should not be delayed unduly.

This chapter uses rotator cuff pathology (tendonitis, impingement and tear) as a model for discussing soft tissue disorders, and reviews normal shoulder anatomy and function. Common soft tissue conditions of the elbow are also briefly considered.

Anatomy of the shoulder

The human shoulder joint's virtually global range of motion exceeds that of any other joint in the body.

Case 2.1 Rotator cuff injury: 1

Case history

Mr Jones, a 50-year-old self-employed carpenter, presented with a 10-week history of gradually increasing right shoulder pain. The pain began when he suddenly took the full weight of a cupboard which he was carrying with his workmate. Initially the pain was of nuisance value only, but more recently it had interfered with sleep and various activities of daily living (washing, dressing, hair care and driving a car). Over the last few weeks, Mr Jones had been unable to continue to work as a carpenter, because of both activity-related pain and, more recently, increasing shoulder weakness when working overhead. Pain was maximal at the front of the shoulder, but occasionally radiated to the deltoid insertion and beyond. The hand was uninvolved.

In quadrupedal animals, the shoulder moves almost purely in the sagittal plane. As arboreal and bipedal apes evolved, so too did the ability to place the arm (and with it the hand) overhead and to the side. This extraordinary multiplanar range of movement distinguishes the shoulder from other joints in the body. The only bony connection between the shoulder girdle and the trunk is via the clavicle and the acromioclavicular joint. The relative unimportance of that joint is illustrated by the ability of those with dislocated acromioclavicular joints to function normally. The attachment of the arm to the trunk is almost totally dependent on musculature.

The scapula is held on and moves on the chest wall. This connection is called the 'scapulothoracic articulation'. The humerus is, in turn, attached to the scapula by the glenohumeral joint, where the head of the humerus sits on the glenoid surface of the scapula (Fig. 2.1A). While this may be seen as a 'ball and socket' joint, the socket is very shallow, almost a plate. Shoulder movement occurs simultaneously at both the glenohumeral and the scapulothoracic joints, in a ratio of approximately two to one.

The articular surfaces of the glenoid and the humeral head are lined by articular cartilage. The glenoid socket is deepened by a fibrocartilaginous labrum or rim which surrounds its edge. The joint is lined by synovium and enclosed by a fibrous capsule.

Interesting facts

Although many animals have supra- and infraspinatus tendons, true rotator cuffs (the fusion of supra- and infraspinatus tendons to form a single 'tendon sheet') are unique to animals which are able to reach overhead—mainly the advanced primates.

Muscles

The scapular motors are large muscles which stabilize and move the scapula on the chest wall. They include the serratus anterior, which protracts the scapula, and the trapezius, levator scapulae and rhomboids which elevate and rotate it (Fig. 2.1B). Paralysis of the serratus produces 'winging' of the scapula. Paralysis of the trapezius allows the shoulder to 'drop', and this may stretch the brachial plexus.

Two large muscles, latissimus dorsi and pectoralis major, cross from the trunk to the humerus, bypassing the scapula. Both adduct the arm to the trunk and can rotate it internally. The scapulothoracic motors, together with latissimus and pectoralis major, provide the gross control of the shoulder.

A number of other muscles connect the humerus to the scapula and provide fine control. The largest of these are deltoid and subscapularis. The deltoid can be regarded in three parts: anterior, middle and posterior. Anterior deltoid (between clavicle and acromion superiorly and humerus inferiorly), can forward-flex the humerus. The lateral deltoid (arising from the side of the acromion), helps abduct the arm. The posterior deltoid extends the arm. All three parts acting together pull the arm up and abduct it. The subscapularis, arising on the deep surface of the scapula, runs across the front of the gleno-humeral joint to attach to the (lesser tuberosity of the) humeral head.

The supraspinatus muscle comes from the dorsal (superficial) surface of the scapula above its spine (hence *supra*spinatus). Its tendon passes over the *top* of the glenohumeral joint to the front of the greater tuberosity of the humeral head (Fig. 2.1C). Infraspinatus and teres minor arise from the dorsal surface of the scapula *below* its spine, and cross over the back of the gleno-humeral joint to the back of the (greater tuberosity of the) humeral head. The supraspinatus helps with forward flexion and abduction, subscapularis with internal rotation, and infraspinatus and teres minor with external rotation.

Various other muscles also affect shoulder function. The tendon of the long head of biceps arises inside the glenohumeral joint, at the top of the glenoid, and crosses over the humeral head before leaving the joint and passing into the biceps groove. It helps hold the humeral head down, but its main function is in elbow flexion and supination. The long head of the triceps arises outside the joint capsule, from the lower pole of the glenoid. While contraction of its muscle belly obviously pulls the arm upwards a little, its main function is to extend the elbow.

The rotator cuff

Although supra- and infraspinatus and teres minor are separate muscles, their flat sheet-like tendons of insertion blend with each other as they approach the humeral head to form a cuff that holds the humeral head in place and assists with active elevation and rotation of the shoulder. This blended combined tendon is referred to as the rotator cuff.

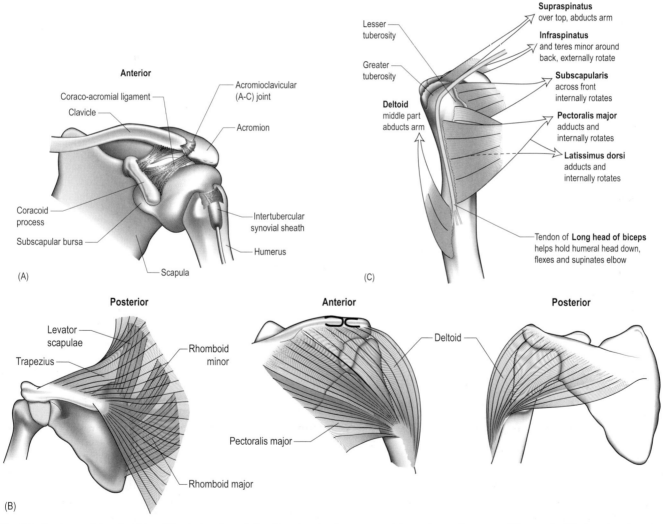

Fig. 2.1 Anatomy of the shoulder: (A) anterior view of shoulder showing bones, synovial membrane, bursae and ligaments; (B) view showing serratus anterior, trapezius, levator scapulae, rhomboids, latissimus dorsi and pectoralis major; (C) diagram of rotator cuff.

Capsule

Like other joints, the glenohumeral joint is closed off by a fibrous capsule. Some parts of the capsule are thicker than other parts. The thickest parts of the capsule are called glenohumeral ligaments (GHLs). The inferior GHL in particular plays an important role in stabilizing the joint. When it is avulsed from its glenoid attachment—the so-called 'Bankart lesion'—anterior instability occurs.

Nerves

The nerve control of the shoulder arises mainly from the fifth cervical nerve root. The axillary nerve supplies the deltoid and the suprascapular nerve supplies the spinati.

Pathophysiology of rotator cuff disease

The commonest site of pathology is in the supraspinatus tendon. The supraspinatus runs under an arch formed by the coracoid, the coracoacromial ligament and the anterior acromion (Fig. 2.2). Rubbing of the tendon on the undersurface of this arch produces the 'subacromial impingement syndrome', which is common in patients over the age of 40. Typically, impingement is related to repetitive overhead activity causing repeated pinching of the cuff beneath the arch. This may be exacerbated by an associated bone spur on the undersurface of the anterior acromion. The repetitive activity may be sports-related (golf swing, tennis serve

or throwing) or work-related, but many impingement cases appear entirely idiopathic. It is not clear whether acromial spurs are the primary cause of impingement or whether they form in response to impingement.

Clinical features of rotator cuff disease

Because the impingement syndrome is usually related to repetitive use, the onset of pain is often insidious, but some cases may begin suddenly following a single, isolated incident or period of overuse activity. Patients (typically) complain of pain over the lateral aspect of the upper arm, possibly as far distally as the deltoid insertion. The pain is often worse at night, and disruption of sleep is common. Patients find it difficult to lie on the affected arm. Reaching overhead and behind the back is also usually painful.

Clinical aspects of shoulder pain

In considering a patient's history, the patient's age, the mechanism of pain onset, the progression of the symptoms, the site of pain and the nature of any resultant disability all provide an insight into the responsible pathology. Different conditions occur at different ages. Musculoskeletal shoulder problems before the age of 30 often relate to shoulder instability, with associated secondary impingement and inflammation of the rotator cuff tendons (discussed below). Over the age of 40, chronic tendonitis of the rotator cuff, especially the supraspinatus tendon, is common. This too is often associated with subacromial impingement (discussed below), and may progress to tearing of the rotator cuff. Over the age of 60, partial and full thickness tears of the supraspinatus tendon are common. Osteoarthritis of the glenohumeral joint is also more common in this age group.

The mechanism of onset provides some clues. Sudden onset, associated with a single traumatic event (such as trying to catch a falling cupboard), suggests a mechanical event, such as a tendon tearing. A more insidious onset suggests degenerative disease, or possibly repeated micro-trauma.

In cases of sudden onset, the position of the arm and the nature of the initial injury may provide some clue. If the arm was forced into abduction and external rotation, anterior subluxation is a real possibility. If the arm was at or near the side at the time of onset, or if the mechanism involved contraction of the shoulder muscles against resistance, an injury to the rotator cuff mechanism is more likely.

The progression of symptoms helps diagnosis. Increasing pain implies progressive pathology. Increasing weakness may be due to painful inhibition of shoulder activity. If the loss of strength is profound, this suggests progressive disruption of a muscle–tendon unit, possibly the rotator cuff. Increasing stiffness (loss of range) suggests an inflammatory process, possibly adhesive capsulitis (frozen shoulder).

The site of pain is important. Subacromial pain is usually felt at the front of the shoulder. Radiation of pain

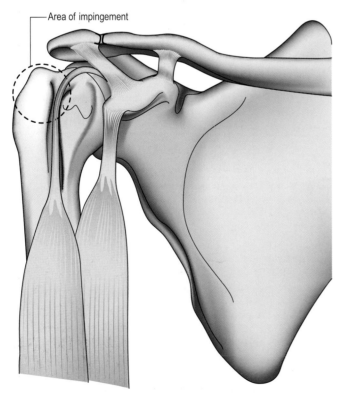

Fig. 2.2 Mechanism of impingement.

Area of impingement

to the deltoid insertion is common but non-specific, as it also occurs with glenohumeral pathology and cervical pathology, especially a C5 radiculopathy (nerve root lesion). Involvement of the trapezius, the parascapular muscles and the side of the neck are also common but relatively non-specific. Pain over the posterior joint line is frequently glenohumeral in origin. Involvement of the hand may suggest neurological or neurovascular pathology, including neck pathology, thoracic outlet syndrome or even carpal tunnel syndrome (see Ch. 3). Regional pain syndromes may also involve both shoulder and hand.

It is important to assess the patient's degree of disability. An inability to attend to activities of daily living, and particularly an inability to sleep at night, warrants serious attention, as does any condition which affects the patient's occupation. For a keen sportsperson, an inability to throw or to serve at tennis may be equally distressing. The use of patient questionnaires and visual analogue scales aids assessment. A typical patient-questionnaire directed at the assessment of shoulder pain is shown below (Fig. 2.3). Questionnaires do not replace history taking. They can be repeated at later dates to help assess progress.

SHOULDER QUESTIONNAIRE   Date: / /

Name: ....   Date of Birth: / /

Are you right-handed ☐ / left-handed ☐ / ambidextrous ☐ ?

Which shoulder is currently troubling you? Right ☐ / Left ☐ / Both ☐

Usual Occupation.. Sports..

Is your shoulder comfortable when your arm is by your side when using a knife and fork?   Yes ☐ / No ☐

Can you lie on affected shoulder at night without waking?   Yes ☐ / No ☐

Can you reach your back pocket and/or tuck your clothes in?   Yes ☐ / No ☐

Can you comb your hair/reach your head with affected arm?   Yes ☐ / No ☐

Can you use your arm (for example, put a coin in a slot) with your arm straight (elbow not bent) at shoulder height

(A) In front of you?   Yes ☐ / No ☐

(B) To your side?   Yes ☐ / No ☐

Can you lift a full 600ml milk container (or equivalent) to shoulder height without bending your elbow?   Yes ☐ / No ☐

Can you carry a suitcase or a heavy shopping bag with your arm by your side (without help from the other hand)?   Yes ☐ / No ☐

Can you throw a tennis ball overarm or use a hair dryer?   Yes ☐ / No ☐

Can you wash the opposite shoulder and armpit?   Yes ☐ / No ☐

Please circle the number on the scale at the point which best depicts your situation.

Shoulder comfort with arm at rest

No pain   1 2 3 4 5 6 7 8 9 10   Very painful

Shoulder comfort during sleep

No pain   1 2 3 4 5 6 7 8 9 10   Painful/wakes me

Ability to use arm at work or play

Little or no problem to use it   1 2 3 4 5 6 7 8 9 10   Painful/cannot

Effect of shoulder on overall quality of life

Little or no problem   1 2 3 4 5 6 7 8 9 10   Very bad

Fig. 2.3 Shoulder questionnaire.

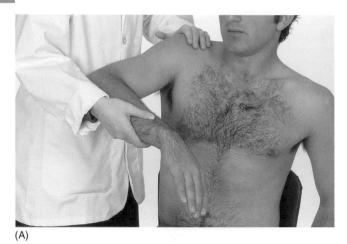

(A)

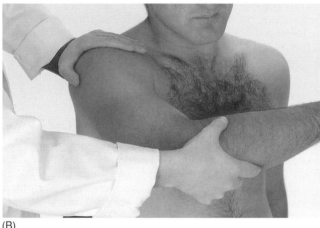

(B)

Fig. 2.4 Neer and Hawkins tests: The Neer test is performed by the examiner lifting the patient's arm in front of the patient with the elbow bent. At the same time the examiner presses up on the elbow with one hand and places counterpressure on the top of the shoulder. In the Hawkins test, the arm is brought by the examiner into the Neer position and then internally rotated (the hand of the patient is brought downward) as the elbow is pushed up. Both should 'pinch' the rotator cuff tendons if impingement is present.

Inspection and palpation are best carried out with the examiner standing behind the seated patient. When present, significant wasting of the spinati muscles will be obvious in all but the most obese patients. The best-known tests for subacromial impingement are the Neer and Hawkins tests (Fig. 2.4). In both, the greater tuberosity, the attached supraspinatus tendon, the overlying bursa and the adjacent biceps tendon are compressed beneath the coracoacromial arch. If either manoeuvre recreates typical symptoms, this suggests cuff impingement, but may also reflect biceps pathology. Yergason's test for biceps tendinitis is less sensitive but moderately specific (Fig. 2.5).

Differential diagnosis

The painful arc suggests subacromial pathology, as did Mr Jones' age and the history of nocturnal pain. Specific

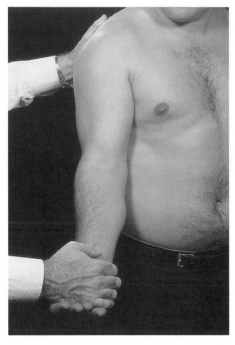

Fig. 2.5 Yergason's sign: with the patient's elbow held at his side and flexed to 90°, the forearm is supinated against resistance while shaking hands.

tests for bicipital tendonitis were negative. Other common pathologies to consider in a patient with shoulder pain are shown in Box 2.1.

Calcific tendonitis of the supraspinatus tendon can cause acute onset of severe pain. It usually occurs between the ages of 40 and 60 but can occur in younger patients. X-rays usually demonstrate calcium deposits. Laboratory tests usually do not reveal any abnormality of calcium or phosphate metabolism. A bursa is a sac lined by synovium. Bursae normally contain small amounts of synovial fluid. They lie between tissues which might otherwise rub against each other repeatedly, reducing friction. For example bursae are found overlying the olecranon in the elbow, the patella in the knee and greater trochanter in the hip. In the shoulder, an extensive bursa lies between the acromion, the coracoacromial arch and the deltoid muscle 'above' and the underlying humeral head and attached rotator cuff tendons 'below'. Chronic irritation (rubbing) of a bursa produces inflammation (called bursitis) in the bursa which becomes swollen with synovial fluid. In the shoulder, this bursa (known variously as the subacromial or subdeltoid bursa) may be irritated by subacromial impingement or other pathologies affecting synovial tissues.

Polymyalgia rheumatica, an inflammatory condition predominantly affecting the proximal limb girdles (shoulders and hips), usually occurs in older subjects. It is usually associated with bilateral shoulder symptoms, prominent early morning stiffness and often fever and weight loss. Adhesive capsulitis or frozen shoulder is characterized by chronic pain and marked global

Case 2.1 Rotator cuff injury: 2

Case history

On examination, Mr Jones appeared a healthy man, slightly overweight, who held his right arm carefully by his side. Shaking hands was painful. With Mr Jones seated, inspection from above and behind revealed obvious wasting of the right supraspinatus muscle belly. Gentle palpation suggested that infraspinatus was also significantly smaller on the right than on the left, despite Mr Jones' right-handedness. Examination of range of movement produced pain in the mid-arc of forward flexion. The pain settled in part, but not completely, as flexion progressed to its limit of 160° (180° on the left). Abduction was similarly painful, but full. The range of external rotation in both adduction and abduction was almost normal, but internal rotation was markedly limited. Active range of movement was more limited, with Mr Jones unable to actively flex more than 80° against gravity, even with the elbow bent to reduce the lever-arm. Strength of external rotation in adduction was markedly weaker on the right than on the left. Pain precluded testing internal rotation. Palpation of the shoulder revealed exquisite tenderness over the greater tuberosity and some tenderness over the biceps groove at the front of the humeral head. A number of specific tests were carried out, including the impingement test (which was severely painful), and various biceps provocation tests which were also somewhat uncomfortable. There was however no evidence of biceps disruption, and the subscapularis appeared intact.

A tentative diagnosis of subacromial pathology, possibly subacromial impingement or a full thickness cuff tear, was made.

Box 2.1 Common causes of shoulder pain

- Rotator cuff impingement (with or without cuff tear)
- Subacromial bursitis
- Bicipital tendonitis
- Calcific tendonitis
- Polymyalgia rheumatica
- Adhesive capsulitis
- Cervical disc disease

restriction of shoulder movement. While most cases are idiopathic, some are secondary to conditions that cause immobility such as a stroke or occur as a late complication of rotator cuff lesions. Three phases are usually recognized: 'freezing' (capsulitis causing pain, especially at the extremes of range when the capsule is stretched, and progressive restriction of movement); 'frozen' (capsulitis causing mainly immobility with lessening of pain); 'thawing' (involving gradual recovery of the range of movement).

The distinction between cervical and shoulder pathology is not always easy. Pain involving the upper arm, especially the region of the deltoid muscle insertion, can be due to shoulder pathology or cervical radiculopathy involving the fifth cervical nerve root. Similarly, spondylotic (osteoarthritic) changes involving the cervical spine can also produce pain in the trapezius muscle, the supraclavicular region and the shoulder. Cervical disc degeneration is usually associated with restricted neck movement and also possibly neurological signs, if there is a nerve compression.

Interesting facts

The incidence of 'idiopathic' frozen shoulder (adhesive capsulitis) is much higher in diabetics than in non-diabetics. Any patient presenting with a frozen shoulder should have a fasting blood sugar test to check for underlying diabetes.

Investigations

Plain X-rays of the shoulder are often normal in patients presenting with shoulder pain but are useful to exclude certain pathologies. In general, one should seek at least three standard views: anteroposterior, supraspinatus outlet (lateral) and axillary, taken at right angles to each other. With an incomplete series of radiographic views, one might well miss significant pathology such as an acromial spur or an os acromiale. If posterior dislocation is ever a consideration, the multiple views are mandatory, as it is possible to miss a posterior dislocation on a single anteroposterior view.

When expertly performed, shoulder ultrasound is a valuable modality for assessing the rotator cuff for impingement or tears (Fig. 2.6). It is, however, very operator-dependent. Ultrasound can also give some indication as to the extent of any fatty degeneration of the supraspinatus and infraspinatus muscles, and the extent of retraction of any torn tendons.

This is important information if a rotator cuff repair is contemplated, as an excessively retracted cuff may be irreparable. Double contrast arthrography, the injection of air and dye into the shoulder, followed by radiography, looks for leakage through a cuff tear and has been useful in the diagnosis of full thickness rotator cuff tears. However, MRI scanning is now more widely used. It allows more accuracy in the assessment of tear size, and particularly the extent of any tendon retraction, and is also useful in assessing atrophy and fatty degeneration of the muscles. Combined with intra-articular gadolinium, it is also useful in assessing pathology involving the labrum of the glenoid and the biceps tendon origin. It is, however, an expensive investigation. Before the advent of MRI, CT arthrography (the combination of a CT scan with intra-articular contrast) was often used to assess labral integrity, but CT scan of the shoulder is now

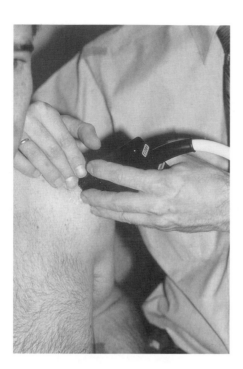

(A)

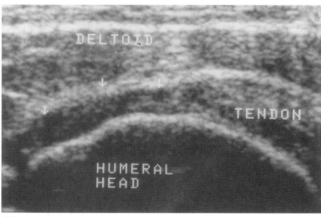

(B)

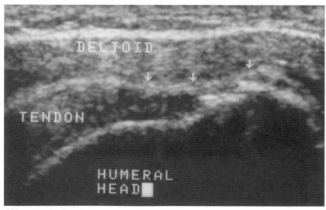

(C)

Fig. 2.6 Ultrasound of rotator cuff tear: (A) ultrasound technique; (B) normal transverse view of supraspinatus; (C) normal longitudinal view of supraspinatus.

mainly used for detailed assessment of bone pathology, or in the planning of surgical intervention. In general terms, soft tissues are better assessed by MRI scan and bone by CT scan.

Radionucleotide bone scan, usually using ^{99m}Technetium, is useful in the assessment of bone vascularity (or avascularity) and areas of increased or decreased osteoblastic activity. It is also useful in localizing metastatic disease. In soft tissue pathology it may show increased activity (vascularity) at sites of enthesopathy (abnormality of bone–tendon junctions).

Treatment

Corticosteroids

Corticosteroid injections are commonly used in the treatment of musculoskeletal conditions. They act by reducing local inflammation, thus directly reducing pain and local swelling. In the subacromial situation, in addition to the corticosteroids' direct effect on inflammation and pain, the reduced swelling of the supraspinatus tendon may be important. The impingement process involves a vicious cycle of 'rub, inflammation, swelling, increased rub, increased inflammation, increased swelling, etc.' By breaking the cycle at the inflammation/swelling stage, corticosteroids can sometimes be virtually curative. There are, however, potential problems associated with injectable steroids. First, any steroid injection into a joint or bursal space carries a small risk of infection, and needs to be performed with appropriate attention to sterility. Second, the effects of corticosteroids on connective tissue are well documented. The repeated use of corticosteroids may produce atrophy and weakening of connective tissues, an obviously undesirable effect in an already damaged structure such as the supraspinatus tendon. There is no consensus regarding how much is safe, but most authorities agree that two injections of steroids to any one site in any 6-month period are not deleterious. As there is a suggestion that steroids produce particular weakening of the soft tissues in the first 24–48 hours after injection, it may be wise to avoid strenuously exercising the injected area for a day or possibly two after a steroid injection.

Interesting facts

Small and medium-sized cuff tears are often compatible with pain-free function. Many older citizens have such tears in one or both shoulders without being aware of 'anything wrong'. Large cuff tears predispose to 'cuff arthropathy', a form of severe secondary shoulder osteoarthritis.

Physiotherapy and exercises

A strong rotator cuff helps hold the humeral head down and away from the coracoacromial arch, reducing the risk

Case 2.1 — Rotator cuff injury: 3

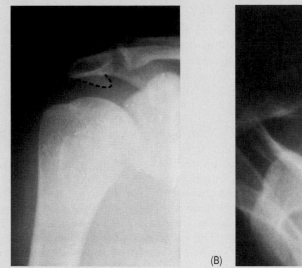 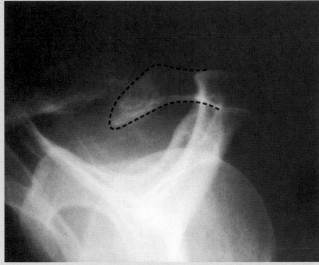

(A) (B)

Fig. 2.7 Plain radiographs of the shoulder: (A) anterior view of acromial spur; (B) outlet view of acromial spur.

Case history

In Mr Jones' case, there was a full and pain-free range of cervical spine movement, and no neurological abnormality (motor, sensory or reflex) in the upper limb.

Plain radiographs of the shoulder were obtained (Fig. 2.7). The anteroposterior view showed chronic changes at the site of cuff insertion to the greater tuberosity, and some minor degenerative arthritis of the acromioclavicular joint. Specifically, there was no evidence of supraspinatus or subscapularis calcification, and acromiohumeral height (the distance between the acromion and the humeral head) was not reduced, as might have occurred in the presence of a major cuff disruption. Nor was there any obvious osteophyte formation or reduction in glenohumeral joint space, to suggest glenohumeral arthritis.

The lateral view did show a spur on the undersurface of the anterior acromion, consistent with possible subacromial impingement. The axillary view (not shown here) showed no evidence of os acromiale, a relatively common congenital variant often associated with subacromial impingement and cuff pathology.

Since the local radiologist had no particular expertise in dynamic ultrasound of the shoulder, an MRI was obtained.

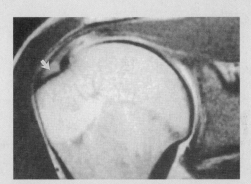

Fig. 2.8 MRI showing a partial-thickness tear of supraspinatus.

This showed a partial thickness deep surface tear of the cuff, without any full thickness extension (Fig. 2.8).

Because of a family history of rheumatoid arthritis, Mr Jones was referred for a full blood count, ESR and rheumatoid factor (Ch. 1), but these were all normal. A high ESR would also be expected in polymyalgia rheumatica.

A definitive diagnosis of partial thickness deep surface cuff tear was made.

Rotator cuff injury: 4

Case history

With a provisional diagnosis of subacromial pathology, including but not necessarily limited to a partial thickness deep surface rotator cuff tear, Mr Jones was given an injection of local anaesthetic and corticosteroid to his subacromial space. The corticosteroid was included to help relieve, at least temporarily, the subacromial impingement component of Mr Jones' symptoms. Within minutes, the local anaesthetic produced almost complete pain relief and, with the pain gone, Mr Jones was able to demonstrate a virtually full active range of shoulder movement. Some secondary inflammation and tightness of the posterior capsule of the shoulder joint prevented full internal rotation. However, strength of forward flexion and abduction was noticeably less than on the asymptomatic side. The pain relief confirmed the presence of subacromial pathology and the normal strength of external rotation indicated that the infraspinatus tendon was almost certainly intact. The significance of this is that the infraspinatus and teres minor tendons form the posterior half of the rotator cuff. If they are intact, any cuff tear is limited to the anterior half of the cuff, and thus not massive, and if necessary, is surgically reparable.

of further impingement and improving overall shoulder function. The lines of pull of both infraspinatus and subscapularis are downwards and medial. Increasing the tone of these muscles may produce an increased downward force vector on the humeral head, further reducing subacromial impingement between the acromion and the humeral head ('inner range internal and external rotator strengthening'), at least while the muscles are 'firing'. Exercises designed to strengthen external rotators (especially infraspinatus) and internal rotators (especially subscapularis) can be performed by keeping the elbow flexed at 90° by the side and rotating the shoulder outwards or inwards, respectively, while holding onto the end of an elasticized band of suitable thickness for resistance. Anatomical studies have shown that the posterior capsule of the glenohumeral joint holds the humeral head up, and that a tight posterior capsule exacerbates subacromial impingement of the rotator cuff. Posterior capsule stretching exercises help lower the humeral head and reduce subacromial impingement.

Increasing the strength of those muscles which move the scapula is of particular help. Shoulder movement occurs at both the glenohumeral and scapulothoracic articulations in an approximate ratio of two to one. By increasing the strength of the scapular muscles ('scapular stabilizing'), better shoulder flexion and abduction can be achieved with scapulothoracic movement, placing less demand on the glenohumeral component of shoulder function,

resulting in less subacromial impingement and pain. The stretching of injured joint capsules, ligaments and tendons is an integral part of systematic rehabilitation.

Physiology

Connective tissues, which include joint capsules, tendons, ligaments and the fascia covering muscles, contain collagen and elastin fibres. Collagen provides tensile strength and elastin provides elasticity. The higher the ratio of elastin to collagen in the capsule of a joint, the greater that joint's range of movement. The basic unit of contraction in muscle is the sarcomere (see Ch. 8). Once a muscle is maximally stretched, with the sarcomere fully stretched, connective tissues take up the slack. In this process, fibres are aligned in the direction of tension. Proprioceptors relay information from the tendon and the muscle–tendon junction to the central nervous system. One important proprioceptor is the Golgi tendon organ, which is sensitive to changes in tension (see Ch. 8). The mechanical behaviour of non-contractile tissue depends on the proportion of collagen and elastin present. In general terms, increased age is associated with decreased maximal tensile strength and increased risk of injury and tear in soft tissues, including tendons and ligaments. Active muscle contraction and passive stretching of muscles is associated with elongation of the connective tissue elements at the ends of the muscle (i.e. tendon and muscle–tendon junction). Regular stretching of connective tissue such as a joint capsule helps alter static (resting) forces on a joint and may actually alter the resting position of the joint and enhance proprioception and joint control.

Surgery

Rotator cuff tears may be repaired arthroscopically or by open surgery. Impingement beneath an acromial spur is often part of the pathology and it may be worthwhile removing the subacromial spur early, by arthroscopic acromioplasty. This is a relatively benign procedure, performed as day surgery and requires a short convalescence and which may allow return to work within 2 weeks of surgery. However, this procedure does not correct any partial thickness cuff tears, which will continue to predispose to further cuff pathology.

The inflammation of the biceps tendon is instructive. The biceps tendon runs immediately in front of the anterior margin of the supraspinatus, between it and the subscapularis, until it exits the shoulder joint. It too can impinge on the undersurface of the acromion and the coracoacromial ligament, and the clinical picture of subacromial impingement is often that of combined supraspinatus and bicipital tendinitis. Supraspinatus changes usually predominate, but occasionally isolated biceps tendinitis occurs, sometimes even progressing to rupture of the tendon of the long-headed biceps, with the resultant well-recognized 'popeye sign' (Fig. 2.9). Biceps rupture is a good example

Rotator cuff injury: 5

Case history

Two days after the steroid injection, Mr Jones was started on a programme of shoulder exercises. A physiotherapist instructed him in a home programme of posterior capsule stretching, inner range internal and external rotator strengthening and scapular stabilizing exercises. He was also instructed in supraspinatus-tendon-stretching techniques.

Mr Jones' shoulder was surprisingly comfortable for 4 days after the steroid injection. Two days after commencing his home exercise programme (5 min, three times a day), Mr Jones again developed shoulder discomfort and nocturnal pain. These increased for a week or so, but just as Mr Jones was about to give up his exercise programme, the pain started to settle. Mr Jones was still not able to return to work, but 8 weeks after starting his exercise programme, his symptoms were at least 75% less severe than they had been. He was given another subacromial corticosteroid injection, and increased the strengthening component of his exercise programme. At 10 weeks after the first corticosteroid injection, Mr Jones returned to work on restricted duties, working mainly at a bench top, and avoiding strenuous and repetitive forward reaching and overhead activity, especially lifting.

He managed well for about 2 months, but then developed sudden severe pain while lifting his toolbox from the boot of the car one evening. The next day, Mr Jones noticed quite marked weakness of forward flexion and especially of external rotation. He had developed a full thickness cuff tear. The surgeon discussed the various treatment options with Mr Jones. Potential advantages of cuff repair included definitive pain relief and return of strength. Disadvantages included the lengthy convalescent period required and a further 2–3 months of physiotherapy and exercise before Mr Jones could return to even light duties as a carpenter. Mr Jones initially opted for ongoing non-operative treatment. Non-steroidal anti-inflammatory medication was added to his regime, and after several days of rest, Mr Jones returned to his exercise programme. Because of a past history of peptic ulcer, Mr Jones was prescribed a specific COX-2 inhibitor anti-inflammatory drug (see Ch. 1). This produced some reduction in pain, but Mr Jones remained frustrated by shoulder weakness and, after a further month, opted for rotator cuff repair.

At surgery, the acromial spur seen on preoperative radiographs was resected as part of an anterior acromioplasty (removal of the under-surface of the anterior acromion to enlarge the space between the bone and the underlying rotator cuff, reducing the risk of tendon-on-bone impingement). There was a large amount of synovial fluid present in the subacromial space, subdeltoid bursa and the shoulder joint, reflecting an ongoing inflammatory process. The full thickness rotator cuff tear was only 2 cm in diameter, but it was in continuity with an interlaminar defect which extended a further centimetre into the rotator cuff tendon posteriorly. The biceps tendon, seen at the front of the rotator cuff defect, was very inflamed. So too was part of the adjacent subdeltoid bursa. Part of the inflamed bursal tissue was resected, together with the inflamed edges of the cuff defect. The interlaminar defect was repaired and the cuff was reattached to the bone of the greater tuberosity.

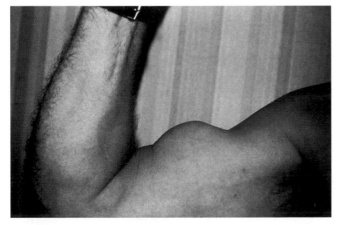

Fig. 2.9 Popeye sign.

of a tendon rupture which does not always require repair. A progressively painful biceps tendinitis suddenly becomes pain-free when the tendon finally ruptures. The resultant weakness affects mainly supination, and elbow flexion is often surprisingly little affected.

Rehabilitation and outcome

Socioeconomic factors are important in the management of 'soft-tissue rheumatism'. An uninsured self-employed contractor may be more willing or likely than some to return to work early, or before complete resolution of symptoms. The use of specialized rehabilitation services is now widespread in industry, and in some places mandatory, to help plan return-to-work programmes, with hour modifications, task modification and retraining each being relevant in certain situations.

The benefits of exercise programmes are never instantaneous. The first week or two of an exercise programme is often associated with increased discomfort, and patients need to be forewarned of this and encouraged to persist with their programme for several weeks before assessing its efficacy. They should also be warned of danger signs. In this case, the sudden loss of strength indicated a major extension of the initially incomplete cuff tear. This suggested possible urgency to surgical repair, before cuff retraction and muscle atrophy precluded a good surgical result. Not all rotator cuff tears need surgery. In fact,

Case
2.1

Case 2.1 — Rotator cuff injury: 6

Case history

Mr Jones' first postoperative week was difficult. To mini-mize postoperative stiffness, especially due to adhesions between the cuff repair and the overlying acromion and deltoid, *passive* mobilization of the shoulder was nec-essary. At the same time, *active* flexion and abduction were avoided to minimize the risk of disrupting the ten-don repair. Six weeks postoperatively, Mr Jones' sling was removed and a programme of *active-assisted* exercises was commenced. In this, Mr Jones employed a pulley, initially raising his right hand with considerable help from the left, but gradually doing more and more of the raising using the muscles of the right shoulder. He also added rotation exercises to his regime. Twelve weeks postoperatively, a more strenuous *'active-resisted'* programme was started, aimed at strengthening the rotator cuff and deltoid muscu-lature in particular. He returned to work 16 weeks postop-eratively, initially avoiding the heaviest of forward-reaching and overhead activities, and minimizing any impact-loading (jarring) on the shoulder. Six months postoperatively, he was coping with unrestricted work activities, sleeping well at night, but vaguely aware of some mild discomfort with overhead activity.

Case 2.1 — Rotator cuff injury: 7

Case history

Mr Jones' physiotherapy regime, was tailored to the expected course of tendon-healing. Initial passive mobilization should not strain the healing bone–tendon junction. By 12 weeks postoperatively, it was hoped that the collagen fibres cross-ing the healing bone–tendon junction, initially haphazardly, would be at least partly 'realigned' perpendicularly to the bone surface, in the 'line of pull' of the tendon. This should provide sufficient strength to allow active and active-resisted exercise.

The success rate of surgery depends on how it is meas-ured. If measured in degrees of motion, or absolute units of strength, recovery is rarely complete. The best measure of success is patient satisfaction. Recent trends in musculoskel-etal outcome studies have been directed towards param-eters determined by the patient (relief of pain, return to normal work and sport activities, ability to perform activi-ties of daily living, etc.) rather than more quantifiable parameters, measured by the examiner, such as range-of-motion or kilopascals of strength. Measured in terms of patient satisfaction, rotator cuff repair is successful in over 90% of non-compensable patients. The reported success rate in compensable patients is significantly lower. In addi-tion to the obvious explanations concerning motivation and secondary gain, this may be in part due to the younger age group and the more strenuous activities required.

---

many rotator cuff tears are asymptomatic. Post-mortem studies suggest that 50% or more of 70-year-olds have partial or full thickness tears involving one or both rotator cuffs. That is, like cervical spondylosis, rotator cuff pathol-ogy is often asymptomatic and may not require treatment, conservative or surgical. The presence of a damaged rota-tor cuff however does increase the risk of further tendon injury.

Anatomy of the elbow

The elbow is a hinge joint composed of three articula-tions, humeroulnar (the principal articulation), radio-humeral and proximal radioulnar. All these articulations are enclosed by the capsule in a common synovial joint cavity. The synovial membrane is usually only palpa-ble posteriorly. One large bursa (olecranon) and several small bursae lie about the elbow (Fig. 2.10). The tendi-nous attachments of muscles to the medial and lateral epicondyles of the humerus are common sites of local-ized tenderness.

Lateral epicondylitis

Lateral epicondylitis or 'tennis elbow' is generally an over-use phenomenon reflecting inflammation of the common

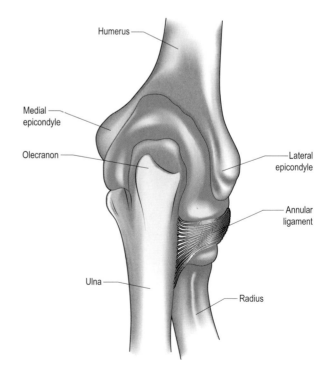

Fig. 2.10 Anatomy of the elbow (posterior view).

Case 2.2 Tennis elbow: 1

Case history

Mrs Smith, 50 years old, gives a history of pain in the lateral aspect of her left elbow, especially when reaching for objects with her left hand, such as when doing the ironing or lifting a kettle of water. She consults her local doctor who elicits tenderness over the lateral epicondyle of the elbow and pain on resisted extension of the wrist. He diagnoses 'tennis elbow'. Mrs Smith asks how could that be, stating that she does not play tennis.

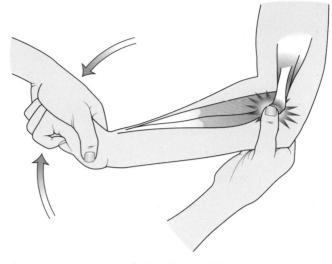

Fig. 2.11 Provocation test for lateral epicondylitis.

extensor tendon, which inserts at the lateral epicondyle of the humerus (Fig. 2.11). The main muscle affected in tennis elbow is extensor carpi radialis brevis (ECRB). Extensor digitorum communis, extensor carpi radialis longus and extensor carpi ulnaris are also often involved. Clinical signs include marked localized tenderness over the epicondyle and pain on resisted extension of the wrist or middle finger. Similar findings at the medial epicondyle, where the wrist flexors arise, are called 'golfer's elbow'. Both syndromes occur commonly without exposure to sports, but often in association with other repetitive wrist activity.

Local corticosteroid injections and stretching exercises are usually effective. Some chronic cases are treated by braces. Diagnostic imaging is rarely needed in the investigation and treatment of lateral epicondylitis. Should conservative measures not suffice however, MRI scan may confirm and localize organic change. Surgical release of ECRB, or occasionally the entire common extensor origin, is sometimes useful. Less frequently, MRI may show the changes to be primarily capsular or intraarticular.

Further reading

Moore, K.L., Dalley, A.F., 2006. Clinically Oriented Anatomy, fifth ed. Williams & Wilkins, Baltimore.

Post, M., Bigliani, L.U., Flatow, E.L., et al., 1998. The Shoulder: Operative Technique. Williams & Wilkins, Baltimore.

NERVE COMPRESSION SYNDROMES

3

Michael Tonkin

Chapter objectives

After studying this chapter you should be able to:

1. Understand normal peripheral nerve anatomy and function including electrophysiological testing.

2. Appreciate the aetiopathogenesis of the most common entrapment syndromes.

3. Assess the risk factors commonly associated with carpal tunnel syndrome.

4. Understand the general principles of medical and surgical treatment of entrapment neuropathies and their complications.

Introduction

Nerve compression (entrapment) syndromes are a common cause of limb pain. The most common of these is the carpal tunnel syndrome in which the median nerve is compressed at the wrist. Other examples include the cubital tunnel syndrome due to compression of the ulnar nerve at the elbow, the tarsal tunnel syndrome due to entrapment of the posterior tibial nerve at the ankle and meralgia paraesthetica due to entrapment of the lateral cutaneous nerve of the thigh in the inguinal region. Understanding these syndromes requires knowledge of nerve anatomy, the classification and pathophysiology of nerve injury and the causes of nerve injury. Electrophysiological examination is the main investigation used to support or clarify clinical diagnoses based upon precise history taking and careful examination. Treatment of individual patients may vary according to the duration and severity of symptoms and signs, age and general medical condition. When present, reversible causes must be addressed.

This chapter will focus on nerve compression syndromes in the diagnosis of hand and upper limb pain and will review normal peripheral nerve anatomy and physiology.

Peripheral nerve anatomy

Peripheral nerves emerge from the spinal intervertebral foramina and travel to their endpoint structures, sensory receptors and neuromuscular junctions. The axon is a peripheral process from the nerve cell body in the anterior horn of the spinal cord (motor neuron) or the dorsal root ganglion (sensory neuron). Excitable cells such as neurons and muscle fibres communicate with each other at special regions called synapses. The first cell communicates with the second by releasing chemicals called neurotransmitters. The synapse between a motor neuron and a skeletal muscle fibre is called the neuromuscular junction, and the neurotransmitter is acetylcholine (see Ch. 8 for further discussion).

The axon is surrounded by Schwann cells and, together, axon and Schwann cells make up a nerve fibre. Myelinated fibres are those in which each axon is surrounded by single Schwann cells arranged longitudinally to form a continuous chain. Non-myelinated fibres contain multiple axons within the cytoplasm of a surrounding Schwann cell.

Peripheral nerve fibres are usually classified into three types in relation to their conduction velocity, which is generally proportionate to size (Table 3.1).

Nerve fibres are gathered into groups called fascicles and are surrounded by a mechanically strong membrane, the perineurium. Within the fascicles, nerve fibres lie within connective tissue called endoneurium. The fascicles themselves are embedded in an internal epineurium surrounded by an external loose epineurial connective tissue layer (Fig. 3.1). Nerves, such as the sciatic nerve, contain a greater percentage of connective tissue in relation to axonal substance. However, most people experience the sensation of leg and foot numbness following prolonged periods of sitting, especially on unyielding objects, when the protective benefit of the connective tissue cushion is overcome.

The nerve trunk receives a segmental vascular supply. Extrinsic vessels run parallel to the nerve providing branches that lie within the epineurium, perineurium and endoneurium in a longitudinal pattern in each layer, with interconnecting branches between layers. Those vessels passing through the perineurium into the endoneurium often lie obliquely, creating a valve mechanism, which is vulnerable to pressure (Fig. 3.2).

Case 3.1 Carpal tunnel syndrome: 1

Case history

Mrs Fotini, aged 55, is a production line worker in a factory with a packaging company. She works an 8-hour day in four shifts divided by half-hour rest periods between shifts.

She presented complaining of pins and needles in both hands, which wake her at night and occur intermittently during the day. She also describes neck stiffness and discomfort with pain radiating from her left shoulder to her hand and swelling in both hands, more so in the early mornings.

She was diagnosed as having late-onset diabetes 2 years earlier, which has been reasonably controlled by diet and oral hypoglycaemic medication. She also takes non-steroidal anti-inflammatory medications for osteoarthritis affecting the small joints in her hands, neck and back.

Examination of her hands reveals no swelling of her joints and a normal range of movement. However, sustained wrist flexion for 1 min reproduced her symptoms of numbness affecting both hands.

The history and examination findings suggest a diagnosis of bilateral carpal tunnel syndrome and her GP recommended she wear a wrist splint at night to keep her wrist in the neutral position.

Table 3.1 Classification of nerve fibres

Group	Function
Group A: up to 20 μm diameter, myelinated, subdivided into:	
α: 12–20 μm	Touch and proprioception (Ia and Ib)
β: 5–12 μm	Touch, pressure and proprioception (II)
γ: 5–12 μm	Fusimotor to muscle spindles (II)
δ: 1–15 μm	Touch, pain and temperature (III)
Group B: up to 3 μm diameter, myelinated	Preganglionic autonomic
Group C: up to 12 μm diameter, unmyelinated	Postganglionic autonomic, and touch and pain (IV)

Nerves span joints with varying ranges of motion. On the outside of the nerve trunk, a conjunctival adventitia allows movement of the nerve trunk within its soft tissue surroundings. In deeper layers, fascicles can slide against each other. This allows movement of approximately 50 mm within the brachial plexus during abduction and adduction of the shoulder, 10 mm of the ulnar nerve at the elbow during flexion and extension, and 9 mm of the median nerve at the carpal tunnel with wrist flexion and extension.

Pathophysiology and classification of nerve injury

The endoneurial environment of the nerve is preserved by a combination of a blood–nerve barrier, in which the endoneurial vessels do not allow extravasation of proteins, and by the diffusion barrier of the perineurial sheath. The tissue pressure inside fascicles is slightly positive, providing a normal and healthy mechanical stiffness of fascicles.

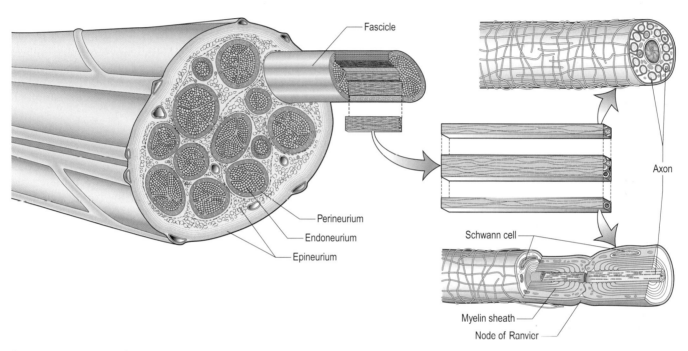

Fig. 3.1 Microanatomy of a peripheral nerve and its components. (A) Fascicles surrounded by perineurium are embedded in a loose connective tissue, the epineurium. The outer layers of the epineurium are condensed into a sheath. The expanded views show the appearance of (B) unmyelinated and (C) myelinated fibres.

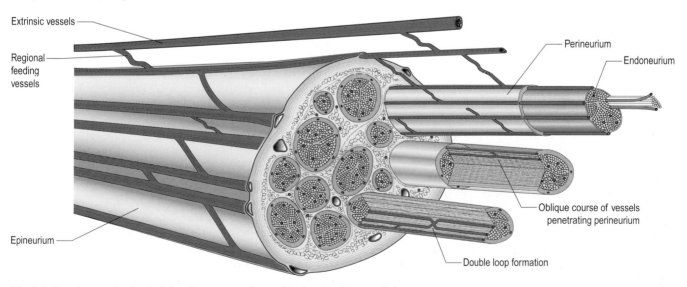

Fig. 3.2 Vascular supply of a peripheral nerve. Vessels are abundant in all layers of the nerve; extrinsic vessels support, via regional feeding vessels, the epineurium, perineurium and endoneurium.

When oedema is introduced into the endoneurial space of the nerve trunk, this may not escape easily owing to the diffusion barrier of the perineurial membrane. Consequently, axonal transport of substances from nerve cell bodies down axons (anterograde axonal transport) and from the periphery to the nerve cell body (retrograde axonal transport) is impaired.

A local metabolic conduction block may be induced by mild compression but is physiological only and without consequences for the structure of nerve fibres. Provided the compression is mild and limited in time, such a metabolic block is reversible. With extended compression, there may be oedema within the fascicles resulting in a local conduction block lasting longer than the duration of the precipitating cause. The myelin sheath is damaged but axonal continuity is preserved. This is termed neurapraxia and is usually spontaneously reversible within 3 months (termed a Sunderland type I lesion).

More severe compression or traction may disrupt the continuity of axons. Provided the endoneurium is intact, regenerating axons are maintained within the correct tubes and are guided to the appropriate sensory receptors and neuromuscular junctions. This lesion is classified as an axonotmesis or a Sunderland type II lesion.

Loss of continuity of axons and connective tissue components result in neurotmesis. This usually is a consequence of an acute stretching of the nerve, a severe crush or traumatic division. Sunderland has subdivided these more severe lesions into three types:

1. Loss of the endoneurial layer (type III)
2. Loss of the perineurial layer (type IV)
3. Complete transection of the nerve with loss of the epineurial layers (type V).

Surgical repair is the only method of returning some function in the last of these. The degree of internal disorganization in types III and IV may result in very poor nerve regeneration and minimal return of function without surgical repair.

Causes of nerve compression

There are a variety of mechanisms that can lead to nerve compression and several factors may be present at the same time, especially at the carpal tunnel.

Anatomical

Unyielding anatomical structures, such as within the carpal tunnel, allow little increase in pressure before the median nerve is compressed.

Inflammatory

Synovial compartments will be affected most commonly by inflammatory diseases such as rheumatoid arthritis. However, any cause of tenosynovitis will increase the size of contents of anatomical compartments and decrease the space for nerves within them.

Metabolic

Common metabolic problems such as diabetes and hypothyroidism can be associated with an alteration in fluid balance. Physiological alterations in fluid balance, such as in pregnancy and premenstrually, may also induce carpal tunnel compression.

Iatrogenic

Tight plasters and dressings or compression during surgery from retraction or other mechanical injury are preventable but all too common causes of nerve injury. Poorly fitted tourniquets, inappropriate pressure within the tourniquet and prolonged tourniquet time, particularly in susceptible subjects, may result in iatrogenic nerve injury.

Postural

Compromise of anatomical spaces occurs when poor posture, perhaps in association with decreased muscle tone, fails to maintain adequate space for the nerve. Repetitive activities placing joints in extreme positions may also compromise the environment of the nerve.

Developmental

Anomalous anatomical structures such as a cervical rib at the level of the thoracic outlet may compress the brachial plexus.

Traumatic

Any injury causing soft tissue swelling or a fracture will affect the pressure, particularly in tight compartments, such as the carpal tunnel.

Swellings

Tumours, of which ganglia are the most common, infections such as an abscess, and vascular tumours such as aneurysm or thrombosis of the median artery, can reduce space for a nerve.

Degenerative

Remodelling of a joint or collapse associated with osteoarthritis, osteophyte formation and instability of joints may result in nerve compression.

Neuropathic

A nerve already damaged, either by a disease such as diabetic neuropathy or by a proximal compressive lesion, renders the nerve more irritable and more likely to be susceptible to compression at other sites. The latter lesion is sometimes called a double crush syndrome, as there are both proximal and distal lesions.

Electrophysiology

Nerve conduction studies and electromyography often provide the only objective evidence of a neuropathic condition. It is necessary to understand the concepts and terminology of nerve physiology, pathology and methods of electrodiagnostic studies in order to evaluate the results of these studies.

Electrodiagnostic studies can help confirm the clinical compression of a compression neuropathy with a high degree of sensitivity and specificity, but there are some pitfalls.

Both nerve and muscle cells have a relative negative electrical charge inside them compared with the extracellular environment by virtue of a much higher concentration of potassium within the cells and a lower concentration of sodium and chloride. Electrical stimulation of the cells causes depolarization and generates an action potential. During depolarization, there is an opening of sodium channels in the cell membrane leading to an increase in sodium permeability and creation of an electric current by this rush of positively charged ions into the cell. Current then flows along the path of least electrical resistance, the length of the axon. Myelinated nerve fibres provide a mechanism for regenerating the charge of current (saltatory conduction). The myelin acts as an insulator to prevent current leakage. The myelin sheath indents at intervals, creating tight gaps that expose the axon, called nodes of Ranvier (Fig. 3.1). The action potential is propagated down the axon and exits at the node completing the electrical circuit through the extracellular fluid. This repeats the process of depolarization and perpetuates regeneration of the longitudinal current. However, there is a delay in the process at each node. Conduction velocity is faster with fewer nodal delays, the large-diameter nerves having the greatest internodal distances and therefore the fastest conduction speeds. These fibres include the alpha motor neurons and the sensory fibres transmitting light touch and proprioceptive (joint position) sensations. Pain and temperature and autonomic functions are conducted by slower, smaller myelinated or unmyelinated fibres.

When the action potential from the motor neuron arrives at the neuromuscular junction, it is transmitted chemically to the muscle. The electrical current is measurable and allows objective measurements of nerve function.

Nerve conduction studies

Motor nerve conduction studies

Motor nerve conduction studies assess the lower motor neurons from the level of the anterior horn to the muscle. The principle will be illustrated by reference to the median nerve (Fig. 3.3). A supramaximal electrical stimulus depolarizes all axons of the nerve and results in an action potential that travels in the normal physiological

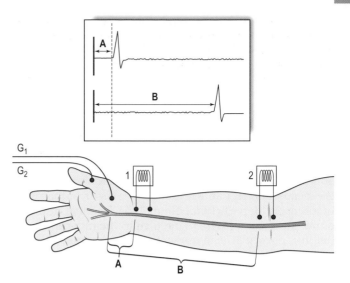

Fig. 3.3 An electrical stimulus is given over the wrist (1) or elbow (2) and measured by recording electrodes at G overlying the abductor pollicis brevis muscle. The time taken to travel from 1 to G is the distal motor latency A; and from 2 to G is the proximal motor latency B (based on Hilburn, 1996, Fig. 4, p. 212).

direction (orthodromically) down the nerve and is measured by recording electrodes overlying the thenar muscle belly. The distal motor latency is the time in milliseconds that it takes the impulse to travel from the stimulation point at the wrist to the recording electrode, say 3 milliseconds (ms). If the nerve is then stimulated at the elbow and the response follows after 7 ms, the motor conduction velocity is estimated by subtracting the distal motor latency from the proximal motor latency (i.e. $7 - 3 = 4$ ms) and dividing the result by the distance between the two stimulating points (240 mm), i.e. a motor conduction velocity of 60 m/s. The shape of the wave is also important. A drop in amplitude indicates a conduction block, whereas an increase in duration indicates a lack of uniform conduction along the axons.

Sensory nerve conduction studies

The sensory nerve action potential is usually recorded by stimulating a distal sensory site and recording proximally over a mixed or sensory nerve (orthodromic conduction). It is also possible to stimulate a mixed nerve proximally and record at a distal site where only sensory axons are present (antidromic conduction, or opposite to the normal physiological direction of impulse transmission). As with motor conduction studies, the sensory nerve action potential is recorded from only the largest 15–20% of myelinated axons within the nerve. With loss of axons (axonal degeneration), or blocking of conduction owing to demyelination, the amplitude of the action potential decreases.

Estimation of the F wave and H reflex provides additional information. The F wave is a late muscle response from the anterior horn cells in response to the same stimulus that evoked the early direct muscle response. It results in a discharge that sends an impulse back down the same motor axon. Thus the stimulus to the median nerve at the wrist resulted in a direct thenar muscle response after 3 ms and a later response, the F wave, giving the conduction time from the wrist to the spinal cord and back again. The F-wave latency gives an indication of the state of the nerve proximally and, if prolonged significantly, one may suspect proximal compression.

The F wave should not be confused with the H reflex, another late response. This is obtained by a submaximal stimulation of the nerve (i.e. a stimulus too low to excite the nerve directly) and results in proximal propagation of a sensory nerve action potential to the spinal cord and a measurable monosynaptic return to the muscle. This is helpful, particularly, in assessing radiculopathies (spinal nerve root lesions).

There are pitfalls of nerve conduction studies. Both motor and sensory studies measure velocity in the largest-diameter and fastest-conducting nerve fibres only. Measurements will be normal if these nerve fibres remain intact. In addition, there is a wide range of normal values for motor conduction velocity of nerves. Operator error may be a factor. Some nerves are located within deep tissues and are less accessible for surface electrode stimulation. The stimulus intensity necessary to depolarize these nerves causes such a spread of current through the intervening tissues that the exact point of stimulation cannot be determined and the measurements are thus less reliable. Radiculopathies (compression at the nerve root origin) and plexopathies (compression of junctions or networks of several nerve roots, e.g. the brachial plexus) are poorly demonstrated on nerve conduction studies. Nerve conduction velocity diminishes with lower temperatures, with increased height of the individual and increased finger circumference. Age is also a factor in determining nerve conduction speed, which is slower in newborns–3 years of age and in older age groups.

Electromyography (EMG)

Motor unit potentials can only be recorded accurately by means of a needle electrode inserted within the muscle tested. Even with fine needles, the associated discomfort may compromise the ability to achieve reliable information. The technique does, however, offer significant information, particularly in proximal lesions in which nerve conduction studies may poorly demonstrate a radiculopathy or plexopathy.

It is possible to measure insertional activity (see below), activity at rest, the size and configuration of the motor unit potentials elicited by minimal voluntary muscle contraction, and the abundance of active motor units (recruitment) at maximal contraction.

Insertional activity is the electrical activity caused by injury to the muscle by movement of the needle electrode. In normal muscle this persists only as long as the needle is being advanced. With denervation, insertional activity is increased and prolonged.

Activity at rest is normally that of relative electrical silence or of endplate noise. Fibrillation potentials are action potentials of single muscle fibres that occur spontaneously and with needle insertion. They appear several weeks after a nerve injury and are also seen in myopathic disorders. Fasciculation potentials have the dimensions of motor unit potentials and can be benign spontaneous discharges or a sign of anterior horn cell disease. Polyphasic motor units, if numerous and of increased duration and amplitude, are indicative of chronic denervation with reinnervation by adjacent sprouting nerve terminals. The nerve injury is relatively chronic but there is some reinnervation. Recruitment of motor units is a measure of the number of motor units activated (recruited) by maximum muscle contraction. Reduction is present with denervation (Fig. 3.4).

Electromyographic investigation is dependent upon the experience of the electrophysiologist and there is significant interobserver variability in interpretation. Anatomical placement of the needle needs to be precise and it may be necessary to sample multiple areas of each muscle to describe a muscle abnormality. It is important to realize that the EMG will be normal in neurapraxic lesions because of the absence of denervation and that the changes measured by EMG are delayed for 3 weeks

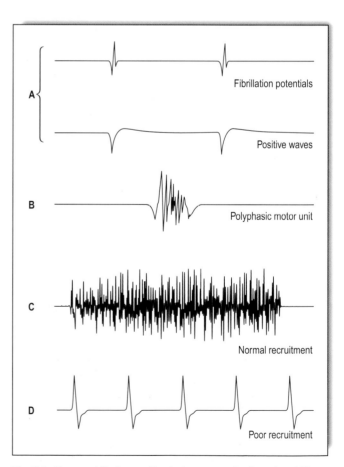

Fig. 3.4 Abnormal findings with electromyography (based on Hilburn, 1996, Fig. 3, p. 211).

following axonotmesis or neurotmesis when anterograde (Wallerian) degeneration of the axons detached from their cell bodies has occurred. The use of EMG for diagnosis of muscle disorders is discussed again in Chapter 8.

Carpal tunnel syndrome

Carpal tunnel compression is the most common of the nerve compression syndromes, with an incidence of approximately 99 in 100000. It is more common in females (65–75%), more common in middle age, and bilateral in up to 50% of cases.

Anatomy of the carpal tunnel

The floor of the carpal tunnel is formed by the concave arch of the carpal bones covered by the extrinsic palmar wrist ligaments. The roof is the transverse carpal ligament (flexor retinaculum), which is attached to the scaphoid and trapezium bones radially and on the ulnar side to the pisiform and the hamate (Fig. 3.5).

The tunnel contains nine flexor tendons and their vascular synovium, and the median nerve, which may be accompanied by a persistent median artery. Within the carpal tunnel, the nerve lies superficial to the flexor tendons beneath the flexor retinaculum in the radial aspect of the tunnel. The ulnar nerve and artery do not lie within the carpal tunnel but are covered by the palmar carpal ligament extending from the superficial aspect of the flexor retinaculum to the pisiform.

The palmar cutaneous branch of the median nerve takes origin from the radial side of the nerve approximately 5cm above the wrist, pierces the antebrachial fascia at the distal wrist crease and lies superficial to the flexor retinaculum, supplying sensory fibres to the skin overlying the thenar eminence (Fig. 3.6). The median nerve proper usually divides at the distal end of the carpal tunnel into radial and ulnar portions and then lies deep to the palmar aponeurosis and the superficial palmar arch. The radial division of the nerve gives rise to the thenar motor branch, which innervates the abductor pollicis brevis muscle, opponens pollicis muscle and usually a large part of the flexor pollicis brevis muscle.

Interesting facts

The role of occupational factors in the aetiology of carpal tunnel syndrome remains controversial in the worker's compensation setting, but systematic reviews of the literature have generally shown that use of vibratory tools and highly repetitive flexion and extension, especially in association with forceful grip, is associated with an increased risk of symptomatic carpal tunnel syndrome.

Pathophysiology and causes

Any one of the causes of nerve compression outlined previously may be responsible for carpal tunnel syndrome. On occasions, the aetiology is multifactorial. However, in most, the cause is unknown and is termed idiopathic.

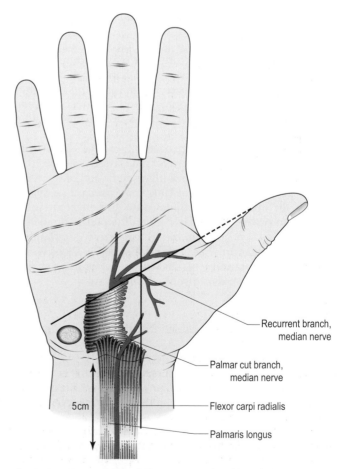

Fig. 3.6 Anatomy of the palmar cutaneous branch and thenar branch of the median nerve.

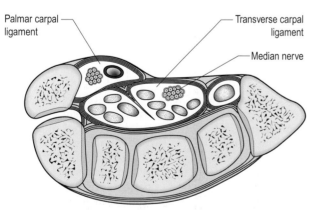

Fig. 3.5 Cross-sectional anatomy of the carpal tunnel. The tunnel contains the median nerve and nine flexor tendons. The transverse carpal ligament forms the palmar surface of the carpal tunnel and the dorsal boundary of the distal ulnar tunnel. The palmar carpal ligament forms the volar boundary of the distal ulnar tunnel.

Carpal tunnel syndrome: 2

Case note: Surgical referral

Mrs Fotini had only partial relief of her symptoms from the wearing of night splints and she was referred to a hand surgeon. On further history taking, she stated that she woke nightly, on at least one occasion with numbness in both hands. She was unable to define which parts of the hands were affected but indicated that she often rose to make herself a cup of tea, during which time the symptoms disappeared.

Her hands were puffy in the mornings, as if 'full of fluid'. Stiffness in the hands improved during the day but was replaced by an aching pain, which was diffusely related to the left wrist and increased towards the end of her working day. Pins and needles occurred in both hands when driving home from work. She also described an aching pain in the neck with radiation to the left shoulder and arm during packaging, particularly towards the end of her working day.

The increased incidence in females, particularly perimenopausally, suggests an alteration in hormonal balance as a causative factor, perhaps in association with alteration in fluid balance.

Carpal tunnel syndrome is not uncommonly associated with distal radial fractures but may accompany any traumatic oedema of the wrist and hand, including that following surgery. The most common tumorous swellings are those of ganglia and lipomata and the most common inflammatory conditions are rheumatoid arthritis, gout and, rarely, amyloidosis.

The association between occupation and carpal tunnel syndrome remains controversial. Those activities that involve repetitive flexion and ulnar deviation of the wrist over a prolonged period of time may precipitate symptoms in an 'at-risk' individual. Cause and effect are more difficult to prove, particularly given the predominance of carpal tunnel syndrome in older, less active populations. However, a clear link has been established in those workers who use vibration tools, in whom symptoms develop during or just after their use.

Clinical diagnosis

History

By far, the most important aspect of diagnosis is the history. Those patients who wake at night with pain and numbness in the distribution of the median nerve, which is alleviated by various physical actions, such as hanging the hands over the edge of the bed, wringing the hands, placing the hands in water, usually have carpal tunnel syndrome.

Symptoms of pain and numbness or tingling in the palmar aspect of the radial three digits may occur when driving a car or holding a newspaper, book or telephone for prolonged periods of time. Patients may not be able to describe a precise distribution of discomfort and may include the little finger in their description and the palm of the hand overlying the thenar eminence as being symptomatic. The former is supplied by the ulnar nerve and the latter by the palmar cutaneous branch of the median nerve, which does not pass through the carpal tunnel.

Patients with carpal tunnel syndrome may describe discomfort radiating proximally as far as the shoulder. Clumsiness and the complaint of dropping objects are more often associated with sensory disturbance than motor weakness, but may be a consequence of both. Those who do not present with the above symptoms are much less likely to have carpal tunnel syndrome. Clinical examination and electrophysiological testing are used to confirm the diagnosis. Although carpal tunnel syndrome is usually idiopathic, the examining physician should consider the multiple but less common causes that are described above.

Examination

In severe cases, the patient may be able to precisely map an area of numbness—the radial three digits and radial half of the ring finger on the palmar aspect to perhaps the distal palmar crease proximally and the level of the proximal interphalangeal joint dorsally. The examiner should attempt to differentiate normal and abnormal sensation within the distribution of the median nerve proper and that of the ulnar nerve, the palmar cutaneous branch of the median nerve, the superficial radial nerve and the lateral cutaneous nerve of the forearm.

Both hands should be examined for wasting, particularly within the thenar musculature. Wasting, if present, should be differentiated from combined thenar and finger intrinsic wasting, indicating a first thoracic (T1) nerve root lesion or a combined median and ulnar nerve lesion. Degenerative osteoarthritis of the basal thumb joints may cause thenar wasting, despite normal median nerve function. Generalized wasting may indicate a peripheral neuropathy or systemic condition. Assessment of motor power may confirm weakness of muscles innervated by the median nerve. Weakness of muscles not supplied by the median nerve should alert the physician to an alternative diagnosis.

Various provocative tests aid in the diagnosis of carpal tunnel syndrome. A positive Tinel's sign overlying the median nerve within the carpal tunnel, just proximal or just distal to the carpal tunnel indicates sensitivity of the nerve (Fig. 3.7). However, percussion over the median nerve may elicit paraesthesia within the median nerve distribution in patients without carpal tunnel syndrome and may be negative in those with more advanced compression. Tinel's sign has a sensitivity of 67%. The Phalen test places the wrist in acute flexion and should be performed bilaterally (Fig. 3.8). This is the test performed by Mrs Fotini's GP (see Case 3.1:1, p. 34). The timing of the development of symptoms is

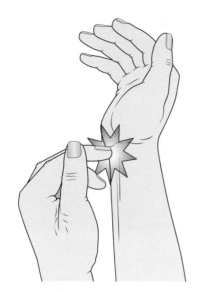

Fig. 3.7 Percussion over the median nerve to elicit Tinel's sign. Tinel's sign is positive when percussion over the nerve elicits a tingling sensation distally.

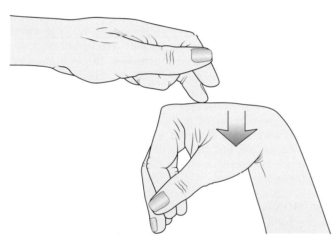

Fig. 3.8 The patient is asked to flex both wrists maximally and keep them flexed for at least 60s—Phalen's test.

of value, particularly in comparison. Onset of numbness in less than 1 min is suggestive. The reversed Phalen test may produce symptoms by placing the nerve on stretch.

Other provocative tests include sustained thumb pressure on the carpal tunnel and the placement of a sphygmomanometer cuff, inflated at the wrist to 150 mm Hg for 30 s.

Investigations

Radiographs of the wrist are usually unhelpful but may demonstrate degenerative arthritis or calcified tumours. The carpal tunnel radiological view is of value in demonstrating the presence of abnormal radiopaque structures within the carpal tunnel. Ultrasound, CT and MRI examination may be appropriate when space-occupying

Case 3.1 | **Carpal tunnel syndrome: 3**

Case note: Examination

On examination, diffuse swelling was present around the dorsal aspect of Mrs Fotini's left wrist. Bony swelling (Heberden's nodes) was present in the distal interphalangeal joints. The bases of both thumbs were swollen and the thenar eminence was wasted bilaterally. Sensory testing indicated a constant alteration in touch sensibility in the thumb, index and middle fingers of the left hand, but not elsewhere. The Tinel and Phalen tests were positive bilaterally. Muscle power of the thenar eminence muscles was considered normal in spite of the thenar eminence wasting.

There was no evidence of a generalized lymphoedema in the feet or hands; however, Mrs Fotini was significantly overweight.

lesions are suspected. Measurements of the carpal tunnel volume and pressure are rarely indicated.

It is uncommon for electrophysiological investigations to make a diagnosis of carpal tunnel syndrome in a patient whose history taking and physical examination have not done so. However, it is interesting that as many as 38% of patients presenting with unilateral carpal tunnel syndrome may be asymptomatic on the opposite side but have abnormal nerve conduction tests.

Baseline electrophysiology is still appropriate to distinguish a compressive lesion from a peripheral neuropathy secondary to diseases such as diabetes; to provide objective evidence of a nerve disorder and its site of compression; and to provide comparative figures against which to measure improvement or lack of improvement. In general, distal motor latencies of more than 4.5 ms and distal sensory latencies of more than 3.5 ms are considered abnormal.

Treatment of carpal tunnel syndrome

Conservative therapy

If a reversible cause of carpal tunnel syndrome can be identified, attention must be directed to this. The use of diuretics and vitamin B_6 (pyridoxine) may be useful, the former when fluid retention is considered to be an aetiological factor, and the latter for patients not responsive to other methods of conservative therapy. Vitamin B_6 deficiency has been associated with carpal tunnel syndrome. Furthermore, resolution of carpal tunnel syndrome symptoms may occur following vitamin B_6 administration. Its actions are numerous, being involved in the structural and functional integrity of many aspects of the nervous system. However, the literature does not give convincing evidence for the use of vitamin B_6 as sole treatment in patients with idiopathic carpal tunnel syndrome.

Carpal tunnel syndrome: 4

Case note: Investigations

The symptoms and signs indicated that Mrs Fotini was suffering from bilateral carpal tunnel syndrome and that this was the primary cause of her presenting complaints. However, the presence of possible contributory factors such as diabetes and the association of pins and needles in the hands with neck, wrist and thumb pain and generalized osteoarthritis required further investigation.

The following investigations were therefore requested. X-rays of the cervical spine and hands revealed a generalized degenerative arthritis affecting the cervical spine, particularly the C5/6, C6/7 and C7/T1 intervertebral disc spaces and foraminal spaces. However, there was no significant encroachment of osteophytes or narrowing of the intervertebral foramina. X-rays of the hands revealed osteoarthritis.

Nerve conduction tests revealed a delay in sensory and motor conduction velocities bilaterally, moderate on the left side and mild on the right. There were prolonged motor and sensory latencies bilaterally. Electromyography did not reveal motor axonal degeneration. Normal studies of radial and ulnar nerves and of the common peroneal nerve of the right lower limb ruled out the possibility of a diabetic neuropathy.

Tests of serum iron and ferritin levels, performed to rule out haemochromatosis, were normal. This condition is characterized by excessive deposits of iron in the body and is associated with liver insufficiency and degenerative arthritis affecting the metacarpophalangeal joints of index and middle fingers, in combination with skin pigmentation and diabetes.

Following the above investigations, the hand surgeon was able to inform Mrs Fotini that there was clinical and electrophysiological evidence of bilateral carpal tunnel syndrome. The neck stiffness and shoulder discomfort were probably consequent upon the cervical spondylosis (degenerative arthritis). It is interesting that bilateral thenar eminence wasting was present. However, motor power was retained and therefore this wasting was apparent rather than real and consequent upon the carpometacarpal joint degenerative arthritis.

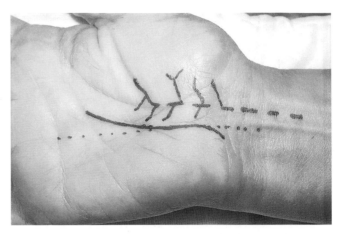

Fig. 3.9 Incision for open carpal tunnel release avoiding the palmar cutaneous branch of the median nerve.

Surgery

In patients unresponsive to the above measures, the mainstay of treatment is surgery. The indications for this are symptoms that interfere with sleep and activities, clumsiness associated with numbness and weakness and the prevention of progressive axonal degeneration.

Classically, the surgery is performed through an open longitudinal incision (Fig. 3.9). More recently, the procedure has been performed endoscopically through one or two portals. Endoscopic carpal tunnel release may decrease postoperative pain, diminish the loss of grip strength and allow patients to return to work and full activities earlier, but most studies suggest there is little difference between open and endoscopic techniques 6 months after surgery. One disadvantage of endoscopic carpal tunnel release is the inability to assess the anatomy of the carpal tunnel and to visualize effectively the nerve itself.

During the open technique, it is appropriate to check the floor of the carpal tunnel for any space-occupying lesions such as ganglia, lipomata or gouty deposits, or the presence of degenerative arthritis with protrusion of carpal bones into the carpal tunnel. A synovectomy in inflammatory arthropathies will debulk the canal and some advocate a routine flexor synovectomy, even in the absence of synovial disease, considering that oedema and fibrosis of the synovium play an important aetiological role in the development of carpal tunnel syndrome. The success of endoscopic carpal tunnel surgery, in which the only structure dealt with is the flexor retinaculum, indicates that the excision of otherwise normal synovium is not necessary.

Splinting of the wrist is effective, particularly in milder cases with nocturnal symptoms. Placement of the wrist in a neutral position avoids extreme positioning during sleep, preventing the increase in carpal tunnel pressure. It is most effective if applied within 3 months of onset of symptoms. Most pregnant women who develop carpal tunnel syndrome gain relief after giving birth. A corticosteroid injection in combination with local anaesthetic is a reasonable method of treatment in many patients. Its method of action is unclear but it will be effective in any inflammatory conditions through its anti-inflammatory effect.

Cubital tunnel syndrome

Cubital tunnel syndrome is the second most common upper limb nerve compression syndrome. As in carpal

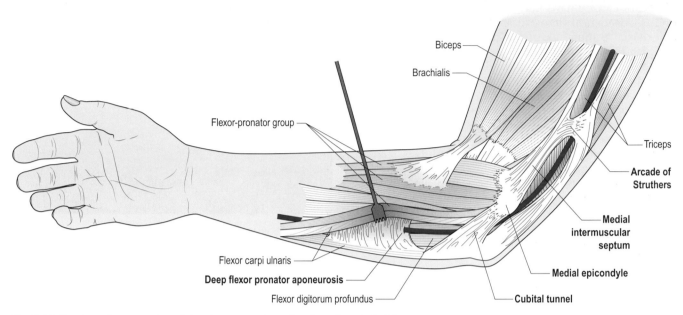

Fig. 3.10 Five sites of compression of the ulnar nerve about the elbow (seen in bold).

tunnel syndrome, the anatomy of the ulnar nerve renders it susceptible to pressure and injury. Pain and dysfunction can be significant.

Anatomy of the cubital tunnel

The ulnar nerve is the main branch of the medial cord of the brachial plexus, arising from the C8 and T1 nerve roots. The nerve reaches the elbow lying behind the medial epicondyle and enters the forearm through the cubital tunnel (Fig. 3.10). The cubital tunnel is formed by the tendinous arch joining the humeral and ulnar heads of attachment of flexor carpi ulnaris. The ulnar nerve branches in the forearm into superficial and deep branches, the former predominantly providing sensory fibres to the ulnar one and one-half digits and the latter providing motor fibres to the intrinsic muscles of the fingers, adductor pollicis, and often part of flexor pollicis brevis. In the forearm, the nerve supplies motor fibres to flexor carpi ulnaris and flexor digitorum profundus of the ring and little finger.

Pathophysiology and causes

There are five common sites of ulnar nerve compression (Fig. 3.10), but there may be no obvious reason for compression at any of these five sites (idiopathic). However, direct injury, external compression, space-occupying lesions, degenerative or inflammatory arthritis, a valgus-flexion deformity of the elbow or systemic diseases such as diabetes, chronic alcoholism, or renal failure may render the nerve at risk.

Normally, the ulnar nerve is subject to compression, traction and friction. Pathology about the elbow may

---

Case 3.1

Carpal tunnel syndrome: 5

Case note: Management

The surgeon advised Mrs Fotini to consider surgical decompression of her left carpal tunnel. In view of the moderately severe pressure in the left wrist, it was thought unwise to consider non-surgical management for fear of possible axonal degeneration if the pressure were not removed from the median nerve. However, the surgeon considered that surgery to decompress the right median nerve was not necessary as the symptoms and electrophysiological change were mild.

The surgeon advised Mrs Fotini that her night symptoms should be relieved by surgery, but that the neck pain and stiffness would not respond and that the discomfort she had at the base of both thumbs and within the small joints of the hand would continue, because they were associated with her degenerative arthritis.

The surgeon requested Mrs Fotini to stop taking aspirin 12 days prior to surgery and to discontinue her non-steroidal anti-inflammatory medication 2 days prior to surgery to prevent the possibility of postoperative bleeding.

---

affect the nerve by limiting its excursion, increasing its required excursion and destabilizing or constricting it.

Dynamic irritation of the nerve occurs during repetitive elbow flexion and extension as the nerve is compressed by the medial epicondyle. During flexion of the elbow, the cross-sectional geometry of the cubital tunnel alters from a circular configuration to a flattened and triangular configuration, decreasing the volume of the tunnel by 55% and increasing intraneural pressure. Contracture of the flexor carpi ulnaris may further increase the pressure and if extraneural fibrosis is present, usually secondary to external trauma, excursion of the nerve will be limited, leading to compression associated with stretching of the tendon. Anterior subluxation (partial dislocation) over the medial epicondyle during flexion may injure the nerve. This is a normal finding in a small percentage of the population (16.2%) without symptoms; however, chronic changes can occur within the nerve secondary to trauma from repetitive subluxation. Alterations in pressure, resultant ischaemia, oedema and fibrosis lead to ulnar nerve symptoms and signs.

A valgus deformity of the elbow may be a normal variant or secondary to previous injury around the elbow, particularly in childhood with growth deformation. Osteoarthritis may result in a flexion deformity. Furthermore, osteophytes may intrude into the cubital tunnel.

Failure to protect the elbow during surgery, in a comatose patient or in those confined to bed may result in irritation of the ulnar nerve because of either a persistent flexion position or external pressure.

Clinical diagnosis

History

The most frequent complaint is that of pins and needles in the little finger and the ulnar half of the ring finger. This may wake the patient at night, particularly when the elbow is bent and may occur during repetitive elbow flexion or when leaning on the elbow. These symptoms are often accompanied by an ache around the elbow. Intermittent symptoms may become constant with the patient complaining of numbness and weakness of grip and pinch strength and loss of dexterity.

Examination

Wasting of the intrinsic muscles indicates an established lesion and is associated with loss of intrinsic strength. Strength within the intrinsic muscles of the fingers (abduction and adduction) may be reduced, as may be adduction strength within the thumb when the Froment sign (Fig. 3.11) will be positive owing to diminished strength in adductor pollicis and the first dorsal interosseous. During an attempt to maintain adduction of the thumb against the index finger, flexor pollicis longus flexes the interphalangeal joint to compensate for loss of power in these two muscles. Intrinsic weakness may be accompanied by diminished power in flexor digitorum profundus to the little finger and perhaps the ring finger. Loss of intrinsic finger function causes clawing of the ring and little fingers because the primary metacarpophalangeal joint flexors are absent (Fig. 3.12).

In those with constant sensory symptoms, it will be possible to demonstrate altered sensibility in the ulnar one and one-half digits supplied by the digital nerves

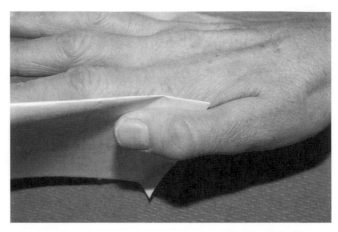

Fig. 3.11 Froment's sign: a sheet of paper can be gripped between index finger and thumb only by flexion of the thumb at the terminal joint.

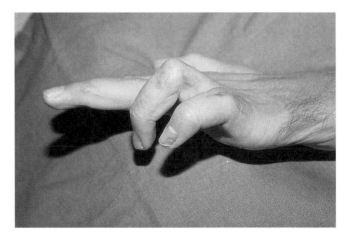

Fig. 3.12 Ulnar claw.

proper, and the dorsal branch of the ulnar nerve will be affected, with alteration in sensation over the dorsal ulnar aspect of the hand and fingers.

The nerve is often tender at the elbow and there may be evidence of flicking (subluxation) of the nerve over the medial epicondyle during flexion. The Tinel sign is positive when the ulnar nerve is percussed at the site of compression. Maintaining both elbows in the flexed position for up to 3 min is equivalent to the Phalen test for carpal tunnel syndrome and may reproduce symptoms.

The symptoms and signs of cubital tunnel syndrome must be differentiated from those accompanying cervical disc disease, thoracic outlet syndrome and compression of the ulnar nerve at the wrist. Cervical disc disease affecting the C8 and/or T1 nerve roots will usually present with a sensory deficit in a dermatomal distribution, weakness in the intrinsic muscles innervated by the median nerve as well as in muscles innervated by the ulnar nerve, neck discomfort and restriction of motion.

Investigations

Electrodiagnostic studies should be performed in an attempt to provide objective evidence of nerve compression at the elbow and to rule out more proximal or distal lesions. However, normal electrodiagnostic studies do not exclude a diagnosis of cubital tunnel syndrome, nor prevent consideration of surgery.

Radiological examination will indicate the presence of degenerative changes. A cubital tunnel projection provides good imaging of the cross-section of the tunnel. Ultrasonography is helpful in delineating nerve swelling and significant areas of constriction, as also is nuclear magnetic resonance imaging.

Treatment

Splinting appears to be effective in patients with mild to moderate symptoms and signs. The splint aims at preventing repetitive flexion of the elbow and resting the nerve in an optimal position, preventing friction, tension or compression, maintaining the elbow at 30° of flexion from the fully extended position. The splint should be worn at night and as often as possible during the day for a period of 4 weeks. The patient should avoid leaning on the elbow. Aggravating factors such as repetitive elbow flexion are avoided. Modification of the work environment may be necessary.

Most would consider that those with severe signs and symptoms, those with electrodiagnostic evidence of nerve damage and those who fail to respond to nonsurgical methods should undergo operative treatment to prevent long-term nerve damage and dysfunction. Many surgical procedures have been described. The least invasive is a simple decompression of the ulnar nerve within the cubital tunnel.

Further reading

Hilburn, J.W., 1996. General principles and use of electrodiagnostic studies in carpal and cubital tunnel syndrome: with special attention to pitfalls and interpretation. Hand Clinics 12 (2), 205–221.

Louis, D.S., Calkins, E.R., Harris, P.G., 1996. Carpal tunnel syndrome in the work place. Hand Clinics 12 (2), 305–308.

Lundborg, G., 1988. Nerve Injury and Repair. Churchill Livingstone, Edinburgh.

Phalen, G.S., 1966. The carpal-tunnel syndrome: seventeen years' experience in diagnosis and treatment of six hundred and fifty-four hands. Journal of Bone and Joint Surgery 48A (2), 211–228.

Seddon, H., 1943. Three types of nerve injury. Brain 66, 237–288.

Stevens, J.C., Sun, S., Beard, C.M., et al., 1988. Carpal tunnel syndrome in Rochester, Minnesota, 1961 to 1980. Neurology 38 (1), 134–138.

Sunderland, S., 1951. A classification of peripheral nerve injuries producing loss of function. Brain 74, 491–516.

Tetro, A.M., Pichora, D.R., 1996. Cubital tunnel syndrome and the painful upper extremity. Hand Clinics 12 (4), 665–677.

von Schroeder, H.P., Botte, M.J., 1996. Carpal tunnel syndrome. Hand Clinics 12 (4), 643–655.

BACK PAIN

Les Barnsley

Chapter objectives

After studying this chapter you should be able to:

1. Understand the normal anatomy and function of the key components of the lumbar spine.

2. Understand how pain may be produced from lumbar spinal structures.

3. Recognize 'red flags' indicating lumbar spinal pain arising from serious medical disorders.

4. Appreciate the significance of leg pain in the setting of lumbar spinal disorders.

5. Understand the known natural history of low back pain.

6. Understand the general principles of management of acute and chronic low back pain.

Introduction

Back pain is a near universal human experience. Despite this, our understanding of low back pain has languished behind that of other spheres of medicine, in part because of the paucity of pathological material and the generally benign nature of the condition. Simply put, very few people die of low back pain. On the other hand, low back pain represents a significant burden of illness in the community because of its frequency and propensity to keep people away from their work and usual activities.

The overwhelming majority of low back pain is due to unspecified mechanical or musculoskeletal causes, and these will be the focus of this chapter. However, low back pain may be the presenting symptom of a number of serious medical conditions. Consequently, a clear understanding of the presentation of different types of back pain is highly desirable.

Case 4.1 Low back pain: 1

Case history

Mr Kotsakis is 54 years old. He owns and runs a small fruit and vegetable shop. He has been quite well in the past and rarely sees his local doctor. Three days ago, while lifting a bag of carrots, he had sudden onset of pain in his lower right lumbar spine. He dropped the carrots and had to lie down. The pain settled a little over the next 2 h but still hurts today, although it is probably settling a little each day. He describes the pain as a deep-seated dull ache that is worse when he bends forward. When severe, it seems to spread into his right buttock and down the back of the thigh, about halfway to his knee, where it has the characteristics of a dull ache. He has been able to sleep with the pain, and has kept working despite it. He has not had any weakness, numbness or tingling in his leg, and has had no change to his bladder or bowel function. He denies any other recent symptoms. In particular, he has not lost weight and has had no temperatures, fevers or night sweats.

On examination, he sits uncomfortably in the surgery and appears to be in some pain. He has restriction of forward flexion of his lumbar spine, only being able to get his fingertips to his knees. Extension of the lumbar spine is also restricted. There are no power or reflex changes in his legs, and sensory examination of his lower limbs is normal. He is quite tender over the right iliac crest posteriorly. The rest of his general physical examination is quite normal.

This history is important for the relevant negatives as much as for any positive feature. This patient has acute (lasting less than 3 months) low back pain. The history suggests a mechanical cause, a lifting injury, and there is no historical or examination evidence of any underlying disorder or disease. Furthermore, there is no evidence of any neurological impairment in the history or on examination.

Normal lumbar spine anatomy

Vertebrae and sacrum

There are five lumbar vertebrae, numbered from the top down. Traditionally, each vertebra is divided into its anterior and posterior elements, which are joined by thick pillars of bone called pedicles. The anterior element, or body, of the vertebra is a kidney-shaped prism of bone, with the concavity directed posteriorly and flat superior and inferior surfaces called endplates (Fig. 4.1). A small rim of bone makes up the outer margin of these surfaces. This is where the outer part of the intervertebral disc attaches, and is a secondary ossification centre of the vertebra.

The pedicles are thick projections that originate nearer the superior part of the vertebral body at the posterolateral corners. The posterior elements are those structures that lie behind the pedicles. Viewed from above, posterior elements, pedicles and posterior parts of the vertebral body elements are seen to form a protective ring that encloses the vertebral foramen. The part of this ring not containing the vertebral body is called the neural arch. The vertebral foramen is occupied by the spinal cord above L1/2 level and the spinal nerve roots below this. Two sheets of bone, or laminae, arise from the pedicles and join in the midline to complete the ring. A bony plate

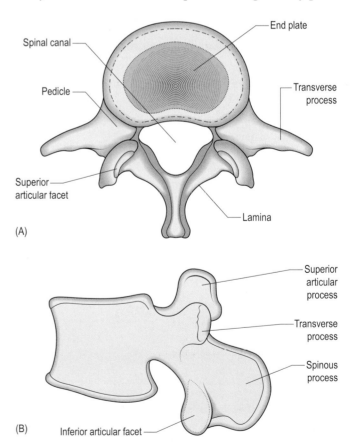

Fig. 4.1 A typical lumbar vertebra viewed (A) from above and (B) from the side.

oriented in the sagittal plane develops from the fusion of the laminae and is known as the spinous process.

Arising superiorly from the junction of each pedicle and its lamina, are two projections known as the superior articular processes. These present a relatively smooth curved surface posteriorly. From the lower corner of each lamina, there are matching projections known as the inferior articular processes, whose smooth curved surface is presented anteriorly. Together, these processes make up the posterior intervertebral joint between adjacent vertebrae. These joints are correctly termed zygapophysial joints, but are commonly and erroneously named facet joints. These joints are identified by side and level, indicating the vertebrae that they link, e.g. the right L4/5 zygapophysial joint (Fig. 4.2). Arising from the side of the lateral aspects of the pedicles are laterally oriented projections of bone known as the transverse processes (Fig. 4.1).

The sacrum is a triangular bone at the base of the spine. It provides a base for the lumbar spine above, and yet is part of the pelvic ring. Its superior components are a flat kidney-shaped surface to match the L5 vertebral body and a superior articular process on each side to form the L5/S1 zygapophysial joints. The vertebral foramen continues into the sacrum, allowing passage of the sacral nerve roots through the bone before they exit through perforations on the anterior and posterior surfaces of the sacrum, known as the sacral foramina (Fig. 4.3).

Intervertebral discs

Between each pair of lumbar vertebrae, and between L5 and S1 lie the lumbar intervertebral discs. These have two components, an outer ring or annulus fibrosus and a central core, the nucleus pulposus (Fig. 4.4). The latter comprises a turgid gel made up of water (70–90%), proteoglycans and some collagen fibres. The proteoglycans are large molecules made up of glycosaminoglycans (GAGs) linked to proteins. The glycosaminoglycans are complex polysaccharides consisting of long chains of repeating units usually made up of a sugar molecule, then a sugar molecule with an amino group attached and so on. These are then linked to proteins. The importance of GAGs both in the disc and elsewhere (such as in articular cartilage) is that they are very hydrophilic, effectively sucking in and holding water. The collagen fibres in the nucleus pulposus are 'protein ropes' that provide some viscosity and tensile strength to the nucleus. There is no blood supply

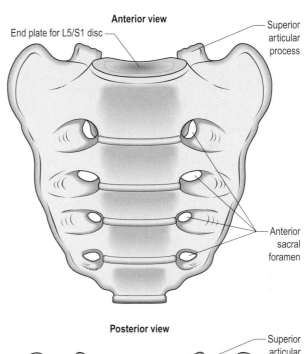

Fig. 4.3 Anterior and posterior views of the sacrum.

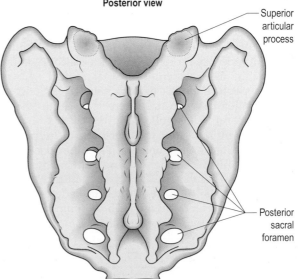

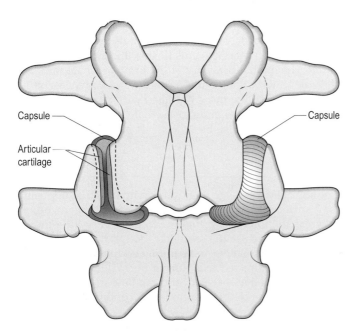

Fig. 4.2 Posterior view of two adjacent vertebrae showing the lumbar zygapophysial joints. On the left, the capsule is drawn intact. On the right, the posterior capsule has been removed to demonstrate the articular cartilage covering the joint surfaces.

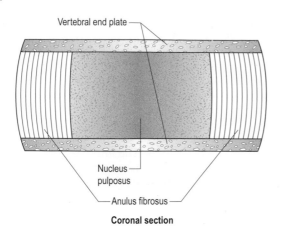

Vertebral end plate

Nucleus pulposus

Anulus fibrosus

Coronal section

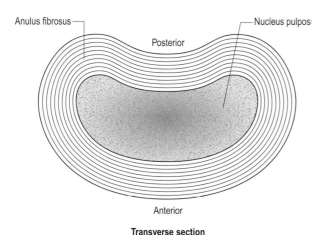

Anulus fibrosus

Posterior

Nucleus pulposus

Anterior

Transverse section

Fig. 4.4 Coronal and transverse sections through a typical lumbar disc, showing the annulus fibrosus surrounding the nucleus pulposus, and limited above and below by the vertebral endplates.

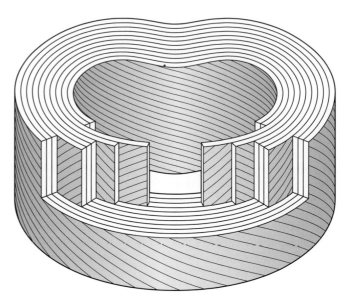

Fig. 4.5 Structure of the annulus fibrosus. The individual collagen fibres are organized into a series of concentric rings. In each ring the fibres are arranged obliquely, at about 25° to the horizontal, with the direction alternating from one ring to the next.

to the nucleus pulposus in the adult, and the nucleus is not innervated and so cannot hurt.

The annulus fibrosus comprises alternating layers of obliquely oriented collagen fibres (Fig. 4.5). Collagens are a group of rope-like proteins. Macroscopic collagen fibres are made of many microfibrils that in turn comprise three polypeptide chains wound helically around each other. Collagen has significant tensile strength (the ability to withstand being pulled apart), which is exploited in numerous musculoskeletal structures, including bone, cartilage, tendons and ligaments. The outer one-third of the annulus fibrosus has nerve fibres and endings, so that this part of the disc may be a source of pain production.

The annulus fibrosus is firmly attached to the outer margin of the vertebral body, with the outer fibres penetrating deep into the bony structure.

Lumbar zygapophysial joints

These joints are formed by the superior articular process of the lower vertebra and the inferior articular process of the upper vertebra. They are synovial joints (see Ch. 1), having a cartilage covering over the bony surface and a capsule lined by synovium (Fig. 4.2). In addition, they have intra-articular structures known as menisci, which help to cover the exposed articular cartilage when the joint moves. It is thought that entrapment of these menisci in the loose ends of the joint capsule may be a cause of an acute 'locked back'.

Lumbar zygapophysial joints are restricted in the type of movements that they can make. The curved, opposing surfaces limit rotation and anteroposterior translation of adjacent vertebrae. However, gliding of the articular surfaces over each other permits flexion and extension of the spine. The medial branches of the lumbar dorsal rami are the sole innervation of the lumbar zygapophysial joints. Their capsules, like those of other synovial joints, contain pain-sensitive nerve endings so that the lumbar zygapophysial joints can also be a source of pain.

Sacroiliac joints

The sacroiliac joints are large joints with irregular opposing joint surfaces. The upper part of the joint is ligamentous, whereas the inferior portion is synovial. Very little movement takes place at the sacroiliac joint, but it is known to provide rotation between the ilium and the sacrum around an obliquely directed axis during normal gait. The sacroiliac joint is well innervated, and can be a source of pain in inflammatory and non-inflammatory conditions.

The lumbar nerve roots and spinal cord

Irritation of the lumbar nerve roots can cause local somatic pain, but more characteristically causes neuropathic

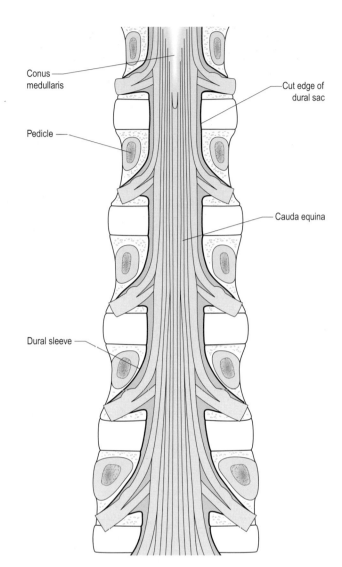

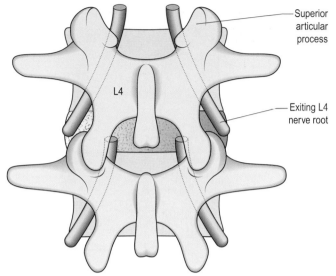

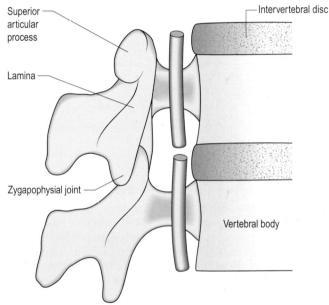

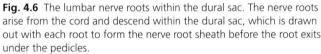

Fig. 4.6 The lumbar nerve roots within the dural sac. The nerve roots arise from the cord and descend within the dural sac, which is drawn out with each root to form the nerve root sheath before the root exits under the pedicles.

Fig. 4.7 The intervertebral foramen, through which the nerve roots exit the spinal canal. Above, the intact vertebra is viewed from the rear, showing the exiting nerve root crossing the posterolateral corner of the intervertebral disc. Below, the nerve roots are viewed from within the vertebral canal demonstrating the structures surrounding and making up the intervertebral foramen.

pain and neurological symptoms and signs in the legs. Knowledge of the relationship of the neural structures of the spine to the vertebral bodies and intervertebral discs is important in understanding nerve root compression due to herniated intervertebral discs, as well as other causes of nerve compression within the spinal column.

The spinal cord itself terminates at the level of L1 or L2. The end of the cord is known as the conus medullaris, and the exiting nerve roots form the cauda equina 'horse's tail', which descends within the dural sac (Fig. 4.6). The nerve roots lie at the back of the sac in the vertebral foramen, before running forward to exit the spinal canal under the pedicle of the vertebra after which they are named, i.e. the L4 nerve root enters underneath the L4 pedicle. They pass through the intervertebral foramen, bounded anteriorly by the vertebral body and the intervertebral disc, and

posteriorly by the zygapophysial joint and lamina of the upper vertebral body (Fig. 4.7).

A posterolateral prolapsed disc can compress the exiting nerve root against the bony structures behind it. Such a prolapse at L4/5 would compress the L4 nerve root. A more central disc prolapse may compress the next nerve root travelling to exit below. This would particularly be the case where there is some narrowing of the vertebral foramen, such as may occur with hypertrophied lumbar zygapophysial joints.

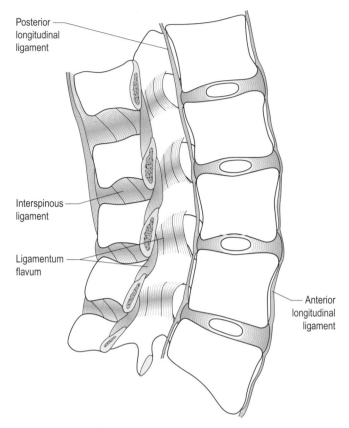

Posterior longitudinal ligament

Interspinous ligament

Ligamentum flavum

Anterior longitudinal ligament

Fig. 4.8 A midline, sagittal section of the lumbar spine demonstrating the principal ligaments. (See text for details.)

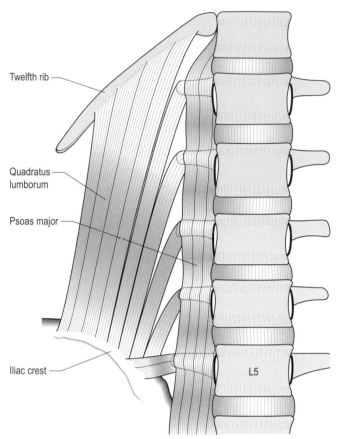

Twelfth rib

Quadratus lumborum

Psoas major

Iliac crest

L5

Fig. 4.9 Anterior view of psoas major, arising from the transverse processes of the lumbar vertebrae, and quadratus lumborum, arising from the 12th rib and inserting into the iliac crest.

Ligaments

The role of the ligaments of the lumbar spine in the production of back pain remains controversial. It has been suggested, by analogy with ligamentous injuries elsewhere, that sprains of these ligaments might cause pain. Knowledge of their basic anatomy is useful, particularly in interpreting imaging. Other than the intervertebral discs, whose annulus fibrosus may be considered a ligament, there are four main ligaments that link adjacent vertebrae (Fig. 4.8). The anterior longitudinal ligament is a thin, flat ligament that covers the front of the spine on the anterior surface of the vertebral bodies and intervertebral discs. The fibres of the anterior longitudinal ligament are oriented vertically, resisting separation of the anterior parts of adjacent vertebral bodies. The posterior longitudinal ligament runs along the posterior surface of the vertebral body, inside the vertebral foramen. Its fibres are also vertically oriented, and it resists separation of the posterior margins of adjacent vertebral bodies. The ligamentum flavum is a series of small ligaments joining the laminae of adjacent vertebrae. They have a very high elastin content, which means that the ligament is more like a rubber band than a rope. Its role seems to be to preserve the shape and smoothness of the vertebral foramen during spinal movements, and prevent compression of the neural structures. In some patients, particularly with zygapophysial joint arthrosis, the ligamentum flavum can become thickened and contribute to a narrowing of the vertebral foramen. The interspinous ligament spans adjacent spinous processes, and restricts separation of the spinous processes, as might occur in forward flexion of the spine.

Muscles

Several muscles act to move the lumbar spine. Flexion and rotation is achieved through contraction of the abdominal muscles. The psoas major muscle arises from the transverse processes of the lumbar vertebrae and the lateral margins of the vertebral bodies. It attaches into the lesser trochanter of the hip, and can either flex the hip or, if the hip is fixed, flex the lumbar spine. Quadratus lumborum is a broad, flat muscle that attaches to the iliac crest, the inferior margins of the 12th rib and the transverse processes of the lumbar spine. This muscle appears to both fix the 12th rib during respiration and facilitate lateral flexion of the lumbar spine (Fig. 4.9). There are several small muscles linking the transverse processes of adjacent vertebral bodies (the intertransversarii). Their function may be to produce proprioceptive information about the position of the lumbar spine, rather than to exert any significant force.

The posterior muscles of the spine act to produce spinal extension, and stabilize the spine during abdominal muscle contraction. The most medial and largest group is multifidus. This consists of many distinct fibres with different origins and insertions. The largest parts of the muscle originate from the spinous processes and course downwards and obliquely to insert into the iliac crest and sacrum. Lateral to the multifidus is the erector spinae muscle, which again is a complex muscle made up of several parts. Part of this muscle group acts between the lumbar transverse processes and the iliac crest, part between the thoracic spine and the sacrum, and part from the ribs to the sacrum and iliac crest. These muscle groups are separated by sheets of fascia. Recent research has suggested that the posterior muscles have very little capacity to rotate the lumbar spine. In addition, their passive elastic recoil even when not actively contracted, helps to extend the spine or resist forward flexion.

Interesting facts

The back muscles themselves do not have the contractile power to lift heavy items. Indeed the exact biomechanics of lifting have not been fully worked out but include a combination of stabilization of the trunk through abdominal muscle contraction, and the elastic recoil of stretched lumbar muscles and the posterior ligamentous structures.

Function of the lumbar spine

Biomechanics of the lumbar spine

The lumbar spine's primary function is weight bearing. This is evidenced by the broad, flat surfaces of the vertebral bodies. However, the spine must also permit movement while fulfilling its weight-bearing function. The intervertebral discs facilitate this through their unique structure. Compression forces will raise the pressure in the nucleus pulposus, which will push the annulus fibrosus out, raising the tension in the annulus. The weight is then borne through the nucleus exerting pressure on the endplates of the vertebrae, and in part by the tense annulus.

Flexion movements between the vertebrae are tolerated through the posterior annulus tightening and the anterior annulus buckling, while the weight continues to be borne by the nucleus pulposus. However, a rise in disc pressure occurs during this manoeuvre. This may put the posterior annulus at risk, as it is tensed from the flexion and is also subject to increased pressure from the nucleus. It is known that it is the posterior annulus of the disc that most commonly fails. Twisting movements are particularly risky for the disc. This is because the arrangement of the fibres in the annulus fibrosus in alternating obliquely oriented layers means that only half of them can resist rotation in one direction. The other half of the fibres are

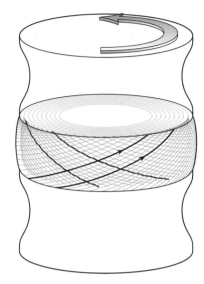

Fig. 4.10 The effects of a twisting motion (axial rotation) on the intervertebral disc. Half of the fibres are being stretched, while the other half are being relaxed.

actually being relaxed during rotation (Fig. 4.10). It is therefore believed that a combination of flexion, lifting and twisting, places the disc in particular jeopardy.

Pain from the lumbar spine

Mechanisms of pain production and transmission

Pain is defined as an unpleasant emotional and sensory experience associated with actual or potential tissue damage or described in such terms. Pain physiology is complex, and since the perception of pain is an individual subjective experience, attempts to measure and interpret pain have been fraught with difficulties.

Primary nociceptive pain arises from a structure innervated by nociceptive neurons. These are neurons that respond to noxious, or tissue-damaging stimuli. They are generally of two types: lightly myelinated (Aδ, mechanoheat) fibres and umyelinated (C, polymodal receptors) fibres. These fibres travel to the posterior horn of the spinal cord, terminating in one of several laminae depending upon their type. Impulses travelling along these afferent neurons have the capacity to excite second-order neurons that travel up the contralateral spinothalamic tract, conveying the pain sensation. Whether the second-order neurons are excited, depends upon a number of complex interactions within the posterior horn. This includes descending influences from the brain. A number of neurotransmitters are known to be involved in this process of descending modulation, including enkephalin, noradrenaline and 5-hydroxytryptamine (5-HT).

Other interactions modulating pain from nociceptive neurons occur with local afferent neurons and interneurons, which are neurons that are wholly within the

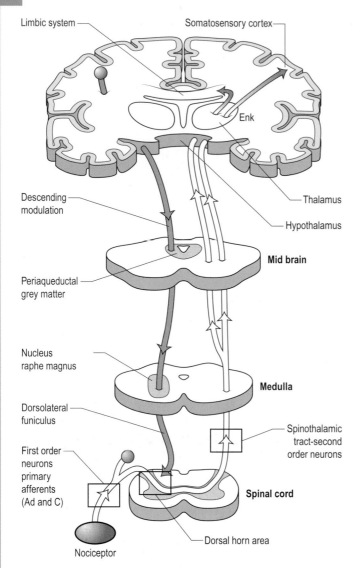

Fig. 4.11 The main nociceptive pathways from a peripheral nociceptor to the brain.

Labels in figure: Limbic system; Somatosensory cortex; Enk; Thalamus; Hypothalamus; Descending modulation; **Mid brain**; Periaqueductal grey matter; Nucleus raphe magnus; **Medulla**; Dorsolateral funiculus; Spinothalamic tract-second order neurons; First order neurons primary afferents (Aδ and C); **Spinal cord**; Dorsal horn area; Nociceptor

spinal cord. Some of these afferent neurons arise from other structures and converge in the dorsal horn, providing a substrate for the phenomenon of referred pain, where pain from one structure is perceived in another. Once excited, the second-order neurons travel up the contralateral spinothalamic tracts, terminating in the contralateral thalamus. Signals from here project to the somatosensory cortex, as well as more diffusely throughout the cortex and the limbic system, accounting perhaps for the emotional impact of pain (Fig. 4.11).

In chronic pain states, there is considerable debate about the relative contribution of peripheral nociception, where there is a persistent peripheral pain generator, and the development of self-sustaining pain arising through disturbance of normal pain pathways that somehow become autonomous producers of pain. In addition, chronic pain is often accompanied by the development of

adverse psychological and social events. Whether these are simply the effect of being in pain or a contribution towards pain is also a matter of debate.

Sources of pain in the lumbar spine

The pattern of pain stemming from the lumbar spine is non-specific. Nociceptive neurons from the various lumbar spinal structures demonstrate a high degree of convergence within the spinal cord. This means that no matter which structure provides the initial nociception, a small repertoire of the ascending neuronal pathways is activated and central perception is much the same. Consequently, there are no distinguishing features that permit a given lumbar structure to be reliably isolated as a source of symptoms. This has been borne out by experimental studies in both patients and normal volunteers that show extensive overlap of pain distributions from both pathological and experimentally induced pain from different structures.

Intervertebral disc

Degenerative changes in the intervertebral disc, sometimes called lumbar spondylosis, occur with ageing, appear to have a significant genetic contribution and are often asymptomatic. Radiologically, the features of spondylosis are disc height loss and adjacent osteophytosis. Internal disc disruption (IDD) provides a cogent explanation for disc pain in the absence of disc prolapse or nerve root compression. The inciting events and pathology are not fully understood, but it is thought that chemical changes within the nucleus pulposus and the annulus fibrosus are both required for the development of IDD. The initial event is likely to be an endplate fracture, permitting vascular access to the nucleus pulposus and the development of an inflammatory, possibly autoimmune-related response affecting the disc. This alters the chemical structure of the nucleus, rendering it less cohesive. Its physicochemical structure deteriorates, putting increased pressure on the annulus, which may also be damaged by the inflammation. This structure then fails, initially fissuring radially, until circumferential fissures develop in the outer annulus, resulting in pain when the innervated outer one-third of the disc is reached. Hence, the disc has a retained external structure, but has internal damage that is painful. Postmortem studies have also suggested that vascular ingrowth into damaged discs is accompanied by nerve fibre ingrowth, providing a substrate for pain from a damaged disc.

Zygapophysial joints

The lumbar zygapophysial joints are susceptible to the conditions that might affect other synovial joints, such as inflammatory arthritis and osteoarthritis, but for unknown reasons are usually spared in rheumatoid arthritis. Studies of osteoarthritis in the hands have shown that there appears to be separate genes for the same process at different joints, rather than a single gene defect that confers the disease process. This may explain the regional differences in disease susceptibility in the spine.

Although pathological data are lacking, these joints would seem to be susceptible to sprains, subchondral fractures, and capsular tears, particularly with rotational injuries. All of these problems might be expected to produce pain.

Sacroiliac joint

The sacroiliac joint has been shown to be a source of pain in normal subjects and patients. It receives both anterior and posterior innervation. Despite an extensive overlap of the pain distribution from the sacroiliac joint and other lumbar structures, the sacroiliac joint has been noted to rarely refer pain higher than the posterior superior iliac spine. Sacroiliac pain can also be perceived in the groin.

Other structures

A number of other structures are potential sources of pain in the low back. Muscle tears at the numerous myotendinous junctions around the lumbar spine would seem likely to be responsible for acute pain following trauma. It is contentious whether muscle injuries lead to chronic pain. It is recognized that local reflexes from both the intervertebral

discs and lumbar zygapophysial joints can cause muscle contraction, which could be a secondary source of pain. Ligamentous sprains could also be a source of acute back pain, but would be expected to heal and seem an unlikely source of chronic back symptoms. Pathological processes causing pain involving the dura and fascia have been proposed but are difficult to prove or disprove.

Leg pain and disorders of the lumbar spine

There are two mechanisms by which leg pain can be related to lumbar spinal disorders. The first is through somatic referred pain, and the second is through radicular pain.

Somatic referred pain

Somatic referred pain occurs when pain is perceived in a region topographically displaced from the region of the source of the pain. It is due to convergence and co-activation of afferents from the lower limbs, buttocks and groin with afferents from the lumbar spinal structures. Therefore, pain

---

Case 4.2 — Radicular pain: 1

Case history

A 40-year-old man presented with excruciating leg pain after working in his garden. He was pulling out a stubborn woody weed when he felt something 'give' in his back. The following day he became aware of a severe, shooting pain down the back of his left leg and into his foot. The outside of his left foot felt tingly and the symptoms were much worse when he strained or sneezed. Neurological examination revealed some mild weakness of extension of his left great toe and a loss of sensation over the lateral aspect of his left foot.

After 4 weeks of treatment with anti-inflammatory drugs and gentle physiotherapy, his symptoms had not improved and he was keen to return to work. An MRI scan was performed that revealed a large focal posterolateral disc herniation at the left L4/5 level compressing the left L5 nerve root as it descended to exit below (Fig. 4.12). The L4 nerve root was able to exit the canal just above the prolapsed disc. A selective epidural injection of corticosteroid was placed around the left L5 nerve root under CT guidance. This resulted in a significant diminution of his symptoms, and he was able to return to work.

This case is a typical story for acute disc prolapse. The delay between the inciting event and the development of radicular pain is characteristic, most likely representing the development of inflammation around the nerve root, sensitizing it so that further mechanical compression results in radicular pain. The natural history is generally favourable. The use of selective epidural or periradicular injections are techniques that have been demonstrated to decrease the need for surgery and hasten recovery.

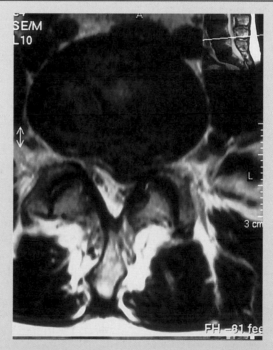

Fig. 4.12 A T2 weighted MRI scan (water appears white) demonstrating a large, left posterolateral disc herniation of the L4/L5 intervertebral disc compressing the descending intervertebral left L5 nerve root and deforming the dural sac. The MRI is reported as being viewed from below. Therefore the left side of the image represents the right side of the patient. Note the descending sacral nerve roots, which appear as black dots in the white CSF within the dural sac. The right L5 nerve root is seen as a black dot in the upper right part of the dural sac (left side of the image).

from the lumbar spine is perceived as radiating down the leg. Somatic referred pain has the characteristics of being dull, deep and aching. It is usually felt in the upper part rather than the lower part of the leg and spreads from the lumbar spine. It usually has an identifiable centroid, or place from which the pain appears to spread. This centroid will typically be over the lumbar spine. This is the type of pain described by Mr Kotsakis.

Radicular pain

Radicular pain occurs because of irritation of a sensitized nerve root, usually but not exclusively because of a prolapsed intervertebral disc. This pain is typically lancinating in quality, shooting down the leg like an electric shock. It affects a narrow band and has both deep and cutaneous components. It is often made worse by coughing or sneezing, which raises intradiscal pressure, and may be associated with neurological signs and symptoms through nerve root compression. The patient has difficulty localizing the pain. The key issue is that lumbar radicular pain is not back pain but leg pain. It requires a different therapeutic approach to back pain, and is included in this chapter to facilitate its separation from low back pain, which is made almost entirely on historical grounds.

Interesting facts

The types of tumour that most commonly metastasize to bone, and therefore the spine, are lung, breast, prostate, thyroid and kidney. This can be remembered by the mnemonic: 'Low Back Precise Tumour Knowledge'.

Lumbar spinal pain due to serious underlying disease

In a small group of patients, back pain is a manifestation of a serious underlying disease such as vertebral or sacral fracture, cancer, infection or an inflammatory arthropathy such as ankylosing spondylitis. The frequency of cancer in patients presenting with back pain varies with age, being 0.14% in patients under 50 and 0.56% in patients over 50. By far the strongest predictor of vertebral cancer is a previous history of malignancy. Other historical features suggesting cancer are a history of significant weight loss, the presence of anaemia, night pain and failure to improve over a 4-week period.

Infection or osteomyelitis is a rare cause of back pain. The presence of fever is by far the most suggestive historical feature for infection. Other important risk factors include previous infection, occupational exposure to infection (such as brucellosis in meat workers), intravenous drug use, infected skin lesions, and the previous use of intravenous and urinary catheters. Vertebral osteomyelitis follows haematogenous spread from an extraosseous source in 40% of patients. Organisms may enter bone from nutrient arteries, or from the venous plexus of Batson, a valveless system of veins that supply

Box: 4.1 'Red flags' in patients with back pain

- History of cancer
- Significant trauma
- Weight loss
- Temperature >37.8°C
- Risk factors for infection
- Neurological deficit
- Minor trauma in patients:
  - over 50 years
  - known to have osteoporosis
  - taking corticosteroids
- Failure to improve over 1 month

the spinal column. Causative organisms include bacteria, mycobacteria, fungi, spirochaetes and parasites, with bacteria being by far the most common. *Staphylococcus aureus* accounts for 60% of cases. The commonest primary sources are the genitourinary tract, respiratory tract and skin. Infections of the musculoskeletal system are discussed in more detail in Chapter 11.

Inflammatory arthropathies of the spine are referred to as the seronegative spondyloarthropathies, and include ankylosing spondylitis, psoriatic arthritis and reactive arthritis. These processes selectively affect the sacroiliac joints. The characteristic history is of insidious onset of low back pain associated with marked stiffness lasting for 1 hour or more after waking in the morning. The pain and stiffness is relieved by exercise, but recurs after resting. These conditions are often associated with the presence of the histocompatibility locus antigen (HLA) B27. Other joints outside the spine can be affected and enthesopathy (inflammation where tendons attach to bone) is common. There may also be extra-articular features such as eye inflammation and skin rash.

It will be appreciated that most of the features identifying those back pain patients with a high risk of a serious underlying cause are historical. This has prompted the development of the so-called 'red flags'. These are features that should be routinely sought on history taking and examination in patients presenting with low back pain. Positive responses to any of the red flag questions should prompt further assessment for serious underlying disorders (Box 4.1). Mr Kotsakis had none of these 'red flags'.

Back pain from extraspinal sources

Low back pain may also be a feature of pathological conditions outside the spine, particularly the pelvis and retroperitoneal space. In women presenting with a history of back pain, a gynaecological history should be taken routinely to exclude pathology of the urogenital tract. Part of the examination of patients with low back pain should include abdominal examination and auscultation of the abdominal aorta and its major branches. Back pain may be the only presenting feature in patients with

Case history

A 72-year-old man presents with the insidious onset of low back pain. He cannot say exactly when it started, but it has got steadily worse over the last 2 months or so. It is worse at night, and has a deep aching quality. He has also felt tired and generally unwell. He has a past history of prostate cancer, which was treated with transurethral resection 3 years ago. On examination he is tender over L5 and looks pale. A bone scan shows multiple hot spots over the ribs and pelvis with an area of increased uptake in the body of L5.

This story is highly suggestive of malignancy as a cause of low back pain. He has the 'red flags' of a past history of malignancy, weight loss and anaemia. His pain has failed to improve and wakes him at night, all signifying an expanding lesion rather than an intermittent mechanical problem.

abdominal aortic aneurysm or dissection. Prompt recognition of these diagnoses may be life-saving. Pain from an extraspinal source should be actively sought when there is any feature in the history that might suggest it, such as hypertension, previous vascular disease and symptoms in other systems. Particular caution should be exercised in assessing patients with no physical findings in their spine. Although their presence is not specific or sensitive for any particular spinal disorder, the *absence* of any signs of restricted movement or tenderness in the lumbar spine should prompt a rigorous evaluation for extraspinal disorders.

Another important differentiation from back pain is hip joint pain. Although hip pain is classically described as being anterior and in the thigh, experimental and clinical data have shown that around 70% of patients with proven hip pathology perceive pain in the buttock. Suspected hip joint pain can usually be confirmed by the clinical examination findings of irritability or restricted movements.

Epidemiology of low back pain

Incidence and prevalence

Back pain is extremely common. Population data indicate an incidence (number of new cases per year) in the order of 1–4%. The prevalence of back pain (number of people in the community at any given time) is 5–10%, with a lifetime prevalence of 80%.

Natural history

Before considering what effect treatment might have on low back pain, it is pertinent to consider what the natural history of the condition is. In the past it has been stated

that 90% of patients with acute low back pain will get better in a few weeks. More contemporary studies suggest a worse outlook, with between 40% and 75% still complaining of back pain 1 year after onset. The pattern would seem to be of relapses and remissions rather than continuous pain. Patients who are destined to recover tend to do so in the first two months. In the case of Mr Kotsakis (Case 4.1: 1), these natural history data can be offered as reassurance that his pain is likely to ease, but that he may expect flare-ups from time to time.

Acute and chronic low back pain

Traditionally, back pain is divided into acute and chronic. Acute back pain is defined as lasting less than 3 months, whereas chronic lasts more than 3 months. This rather arbitrary division makes sense in terms of the natural history that has been observed in follow-up studies. The treatment for back pain is quite different for acute and chronic types. The term 'sub-acute' is used to describe patients who have had symptoms for between 6 and 12 weeks. Attention has focused on this group with the intention of preventing the transition to chronic symptoms. Mr Kotsakis is still in the phase of disease where his problems would be described as acute, so treatment would be guided by studies that have addressed similar patients.

Treatment of low back pain

Acute low back pain

Acute back pain may be due to injuries and derangements of any of the structures mentioned above. However, since many patients will settle over time, there seems to be little value in trying to determine which structure is responsible for the pain. Consequently, the source of pain in most cases of acute low back pain is not known, although simple muscle, ligamentous or capsular strains would seem likely culprits. More chronic symptoms would be expected from injuries to discs or other avascular structures such as articular cartilage that may be expected to heal poorly.

Patient education

Many patients fear back pain, concerned that it may represent serious disease or threaten their independence, work capacity or mobility. Confident reassurance of the generally benign nature of acute back pain and an encouragement to pursue normal activities is a proven strategy for the prevention of future disability. In practical terms, Mr Kotsakis should be asked about any fears, concerns or anxieties that he has about his pain, and be encouraged to resume normal activities as soon as possible. In the sub-acute phase, a single 1-hour consultation with a physician has been shown to decrease by 50% the rate of work disability over a control group of 'usual treatment' at both 12 months and 5 years. The consultation simply provides a cogent explanation of back pain, confident reassurance and a strategy of light exercises and stretches to deal with flare-ups of pain.

Rest and exercise

Various levels of activity have been suggested for low back pain, ranging from strict, prolonged bed rest to specific structured exercises. Systematic reviews of the literature have shown that rest, beyond stopping a specific inciting or aggravating factor, is counterproductive. Specific prescribed exercises showed mixed effects, and the best outcomes are from recommending that patients stay active and resume their normal activities as quickly as they can.

Pharmacological intervention

The use of simple analgesics such as paracetamol/acetaminophen would seem to be appropriate for the management of acute low back pain. If ineffective, non-steroidal anti-inflammatory drugs (NSAIDs) have been shown to offer benefit. The limiting factor in their use is toxicity, particularly gastrointestinal adverse effects such as gastritis, ulceration and bleeding and impaired renal function, discussed in Chapter 1. Muscle relaxants of various types have been shown to be effective, but their adverse effects such as drowsiness and other central nervous system effects severely limit their use.

Injection therapy

Several studies have been undertaken into the effectiveness of local injections into tender structures in the back, typically muscles or muscle attachments. Injections of local anaesthetic along the iliac crest have been shown to be effective in temporarily relieving pain. Decreasing pain with such techniques may facilitate the early restoration of normal movements, and improve longer-term outcomes. The injections are normally with either local anaesthetic or corticosteroid, or both, but there is no reason or empirical data to support the use of corticosteroid over local anaesthetic alone.

> ### Interesting facts
>
> Applying 40 kg of pressure to a single, intact intervertebral disc causes only 1 mm of compression of the disc and 0.5 mm of radial distension of the annulus.

Manipulation

The underlying assumption that there is some part of the back 'out of place' or 'stiff' in low back pain has led to a proliferation of different types of manual therapy techniques that aim to move spinal structures passively by the application of external pressure in various forms. A detailed description of the different types of manipulation and mobilization is outside the scope of this chapter.

Case 4.1   Low back pain: 2

Case note: Management

Mr Kotsakis was most concerned about his back, and detailed questioning suggested that he had particular concerns over becoming paraplegic, as he had a relative with a spinal cord injury. He appeared happier after hearing some detailed information from his doctor. His pain was eased on the spot by some local anaesthetic injections. He was not keen to take tablets and had eight sessions of mobilizing treatments to his spine by a manipulative therapist. Over 4 weeks his pain settled to a dull background ache, and he returned to his work, taking care to avoid lifting and twisting simultaneously.

However, systematic reviews of manipulation have described modest short-term benefits over placebo treatments, but no benefit over conventional physical therapy techniques. Manipulation could reasonably be offered to patients who fail to respond to advice and pharmacological interventions after a few weeks, but should not be relied upon as an isolated treatment, which might encourage passivity and discourage the patient from activity and light exercise.

Chronic low back pain

Mr Kotsakis was fortunate not to develop chronic symptoms. Identified risk factors for the development of chronic low back pain at presentation include female sex, psychological distress, dissatisfaction with employment, a previous history of low back pain, radiating leg pain, widespread pain and restriction of two or more spinal movements. The more risk factors, the higher the risk of developing chronic symptoms.

When confronted with a patient with chronic low back pain, the physician should reassess the history for the presence of 'red flags'. Assuming that there is no historical evidence of serious underlying conditions, one of two approaches can be taken. On the one hand, the back pain is treated as undifferentiated back pain with systemic or empirical treatments. On the other hand, attempts can be made to isolate the source of pain and institute target-specific treatments.

Empirical treatments

Systematic reviews of the empirical treatment of chronic low back pain attest to the efficacy of intensive, inpatient structured exercise programmes with behavioural elements. Chronic use of passive physical modalities of treatment such as ultrasound is ineffective and may be worse than doing nothing. Manipulation has only marginal benefit over simple education. The use of cognitive behavioural techniques, often in the setting of multidisciplinary pain clinics, has been shown to help certain parameters such as the behavioural expression of pain and specific coping skills. Other measures of pain itself are not significantly affected. Involvement of patients in programmes aiming to increase function independently of pain (functional restoration) show little sustained benefit. The use of various analgesic medications including opiates remains an option for patients with chronic low back pain, but trial data are lacking and their use remains controversial for many practitioners.

Target-specific treatments

Target-specific treatments are those which are directed against pain arising from specific structures. These techniques, while proven, are often not generally available, limiting their usefulness.

Injection techniques that selectively and specifically anaesthetize the lumbar zygapophysial joints allow these joints to be evaluated as sources of pain. They involve small amounts of local anaesthetic being precisely placed, under X-ray control, onto the medial branches of the lumbar dorsal rami that supply a particular joint or into the joint itself. If the patient experiences pain relief, the target joint is incriminated as a source of pain. This response can be confirmed with control injections using either different local anaesthetic or a placebo injection such as normal saline. If a painful lumbar zygapophysial joint is identified, studies have shown the effectiveness of 'cooking' the medial branches of the lumbar dorsal rami using radiofrequency energy to denervate the painful joint and provide pain relief, typically for around 12 months.

Painful intervertebral discs can be diagnosed on the basis of provocation discography, in which a needle is placed into the nucleus pulposus of a disc. An injection, usually of contrast medium then distends the disc and the patient's response is noted. Reproduction of a patient's pain at a disc shown to be disrupted (see above), with no response at a control level, constitutes a positive response. Treatment of painful discs remains problematic. A number of mechanisms for creating thermal lesions in the discs have been tested but remain of uncertain utility.

Although sacroiliac joint pain can be diagnosed through intra-articular injection of local anaesthetic, there are, as yet, no proven treatments available for mechanical sacroiliac joint pain.

Surgery

Surgery such as laminectomy (removal of part of the laminae) has an important and established role for the management of disc prolapse and other causes of nerve root and spinal cord compression, such as spinal canal stenosis. However, it has little, if any, application to uncomplicated low back pain. Operations that have been advocated for back pain include posterior fusion of adjacent segments, but there is little evidence and poor justification for such interventions. Anterior fusion, using a transabdominal approach in which the disc is replaced with a bone graft, has been used for patients with proven painful discs where all other options have been exhausted. The long-term results in uncontrolled studies of carefully selected patients suggest at least a moderate benefit. However, these techniques are not generally available and should by no means be considered routine. Their applicability is limited to a very small proportion of patients with chronic low back pain.

Further reading

Bogduk, N., 2005. Clinical Anatomy of the Lumbar Spine and Sacrum, fourth ed. Churchill Livingstone, Melbourne.

Hall, H., McIntosh, G., 2008. Low back pain (acute). Clin Evid (Online).

Hall, H., McIntosh, G., 2008. Low back pain (chronic). Clin Evid (Online).

Van Tulder, M.W., Koes, B., Bouter, L.M., 1997. Conservative treatment of acute and chronic nonspecific low back pain: A systematic review of randomised controlled trials of most common interventions. Spine 22, 2128–2156.

BONE STRUCTURE AND FUNCTION IN NORMAL AND DISEASE STATES

5

Philip Sambrook

Chapter objectives

After studying this chapter you should be able to:

1. Understand normal bone structure and function including bone remodelling and the different hormones that affect calcium metabolism.

2. Appreciate the aetiopathogenesis of the most common metabolic bone diseases.

3. Understand the epidemiology of osteoporosis and its clinical importance.

4. Assess the risk factors commonly associated with osteoporosis.

5. Describe the essential anatomy of the hip joint relevant to femoral neck fractures and other common diseases affecting the hip.

6. Understand the general principles of management of osteoporosis.

7. Understand the general principles of surgical treatment of hip fractures and their complications.

Introduction

The principal functions of the skeleton are mechanical support, maintenance of calcium homeostasis and haematopoiesis in the bone marrow. These can be disturbed in a variety of conditions encompassed by the general term, metabolic bone disease. Osteoporosis is the commonest metabolic bone disease. It is an important public health problem in all developed countries and is becoming one in most developing countries. Osteoporosis means skeletal fragility leading to an increased risk of fracture. Hip fractures are the most important type of osteoporotic fracture, both in terms of direct health costs and social effects on the patient. In western countries, up to one in two women and one in three men will sustain an osteoporotic fracture during their lifetime. The cost of treating osteoporosis has been estimated to be in excess of US$20 billion in the USA and 25 billion Euros in the European Union. Early diagnosis is now possible using precise methods such as bone density measurement.

This chapter will review normal bone structure and function as well as the major metabolic bone diseases. Since this topic will be illustrated by a case in which an osteoporotic hip fracture has occurred, the key anatomy of the hip joint will also be reviewed.

Normal skeletal structure and function

Bones are extremely dense connective tissue that, in various shapes, constitute the skeleton. Although one of the hardest structures in the body, bone maintains a degree of elasticity owing to its structure and composition. Bone is enclosed, except where it is coated with articular cartilage, in a fibrous outer membrane called the periosteum. Periosteum is composed of two layers, an outer fibrous layer and a deeper elastic layer containing osteoblasts that are capable of proliferating rapidly when a fracture occurs, as will be discussed further in Chapter 10. In the interior of the long bones is a cylindrical cavity (called the medullary cavity) filled with bone marrow and lined with a membrane composed of highly vascular tissue called the endosteum.

Types of bone: cortical and cancellous

There are two types of bone: (a) compact or cortical bone and (b) trabecular or cancellous bone. Cortical bone is found principally in the shafts (diaphyses) of long bones. It consists of a number of irregularly spaced overlapping cylindrical units termed Haversian systems. Each consists of a central Haversian canal surrounded by concentric lamellae of bony tissue (Fig. 5.2A). Trabecular bone is found principally at the ends of long bones, and in vertebral bodies and flat bones. It is composed of a meshwork of trabeculae within which are intercommunicating spaces (Fig. 5.2B).

The skeleton consists of approximately 80% cortical bone, largely in peripheral bones, and 20% trabecular bone, mainly in the axial skeleton. These amounts vary according to site and relate to the need for mechanical support. While trabecular bone accounts for the minority

---

Case 5.1 Osteoporosis: 1

Case history

Mrs Jones, a 74-year-old woman living independently in the community, has suffered several recent falls. Today, while out walking, she fell backwards onto her left hip. Her GP has been treating her for cardiac failure, obstructive airways disease and intermittent low back pain. Because of the back pain, she has been sleeping poorly and her GP recently started her on a sedative, to be taken before retiring to bed. On admission to hospital, it is found she is taking 10 different medications. Mrs Jones is uncertain of what these were all for, but is able to remember that she is on 'fluid tablets for her heart', 'a cortisone puffer for her lungs' and 'an anti-inflammatory for her back pain'. Her past medical history reveals several risk factors for osteoporosis. These include an early menopause, a family history of osteoporosis, smoking and poor nutrition.

On examination in hospital, her left leg is noted to be shortened and externally rotated. Mrs Jones is also tender over the lateral aspect of the right hip but without bruising there. X-rays reveal a fracture through the neck of her left femur (Fig. 5.1).

We can see from the details of this case that Mrs Jones has suffered a hip fracture due to osteoporosis. In deciding what investigations are appropriate and how best to manage her, an understanding of calcium metabolism and bone structure and function is necessary.

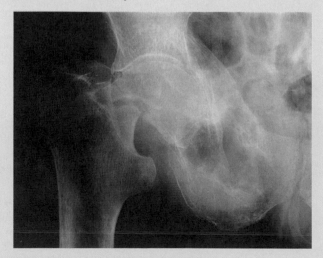

Fig. 5.1 X-ray showing fracture of left femoral neck.

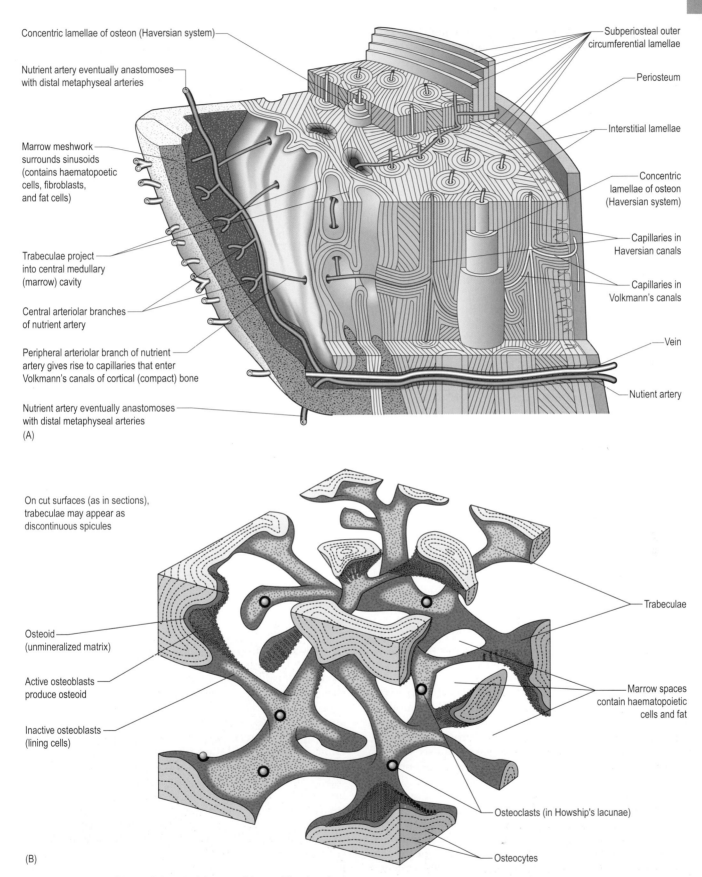

Concentric lamellae of osteon (Haversian system)

Nutrient artery eventually anastomoses with distal metaphyseal arteries

Marrow meshwork surrounds sinusoids (contains haematopoetic cells, fibroblasts, and fat cells)

Trabeculae project into central medullary (marrow) cavity

Central arteriolar branches of nutrient artery

Peripheral arteriolar branch of nutrient artery gives rise to capillaries that enter Volkmann's canals of cortical (compact) bone

Nutrient artery eventually anastomoses with distal metaphyseal arteries
(A)

Subperiosteal outer circumferential lamellae

Periosteum

Interstitial lamellae

Concentric lamellae of osteon (Haversian system)

Capillaries in Haversian canals

Capillaries in Volkmann's canals

Vein

Nutient artery

On cut surfaces (as in sections), trabeculae may appear as discontinuous spicules

Osteoid (unmineralized matrix)

Active osteoblasts produce osteoid

Inactive osteoblasts (lining cells)

(B)

Trabeculae

Marrow spaces contain haematopoietic cells and fat

Osteoclasts (in Howship's lacunae)

Osteocytes

Fig. 5.2 Structure of bone: (A) cortical (compact) bone; (B) trabecular bone.

of total skeletal tissue, it is the site of greater bone turnover because of its different structure and because its total surface area is greater than that of cortical bone.

Blood supply of bone

Bones are generally richly supplied with blood, via periosteal vessels, vessels that enter close to the articular surfaces and nutrient arteries passing obliquely through the cortex before dividing into longitudinally directed branches. Loss of the arterial supply to parts of a bone can result in death of bone tissue, usually called avascular necrosis or osteonecrosis. Certain bones in the body are prone to this complication, usually after injury, including the head of the femur (discussed later in this chapter), the scaphoid bone in the wrist, the navicular in the foot and the tibial plateau. Nutrient arteries to the scaphoid bone are large and numerous at the distal end but become sparse and finer as the proximal pole is approached. Fractures of the scaphoid, especially of the waist or proximal pole, may be associated with inadequate blood supply resulting in necrosis and later secondary osteoarthritis in the wrist. In the foot, the navicular bone is the last tarsal bone to ossify and its ossification centre may be dependent on a single nutrient artery. Compressive forces on weight bearing are thought to be the cause of avascular necrosis of the ossification centre, which usually presents as a painful limp in a child. This condition is also known as Kohler's disease.

Calcium homeostasis and hormonal control

In addition to its role as a support structure, the bone's other primary function is calcium homeostasis. More than 99.9% of the total body calcium resides in the skeleton. The maintenance of normal serum calcium depends on the interplay of intestinal calcium absorption, renal excretion and skeletal mobilization or uptake of calcium. Serum calcium represents less than 1% of total body calcium but the serum level is extremely important for maintenance of normal cellular functions. Serum calcium regulates and is regulated by three major hormones: parathyroid hormone (PTH), 1,25-dihydroxyvitamin D and calcitonin (Fig. 5.3). Parathyroid hormone is an 84-amino acid peptide secreted by the four parathyroid glands located adjacent to the thyroid gland in the neck. Calcitonin is a 32-amino acid peptide secreted by the parafollicular cells of the thyroid gland. Vitamin D, from dietary sources (D_3) or synthesized in skin (D_2), is converted to 25-hydroxyvitamin D in the liver and then to 1,25-dihydroxyvitamin D in the kidney.

PTH and 1,25-dihydroxyvitamin D are the major regulators of calcium and bone homeostasis. Although calcitonin can directly inhibit osteoclastic bone resorption, it appears to play a relatively minor role in calcium homeostasis in normal adults. PTH acts on the kidney to

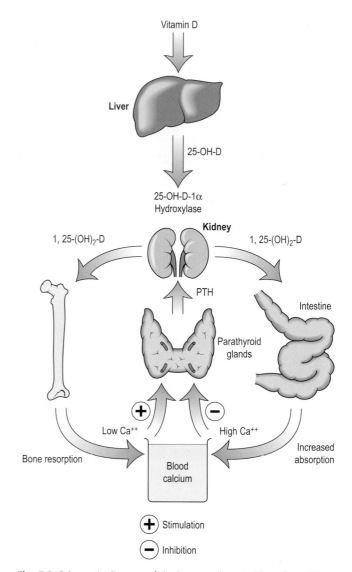

Fig. 5.3 Schematic diagram of the hormonal control loop for calcium metabolism.

increase calcium reabsorption, phosphate excretion and 1,25-dihydroxyvitamin D production. It acts on bone to increase bone resorption. 1,25-dihydroxyvitamin D is a potent stimulator of bone resorption and an even more potent stimulator of intestinal calcium (and phosphate) absorption. It is also necessary for bone mineralization. Intestinal calcium absorption is probably the most important calcium homeostatic pathway.

A number of feedback loops operate to control the level of serum calcium and the two major calcium homeostatic hormones. A calcium-sensing receptor, identified in parathyroid and kidney cells but also found in other tissues, which senses extracellular calcium levels plays a critical role in calcium homeostasis. Low serum calcium levels stimulate 1,25-dihydroxyvitamin D synthesis directly through stimulation of PTH release (and synthesis). The physiological response to increasing levels of PTH and

1,25-dihydroxyvitamin D is a gradual rise in serum calcium level. To prevent an elevated level of serum calcium, a second set of feedback loops operate to decrease PTH and 1,25-dihydroxyvitamin D levels. These feedback loops maintain serum calcium within a narrow physiological range. Disturbances in these control mechanisms or over/underproduction of these three major hormones can lead to various clinical states, discussed in more detail below. A PTH-related peptide (PTHrP) also plays a role in calcium homeostasis, especially in the fetus and in the growing skeleton.

Cellular basis of bone remodelling

The structural components of bone consist of extracellular matrix (largely mineralized), collagen and cells. The collagen fibres are of type I, comprise 90% of the total protein in bone and are oriented in a preferential direction giving lamellar bone its structure. Spindle- or plate-shaped crystals of hydroxyapatite $[3Ca_3(PO_4)_2]\cdot(OH)_2$ are found on the collagen fibres, within them, and in the ground substance. The ground substance is primarily composed of glycoproteins and proteoglycans. These highly anionic complexes have a high ion-binding capacity and are thought to play an important role in the calcification process. Numerous non-collagenous proteins have been identified in bone matrix, such as osteocalcin synthesized by the osteoblasts, but their role is unclear.

The principal cells in bone are the osteoclasts, osteoblasts and osteocytes. Osteoclasts, the cells responsible for resorption of bone, are derived from haematopoietic stem cells. Osteoblasts are derived from local mesenchymal cells. They are responsible directly for bone formation and indirectly, via paracrine factors, for regulating osteoclastic bone resorption. Osteocytes are formed when osteoblasts become entombed within the hard mineralized matrix. More than 90% of all cells within the adult skeleton are osteocytes. Osteocytes are thought to sense mechanical loads on the skeleton and have a dendritic structure that allows communications with other cells via gap junctions so that bone fluid flow shear stress can be translated into biochemical signals that direct bone modeling and remodelling.

Various cytokines control osteoclast recruitment and activity, including interleukin-1β (IL-1β) and IL-6. A transmembrane protein belonging to the tumour necrosis factor superfamily, plays an important role in osteoclast differentiation and activity (Fig. 5.4A). Its receptor is called RANK (receptor activator of NFκB) since, after binding, a transcriptional factor known as NFκB translocates to the nucleus and appears responsible for expression of genes that lead to the osteoclast phenotype. This process is inhibited by a soluble receptor, osteoprotegerin (OPG), which competes for binding of RANK ligand to produce an inactive complex. Control of osteoblast differentiation and function is achieved by integration of a number of pathways. Bone morphogenetic proteins and the Wnt signalling pathway are important modulators of osteoblast function and hence bone formation. Sclerostin,

a product of the osteocyte, antagonizes the Wnt signalling pathway, which can inhibit osteoblast generation.

Interesting facts

Sclerostin is expressed by the SOST gene. Mutations in this gene leading to increased expression are associated with a low bone mass state whereas mutations that lead to decreased expression of the SOST gene lead to a high bone mass phenotype, first described in Dutch subjects and called Van Buchem disease. Van Buchem disease is characterized by overgrowth of bones, especially of the jaw, and enlargement of the skull, ribs, diaphysis of long bones, as well as tubular bones of the hands and feet.

Bone is continually undergoing renewal called remodelling (Fig. 5.4B). In the normal adult skeleton, new bone laid down by osteoblasts exactly matches osteoclastic bone resorption, i.e. formation and resorption are closely 'coupled'. Although there is a lesser amount of trabecular bone than cortical bone in the skeleton, because trabecular bone 'turns over' between 3–10 times more rapidly than cortical bone, it is more sensitive to changes in bone resorption and formation. Most bone turnover occurs on bone surfaces, especially at endosteal surfaces. Moreover, the rate of remodelling differs in different locations according to physical loading, proximity to a synovial joint or the presence of haematopoietic rather than fatty tissue in adjacent marrow.

Bone remodelling follows an ordered sequence, referred to as the basic multicellular unit of bone turnover or bone remodelling unit (BMU). In this cycle, bone resorption is initiated by the recruitment of osteoclasts, which act on matrix exposed by proteinases derived from bone lining cells. In cortical bone, a resorptive pit (called a Howship's lacuna) is created by the osteoclasts. Osteoclasts have a convoluted membrane called a ruffled border through which lysosomal enzymes are released into pockets, causing matrix resorption. This resorptive phase is then followed by a bone formation phase where osteoblasts fill the lacuna with osteoid. The latter is subsequently mineralized to form new bone matrix. This cycle of coupling of bone formation and resorption is vital to the maintenance of the integrity of the skeleton. Uncoupling of the remodelling cycle, so that bone resorption or formation are in excess of each other leads to net bone change (gain or loss).

In clinical practice, it is possible to measure serum biochemical markers of bone remodelling that reflect bone formation and bone resorption (Table 5.1). These markers have been shown to be independent predictors of fracture risk.

Skeletal development

Bones develop by one of two processes, either:

1. From a preformed cartilaginous structure (endochondral ossification), or

2. De novo at specific sites in the skeleton (intramembranous ossification).

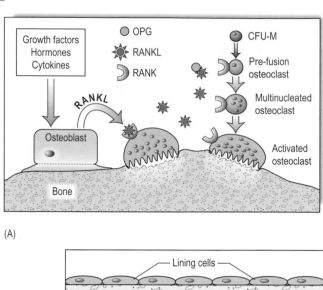

(A)

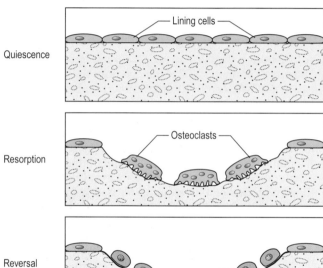

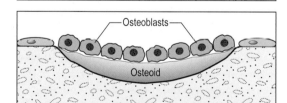

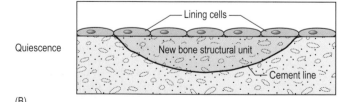

(B)

Fig. 5.4 (A) Osteoblasts and stromal cells produce RANKL. Binding of RANKL to its receptor (RANK) on osteoclast precursor cells results in their differentiation and activation. This process is regulated by an inhibitor of RANKL, osteoprotegerin (OPG), which competes with RANK for binding of RANKL to produce an inactive complex. (B) The bone remodelling sequence is initiated by osteoclasts. Subsequently, osteoblasts appear within the resorption bay and synthesize matrix, which is mineralized later.

Table 5.1	Serum biochemical markers of bone turnover	
Bone formation	**Bone resorption**
Aminoterminal propeptide of type I procollagen (PINP)	Tartrate-resistant acid phosphatase
Bone-specific alkaline phosphatase	Carboxyterminal telopeptide of type I collagen (CTX)

Subsequent skeletal growth involves remodelling of bone. In the growing skeleton, the long bones consist of a diaphysis (or shaft) separated from the ends of the bone (called the epiphyses) by cartilage. The part of the diaphysis immediately adjacent to the epiphysial cartilage is the site of advancing ossification and is known as the metaphysis. Endochondral ossification is a complex process in which the growth plate cartilage is progressively replaced by bone. The growth plate (physis) and bone front steadily advance away from the bone centre, resulting in progressive elongation of bone. Longitudinal growth continues while the growth plate remains open.

Growth plates start to close after puberty in response to the surge in circulating oestrogen. Several hormones including growth hormone, insulin-like growth factor-1 (IGF-1) and PTHrP play a role in bone growth. With growth throughout early childhood, bone size and mass gradually increase in a linear fashion. Then between the onset of puberty and young adulthood, skeletal mass approximately doubles. Most of the increase in bone mass in early puberty is due to increases in bone size. In cortical bone, both the inner (endocortical) and outer (periosteal) diameters increase, owing to enhanced resorption and apposition on these surfaces respectively. Gains in bone mineral density during puberty are dependent on the pubertal stage.

Growth ceases when closure of the growth plate occurs, but bone mass and density may continue to increase beyond this time by a process called consolidation. The maximum skeletal mass achieved is termed the peak bone mass. The age at which this is attained varies in different skeletal sites.

The adult skeleton

In both men and women, bone mineral loss from the skeleton starts from age 40–50, again depending upon the skeletal site. In addition, in women bone loss can be rapid immediately after the menopause. Bone size also contributes to bone strength. Thus men in part have higher bone mineral density (and a lower fracture risk) than women, because they have bigger bones. In clinical practice, osteoporosis is usually defined in relation to the degree to which bone mineral density is reduced. Bone mineral density is usually expressed as a T score (number of standard deviations from the young normal mean) or Z score (number of standard deviations from the age-matched mean). Osteoporosis is usually defined as a T score below −2.5 (Fig. 5.5).

Metabolic bone disease

Metabolic bone disease is a loose term that encompasses diseases of bone in which abnormal bone remodelling results in a reduced volume of mineralized bone and/or abnormal bone architecture. These processes in turn give rise to bone pain and usually an increased risk of fracture. The commonest metabolic bone diseases are osteoporosis, osteomalacia, Paget's disease, hyperparathyroidism, and bone disease associated with renal failure (renal osteodystrophy).

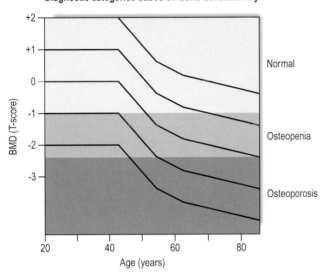

Fig. 5.5 Diagnostic categories based upon bone densitometry according to the number of standard deviations from the young normal mean (a T score of zero). T scores between −1 and −2.5 are called low bone mass or osteopenia. T scores below −2.5 are called osteoporosis.

Case 5.1	Osteoporosis: 2

Case note: Measurement of bone mineral density

In most subjects with hip fractures, bone mineral density is not routinely measured since low bone mineral density is evident in virtually all elderly subjects. However, Mrs Jones sustained her hip fracture at a relatively early age, so measurement is appropriate in her case. Her bone mineral density reveals a femoral neck T score of −4.0 and her Z score is −2.3 (Fig. 5.6). Her T score confirms that she has osteoporosis (being below −2.5). However, since her Z score is also considerably below what is expected for her age, secondary causes for osteoporosis or other metabolic bone disease should be sought.

Osteoporosis

Osteoporosis is characterized by an imbalance in remodelling—a relative increase in resorption that is not matched by a concomitant increase in formation. The bone matrix is normally mineralized but there is simply less bone. In most forms of osteoporosis the loss of bone is not evenly distributed throughout the skeleton. For example some struts of trabecular bone are resorbed completely, resulting in a loss of connectivity between adjacent bone plates (Fig. 5.7). This contributes to markedly decreased bone strength and fracture risk. Because the remodelling surface-to-volume ratio of trabecular bone is high, bone loss tends to affect this type of bone, in the spine and hip, to a greater extent.

An imbalance between resorption and formation occurs with ageing but also in several other circumstances. These include:

- when bone is subject to reduced mechanical loading as a result of bed rest or immobilization

- the presence of reduced sex hormone concentrations such as after the menopause in females

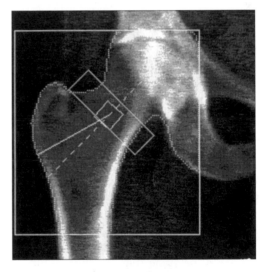

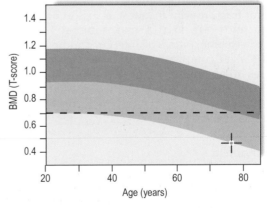

Fig. 5.6 Mrs Jones' right hip scan measured by dual energy X-ray absorptiometry showing her values plotted against the age-related normal range.

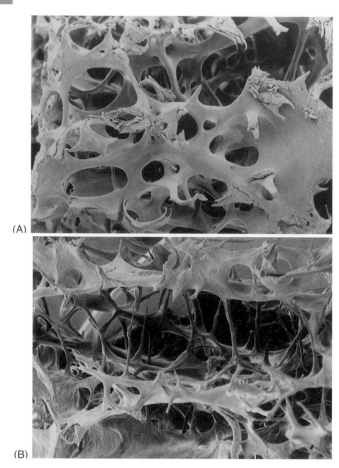

(A)

(B)

Fig. 5.7 Scanning electron micrographs of (A) normal and (B) osteoporotic bone (courtesy of Lis Mosekilde, Institute of Anatomy, University of Aarhus, Denmark).

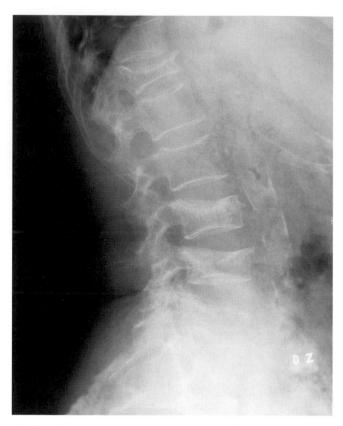

Fig. 5.8 X-ray of patient with multiple vertebral fractures.

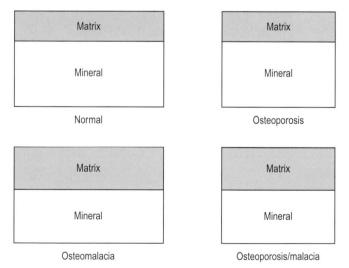

Matrix	Matrix
Mineral	Mineral
Normal	Osteoporosis

Matrix	Matrix
Mineral	Mineral
Osteomalacia	Osteoporosis/malacia

Fig. 5.9 Illustration of the difference between osteoporosis and osteomalacia. In osteoporosis, the amount of bone is decreased but the ratio of matrix to bone mineral is normal. In osteomalacia, the amount of bone is normal but the ratio of matrix to bone mineral is decreased.

- the presence of excess corticosteroids usually given as treatment for a variety of conditions such as arthritis or asthma.

Loss of bone mineral has no clinical effect itself, unless a fracture occurs. Common sites of fracture due to osteoporosis include the spine (Fig. 5.8), wrist, hip or pelvis after minor trauma, but almost any bone can be affected. Vertebral fractures can manifest as loss of anterior height (wedge fractures), loss of mid-vertebral height (called codfish vertebrae) or loss of anterior, middle and posterior height (called compression or crush fractures). Vertebral fractures may present with an acute self-limiting episode of back pain or subclinically (i.e. asymptomatically) as height loss and increasing thoracic kyphosis (forward bending of the spine).

Osteomalacia

Osteomalacia occurs when there is insufficient calcium and phosphate to mineralize newly formed osteoid. Since bone mineral—hydroxyapatite—gives bone its compressive strength, osteomalacic bones are softer and more liable to bend, become deformed, or fracture. Rickets is essentially the same problem—impaired mineral deposition in bone—when it occurs in children or adolescents. Rickets is only seen before the growth plate disappears. Osteomalacia and rickets usually occur as a result of vitamin D deficiency, such as in institutionalized patients, those

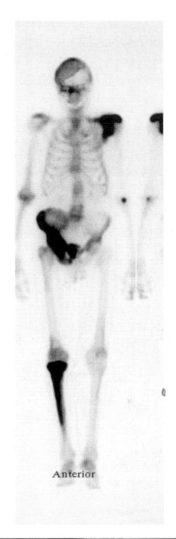

with reduced sun exposure and in patients with gut malabsorption or poor nutrition. Rarely, an inability of the kidney to retain phosphate results in phosphate wasting and chronic hypophosphataemia and osteomalacia/rickets (Fig. 5.9).

Paget's disease

Paget's disease is a condition in which localized areas of bone show markedly increased bone turnover. There is gross disorganization of newly reformed bone, triggered by overactive osteoclasts. These local areas of increased remodelling may cause deformity such as bowing of a limb or enlargement (Fig. 5.10), bone pain, increased fracture risk and, rarely, neoplastic transformation to osteosarcoma. The X-ray appearance often shows a complex pattern of radiolucency (owing to early osteolysis) and bone expansion and sclerosis (generally later). Paget's disease is treated most effectively by drugs called bisphosphonates, which are discussed later in this chapter (p. 75).

Hyperparathyroidism and renal osteodystrophy

Overproduction of parathyroid hormone, usually by a benign tumour (adenoma) of one of the four parathyroid glands, leads to increased bone resorption and elevation of the serum calcium level. Hyperparathyroidism can occur as a discrete condition (primary hyperparathyroidism) or may be secondary to conditions such as renal failure (owing to decreased production of 1,25-dihydroxyvitamin D by the kidney). In patients with renal failure, the mixed picture of secondary hyperparathyroidism and osteomalacia is commonly called renal osteodystrophy.

Osteoporosis: pathophysiology and risk factors

Fracture risk is directly related to bone mineral density. Bone mineral density at any age is the result of the peak bone mass achieved and subsequent bone loss (postmenopausal and age-related). This section will discuss factors contributing to bone loss that are considered important in the aetiology of osteoporosis.

Sex hormone deficiency

Since Albright first observed that the majority of women with osteoporosis were postmenopausal, sex hormone deficiency, resulting from natural or surgical menopause, has been recognized to cause bone loss. Replacement of oestrogen following the menopause prevents bone loss and fractures. In men, testosterone deficiency is similarly associated with bone loss and can be reversed with testosterone replacement.

(A)

(B)

Fig. 5.10 (A) Bone scan showing increased uptake due to Paget's disease involving the right hemipelvis, right tibia, left scapula, skull and eleventh thoracic vertebra. (B) X-ray of the same patient showing Paget's disease characterized by expansion of the right hemipelvis with cortical thickening and coarse trabecular pattern.

Osteoporosis: 3

Case note: Screening for metabolic bone disease

We recall that Mrs Jones had poor nutrition, so vitamin D deficiency should be checked for by measuring serum 25-hydroxyvitamin D. A simple screen for metabolic bone disease can be performed (Table 5.2). The usual tests to exclude a metabolic bone disease include measuring serum calcium, phosphate, creatinine, alkaline phosphatase and PTH. Serum calcium will be elevated in hyperparathyroidism and often low in osteomalacia or renal failure. If the serum calcium is elevated in renal failure, this may be due to so-called tertiary hyperparathyroidism. Phosphorous is the most abundant intracellular anion in the body and 85% is located in the skeleton. Serum phosphate generally has an inverse effect on serum calcium concentration. Serum creatinine will be elevated in renal impairment. Alkaline phosphatase is an enzyme found in human serum, mainly produced by the liver or osteoblasts. Bone-specific isoenzymes can be measured but automated biochemical screens mostly measure total serum alkaline phosphatase (i.e. enzyme from both sources) and it is usually modestly elevated in osteomalacia but much higher in Paget's disease. Serum PTH should be measured when the serum calcium is elevated, to confirm hyperparathyroidism.

Table 5.2 Differential diagnosis of common metabolic bone disorders

Disorder	Blood				
	Ca	P	Alkaline phosphatase	PTH	25-OH-vitamin D
Primary hyperparathyroidism	↑	↓	↑, normal	↑	Normal
Osteomalacia	↓	↓	↑	↑	↓
Paget's disease	Normal	Normal	↑↑	Normal	Normal
Osteoporosis	Normal	Normal	Normal	Normal	Normal

Menopausal status is probably the most important risk factor for osteoporosis. Women with an early menopause (generally considered to be present in women who become menopausal before 45 years of age) or having bilateral oophorectomy have lower bone mineral density and increased risk of subsequent fracture. The earlier the menopause, the greater the risk appears to be.

Race and genetic influences

Racial factors influence bone mineral density. For example, Blacks, whether in Africa or in the USA, appear to have greater bone density than Whites of the same age and sustain fewer related fractures. People of Asian origin often have lower bone densities which may result in higher fracture rates than Whites although other factors such as exercise levels which can influence falls risk can also alter this risk.

Similarly, it is well established that bone mineral density at both the appendicular and axial skeleton is strongly genetically influenced. A family history of a relative sustaining a fracture after age 50 should be viewed as suggestive.

Physical activity and muscle strength

Bone is responsive to physical strain. Changes in the forces applied to bone produce effects in bone. For example, weightlessness and immobilization induce marked degrees of bone loss. On the other hand, athletes tend to have greater bone mineral density, although this effect is often site specific. For example, tennis players have increased bone density in their dominant but not non-dominant arm and weight lifters have greater femoral bone density than other athletes. This is consistent with a local effect of exercise on bone.

Nutrition

Although the majority of body calcium is stored in the skeleton, there is controversy about the role of dietary calcium intake in the aetiology and prevention of osteoporosis. However, there appears to be a role for dietary calcium intake in the attainment of peak adult bone density. Moreover, a daily dietary calcium intake of around 800 mg/day in premenopausal women and 1200 mg/day in postmenopausal women is generally considered appropriate to avoid negative calcium balance.

Other dietary factors have been postulated to play a role in skeletal homeostasis. Sodium intake may have important effects on bone and calcium metabolism. Sodium loading results in increased renal calcium excretion, which has led to the suggestion that lowering dietary sodium intake diminishes age-related bone loss. Excessive protein and caffeine intakes are associated with bone loss.

Glucocorticoids

Glucocorticoids or corticosteroids are commonly used to treat inflammatory diseases, including arthritis and asthma.

Corticosteroids affect calcium metabolism deleteriously in a variety of ways. The most important effect is to inhibit osteoblastic bone formation directly. They also decrease calcium absorption in the intestine, increase urinary calcium excretion and enhance osteoclast activity by inhibiting OPG.

Case note: Risk factors

We recall that on admission to hospital, Mrs Jones' past medical history revealed several risk factors for osteoporosis. These include an early menopause, a positive family history, smoking and poor nutrition.

- An early menopause is one that occurs before 45 years of age.
- A positive family history could include a mother who sustained any fracture after age 50 or early height loss due to kyphosis.
- Smoking exposure can be quantified in terms of pack years. One pack year is smoking 20 cigarettes per day for 1 year. Someone who smokes 10 cigarettes per day for 10 years thus has 5 pack years of exposure.
- Poor nutrition includes avoidance of dairy products, and thus a low dietary intake of calcium, or a poor diet overall.

Mrs Jones' medications also include corticosteroid therapy. Although corticosteroid-induced osteoporosis is dose dependent, even inhaled corticosteroids can cause bone loss if used in excessive doses.

Case 5.1 Osteoporosis: 5

Case note: Preoperative management of hip fracture

After admission to hospital, Mrs Jones is transferred to the Orthopaedic Ward, 24 of whose 30 beds are occupied by elderly subjects recovering from hip fractures. These fractures all occurred following a fall or trivial trauma. Like many older subjects, Mrs Jones is on a large number of drugs (polypharmacy) and her 10 current medications should be critically reviewed to determine if they are all necessary. Her sleeping tablets should be stopped, as these types of medications are commonly associated with falls. Since she also takes diuretics, postural hypotension should be checked for as a cause of her falls. To reduce the risk of morbidity or mortality, Mrs Jones must be assessed by her anaesthetist prior to surgery for co-morbid conditions, and her cardiopulmonary and fluid–electrolyte state should be evaluated. Fluid and electrolyte imbalance is common in an elderly patient taking diuretics and anti-inflammatory drugs and with poor nutrition. Any imbalance must be corrected before surgery.

These mechanisms cause rapid bone loss when corticosteroids are used in high doses for prolonged periods.

Epidemiology of fractured hip

Hip fractures, or fractures of the neck of the femur, are the most serious fractures in older people, at both an individual and population level. Their economic cost is enormous because of the need for hospitalization, surgery and rehabilitation. Complications are frequent, especially in those with co-morbid conditions (which are common in subjects aged >80 years). A total of 20% of those who fracture their hip die within 1 year and most survivors never regain their pre-fracture level of physical function. Hip fractures lead to permanent admission to a nursing home in approximately 20% of patients.

The incidence of hip fracture rises dramatically with increasing age in most countries. Hip fractures are more common in women than in men: epidemiological studies suggest a white woman has a 16% lifetime risk of suffering a hip fracture and a white man has a 5% lifetime risk.

Risk factors for falls

The high rate of hip fracture in older people is due not only to their lower bone strength and but also to their increased risk of falling. Established risk factors for falls and hence hip fracture include impaired balance, muscle weakness, poor vitamin D status and use of psychotropic medication. Although physical activity levels are related to bone density, the benefits of exercise in the elderly may relate more to reduced risk of falling than increases in bone strength.

Essential anatomy of the hip

The hip joint, like most of the lower limb joints, is a synovial joint. Synovial joints are characterized by the following features:

- articular cartilage covering the bony surfaces
- a joint cavity containing viscous synovial fluid
- a surrounding articular capsule that consists of outer fibrous tissue and an inner lining called a synovial membrane.

The hip joint is also a ball-and-socket joint, formed by the articulation of the rounded head of the femur with the cup-shaped acetabulum of the pelvis. It combines a wide range of motion with great stability. This is possible because of the deep insertion of the head of the femur into the acetabulum, the strong articular capsule and the muscles that pass over the joint and insert at a distance below the head of the femur. These anatomical features provide leverage for the femur and stabilization for the joint. When a hip fracture occurs, it is usually at one of three sites (Fig. 5.11): either high in the femoral neck (subcapital), across the neck itself (cervical) or in the trochanteric region (pertrochanteric).

The acetabulum is formed by fusion of three pelvic bones: the ischium, ilium and pubis (Fig. 5.12). There is a circular rim of fibrocartilage, which forms the glenoid labrum inside the acetabular cavity, the lower portion of which is incomplete, forming the acetabular notch. Blood vessels pass into the joint through a foramen formed by a transverse ligament over this notch. The acetabulum is deepest and strongest superiorly and posteriorly, where

it is subject to the greatest strain when a person is in the erect position.

The hip joint has a strong, dense articular capsule. It is attached proximally to the edge of the acetabulum, the glenoid labrum and the transverse ligament passing over the acetabular notch. All of the anterior surface and the medial half of the posterior surface of the femoral neck are intracapsular. The articular capsule is strong and thick over the upper and anterior portions of the joint but becomes thinner and weaker over the lower and posterior portions of the joint.

Important structures around the hip joint

Ligaments

The fibrous tissue of the articular capsule of any joint usually shows localized thickenings, which form the

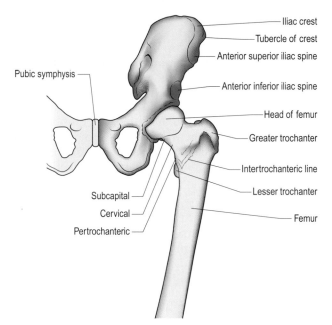

Fig. 5.11 Anterior view of bones of the hip joint showing three main sites of fracture: high in the femoral neck (subcapital), across the neck itself (cervical) or in the trochanteric region (pertrochanteric).

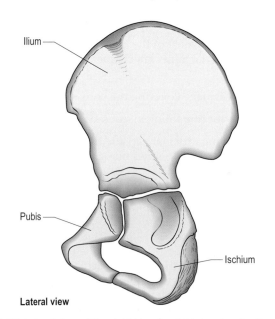

Lateral view

Fig. 5.12 Lateral view of the right hip of a child showing the three bones that form the acetabulum before fusion occurs.

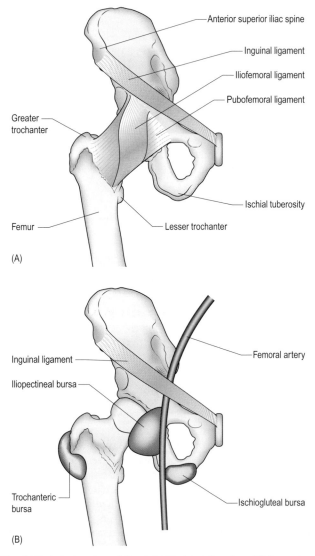

(A)

(B)

Fig. 5.13 Anterior view of the right hip joint showing: (A) the main ligaments; (B) the key bursae.

ligaments of the joint (Fig. 5.13A). There are a number of important ligaments around the hip joint. The iliofemoral ligament is the strongest of these. Crossing the front of the capsule, it extends from the ilium to the anterior portion of the base of the neck. Its lower portion divides into two bands, forming an inverted Y shape. It is relaxed in flexion and taut in extension of the thigh and prevents excessive extension of the hip. In the upright position, the iliofemoral ligament stabilizes the hip by pulling the femoral head firmly into its socket.

The pubofemoral and ischiocapsular ligaments are weaker than the iliofemoral ligament but help reinforce the posterior portion of the capsule. The ligamentum teres is an intracapsular ligament that loosely attaches the femoral head to the lower portion of the acetabulum and adjacent ligaments. It has little effect on the normal motion or stability of the joint but is a channel for blood vessels to the head of the femur. Although the femoral head's blood supply is mainly by other vessels via the femoral neck, these may be damaged in cervical fractures. If the blood supply via the ligamentum teres is insufficient, avascular necrosis of the femoral head may occur.

The iliotibial band is a portion of the fascia lata of the thigh that extends inferiorly from the sacrum, the iliac crest and the ischium, over the greater trochanter of the femur and lateral aspect of the thigh to insert into the lateral condyle of the femur and tibia.

Synovial membrane

A synovial membrane lines the deep surface of the articular capsule. It is a common site of pathology in septic arthritis in children (see Ch. 11) and chronic inflammatory diseases in adults such as rheumatoid arthritis and ankylosing spondylitis (see Ch. 1).

Bursae

In areas of the skeleton where friction occurs, a definite sac lined with a synovial membrane called a bursa is often present. There are several bursae (Fig. 5.13B) around the hip joint that are of clinical importance.

The largest and most important is the trochanteric bursa, situated between the gluteus maximus muscle and the posterolateral surface of the greater trochanter. It is usually a multilocular bursa but is not palpable or visible unless distended. Inflammation of this bursa (called trochanteric bursitis) can occur in various types of arthritis (e.g. rheumatoid arthritis) or as a separate entity. It often occurs in patients with lumbar spine pathology or gait disturbances.

The iliopectineal bursa lies between the deep surface of the iliopsoas muscle and the anterior surface of the joint. It lies over the anterior portion of the articular capsule and since it communicates with the joint cavity in about 15% of normal individuals, swelling of the bursa may present as a synovial cyst of the hip near the inguinal ligament. The ischiogluteal bursa is situated near the ischial tuberosity and overlies the sciatic nerve and the posterior femoral cutaneous nerve.

Muscles

The hip joint is surrounded by powerful and well-balanced muscles (Fig. 5.14) that not only move the extremity but also help maintain the upright position of the trunk. Extension of the femur on the pelvis is performed largely by the gluteus maximus and hamstring muscles. Flexion of the hip is carried out mainly by the iliopsoas, iliacus and rectus femoris muscles. Abduction is achieved by the glutei medius and minimus, and adduction by the adductors magnus, longus, and brevis, the pectineus, and the gracilis muscles.

Femoral triangle

The femoral triangle is a clinically important subfascial space whose main contents are the femoral artery and vein, and branches of the femoral nerve. It is located in the superomedial third of the thigh and appears as a depression below the inguinal ligament when the leg is actively flexed at the hip joint. The boundaries of the femoral triangle are shown in Figure 5.15.

Interesting facts

Of clinical importance, the femoral artery is easily exposed and cannulated in the femoral triangle. Moreover, the superficial position of the femoral artery in the triangle makes it vulnerable to lacerations and puncture from trauma.

The femoral nerve is the largest branch of the lumbar plexus (L2–L4) and passes lateral to the femoral vessels in the triangle.

Adductor canal

The adductor canal is a narrow fascial tunnel in the thigh, providing an intramuscular passage through which the femoral artery and vein pass into the popliteal fossa of the knee (Fig. 5.15).

Case 5.1 Osteoporosis: 6

Case note: Relating clinical features to pathology

We can now understand why Mrs Jones is tender over the lateral aspect of the right hip. Tenderness over the right greater trochanter is likely to be a sign of trochanteric bursitis. Her history includes recurrent low back pain, which is commonly associated with altered gait and trochanteric bursitis. We can also appreciate why Mrs Jones' leg is shortened and externally rotated. Key muscles around the hip such as the iliopsoas muscle are de-functioned by the fracture and the normal lever arm of the femoral neck is disrupted.

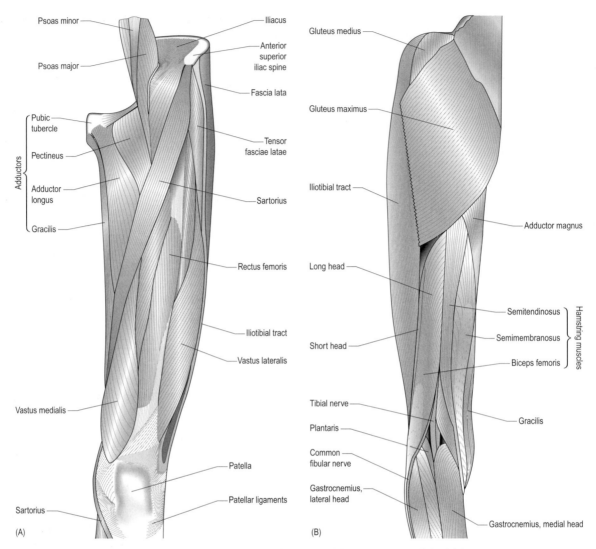

Fig. 5.14 The key muscles of the hip joint: (A) anterior view of the left hip joint; (B) posterior view of the left hip joint.

Surgical management of hip fractures

Surgical management followed by early mobilization is the treatment of choice for hip fractures. Surgical management varies according to the type of fracture and can be broadly divided into two types.

Femoral neck fractures

Undisplaced femoral neck fractures are most commonly fixed with multiple parallel screws or pins. The treatment of displaced femoral neck fractures depends on the patient's age and activity level: young active patients should undergo open reduction and internal fixation; older, less active patients are usually treated with hip replacement (hemiarthroplasty). The ultimate goal is to return patients to their pre-fracture level of function by rapid rehabilitation.

Trochanteric fractures

A sliding hip screw is the device most commonly used for fracture stabilization in both undisplaced and displaced intertrochanteric fractures. Fracture stability is dependent on the status of the posteromedial cortex of the femur. The most important aspect of its insertion is secure placement in the femoral head. Although the sliding hip screw allows postoperative fracture impaction, it is essential to obtain an impacted reduction at the time of surgery.

Medical management of osteoporotic hip fracture

Hip fractures are particularly common problems in the very elderly. After initial surgical management, diagnostic approaches should be directed at a general medical assessment. Elderly patients often have significant

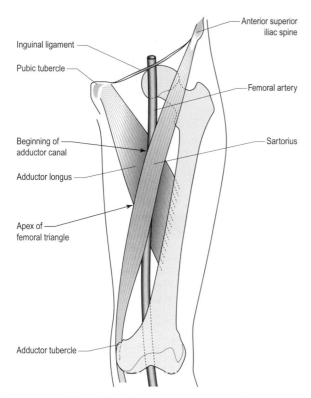

Fig. 5.15 Boundaries of the femoral triangle in the left thigh and the adductor canal.

Labels in figure:
Inguinal ligament
Pubic tubercle
Anterior superior iliac spine
Femoral artery
Beginning of adductor canal
Sartorius
Adductor longus
Apex of femoral triangle
Adductor tubercle

unrecognized multisystem disease that may impair the rehabilitation process. Investigations to exclude different types of underlying metabolic bone disease should include looking for the possibility of subclinical vitamin D deficiency as a contributing factor to falls (due to muscle weakness) and fracture (due to osteomalacia), especially in institutionalized patients.

Measurement of bone mineral density is the best method for confirming the diagnosis of osteoporosis and is commonly used for monitoring the response to therapy. Bone density is usually measured at two sites, most commonly the spine and hip, using the technique of dual energy X-ray absorptiometry. Bone density can also be assessed by quantitative CT scanning. The ability of bone density to predict fracture is at least as good as cholesterol level to predict heart disease and blood pressure to predict stroke. Bone biopsy may rarely be performed to exclude diseases like osteomalacia. Ultrasound measurements, usually of the heel (calcaneus), can also be used to provide an assessment of bone density and structure. Spinal X-rays may be appropriate to examine for vertebral wedge or compression fractures. These fractures may be associated with pain but often occur silently and result in height loss and increased kyphosis.

Treatment of osteoporosis is aimed at preventing further fractures. It is important to select treatment individually for each patient. Treatment options for osteoporosis include calcium, vitamin D, oestrogen, selective oestrogen-receptor modulators, bisphosphonates, strontium, monoclonal

antibodies that affect the RANKL pathway, parathyroid hormone and calcitonin.

Calcium

Calcium is weakly antiresorptive (i.e. a weak inhibitor of bone resorption) and supplementation may reduce negative calcium balance and so reduce bone resorption, particularly in older age. Controlled trials have demonstrated calcium supplementation can prevent bone loss in postmenopausal women and this appears to be associated with a mild reduction in fracture risk. There is also evidence that calcium supplementation augments the effect of oestrogen on bone density.

Vitamin D

Since a substantial proportion of institutionalized (or house-bound) elderly may be vitamin D deficient, vitamin D supplementation is recommended in institutionalized or house-bound elderly subjects.

Oestrogen and selective oestrogen-receptor modulators

In the past, oestrogen replacement therapy was the treatment of first choice in most perimenopausal women. Oestrogen reduces osteoclastogenesis by decreasing production of cytokines such as IL-1 and RANK (Fig. 5.4). However because use of oestrogen therapy has been linked to adverse effects on the cardiovascular system, its long-term use for treating osteoporosis is not advocated.

Controversy exists over whether there may be an increased risk of breast cancer with long-term oestrogen use. This has led to the development of selective oestrogen-receptor modulators or SERMS, which act to decrease bone resorption, like oestrogen, while not stimulating the breast or uterus. Controlled clinical trials have shown modest increases in bone density and significant reductions in spine fractures with SERMs.

Bisphosphonates

Bisphosphonates are potent inhibitors of bone resorption, acting through the inhibition of osteoclast function (Fig. 5.4). Treatment with these agents can significantly increase bone density and reduce further fracture risk at both spine and non-spine sites.

Interesting facts

Because bisphosphonates are retained in the skeleton for prolonged periods, the usual plasma pharmacokinetics do not apply to dosing. Rather, differences between bisphosphonates in binding affinity to hydroxyapatite and their potency of inhibition of the key enzyme, FPPS, mean that regimens can vary from daily oral, to weekly oral, monthly oral, 3 monthly intravenous or once yearly intravenous.

Osteoporosis: 7

Case note: Postoperative management of hip fracture

A multidisciplinary team comprising her orthopaedic surgeon, a physician, a physiotherapist, an occupational therapist and a social worker were all involved in Mrs Jones' postoperative progress. The main goals were re-establishing her independence and early mobilization to avoid pressure sores and thromboembolism.

As falls were involved in Mrs Jones' case, a general medical assessment that included her visual function, and neuromuscular and cardiovascular systems was made. Calcium and vitamin D supplements were added to her treatment and she was transferred to a rehabilitation unit on day 8 after her surgery.

Other considerations

Exercise programmes are most useful in relation to preventing further falls, even though little effect on bone density may be achieved. Serum biochemical markers of bone turnover may be used to monitor compliance with therapy.

A period of weeks to months in a specialist rehabilitation unit may be necessary to improve coordination and gradually strengthen muscle power. However, functional impairment in activities of daily living because of poor mobility will be present in many of these patients. For example, about 50% of hip fracture survivors are discharged to nursing homes. Rehabilitation will enable many patients to regain independence. Prior to discharge, a home visit by the occupational therapist may be necessary to ensure that the home environment is safe. In addition, a variety of aids may be recommended by the occupational therapist to promote independent living.

Further reading

Favus, M.J. (Ed.), 2006. Primer on the Metabolic Bone Diseases and Disorders of Mineral Metabolism, sixth ed. American Society for Bone and Mineral Research, Washington DC.

Marcus, R., Feldman, D., Kelsey, J. (Eds.), 2008. Osteoporosis, third ed. Academic Press, San Diego.

Moore, K.L., Dalley, A.F., 2006. Clinically Oriented Anatomy, fifth ed. Williams & Wilkins, Baltimore.

ARTICULAR CARTILAGE IN HEALTH AND DISEASE

6

Lyn March and Chris Little

Chapter objectives

After studying this chapter you should be able to:

1. Understand normal articular cartilage structure and function, including the delicate balance between synthesis and catabolism performed by cartilage cells (chondrocytes).

2. Appreciate the essential structure and anatomy of the knee joint.

3. Understand the pathological processes of osteoarthritis, including articular cartilage degeneration and changes in the subchondral bone, synovial lining and synovial fluid.

4. Understand the clinical symptoms and signs of osteoarthritis.

5. Understand the epidemiology of osteoarthritis including risk factors for development and progression.

6. Understand the general principles of medical and surgical management of the osteoarthritic knee.

ARTICULAR CARTILAGE IN HEALTH AND DISEASE

Introduction

The principal function of articular cartilage is to act as a protective shock absorber for the underlying bones. When it degenerates or becomes 'diseased', osteoarthritis ensues, with its accompanying pain and disability. Osteoarthritis affects approximately 10% of the population of the western world and is the leading cause of chronic disability in these communities. It increases dramatically with age, with as many as 50% of those over 65 years suffering from musculoskeletal symptoms, the majority of which will be due to osteoarthritis. No 'cure' as such exists for osteoarthritis but much is now known about risk factors that could contribute to prevention of progression, and numerous interventions, including non-pharmacological ones, have proven benefits for symptom relief.

This chapter will review normal structure and function of articular cartilage, as well as the normal anatomy, structure and function of the synovial joint with a focus on the knee joint. The 'diseased' state of articular cartilage describes the pathological process of osteoarthritis and a case will demonstrate the clinical symptoms and signs, risk factors and treatment of this condition.

Case 6.1 Osteoarthritis: 1

Case history

Mrs Campbell is a 64-year-old retired teacher, living independently with her husband in their own home. She is in good health but, although always on the larger side, has become more overweight in recent years. For the past 5 years she has had gradually increasing right knee pain. This initially troubled her after her weekly tennis, with aching felt on the inside aspect of the knee. This has progressed to the point where she no longer wants to play, she is experiencing pain during the games and some low-grade swelling after. She is also having trouble kneeling down to do her gardening and is particularly concerned that she cannot keep up with her grandchildren. The knee has not been catching, locking or giving way but she is now also having trouble getting out of low lounge chairs and feels lack of confidence in the knee when going down stairs and slopes.

She has a strong family history of osteoarthritis with her 88-year-old mother having knobbly arthritic fingers and her father requiring a total knee replacement when he was 70 years of age. Mrs Campbell had played a lot of sport in her youth and recalled numerous knee injuries when playing hockey. She has taken the occasional paracetamol/acetaminophen tablet for pain but generally does not like to take medications. She is on no other regular prescription or non-prescription medications. A provisional diagnosis of osteoarthritis of the knee is made.

Anatomy

The knee is a synovial joint with a surrounding capsule, an internal synovial lining that produces the lubricant joint fluid, internal menisci and stabilizing ligaments, and articular cartilage covering the surface of the bones. In the pathogenesis of osteoarthritis, changes occur in all structures including the synovial lining layer, the synovial fluid, the articular cartilage and the subchondral bone (Fig. 6.1). It is felt that the earliest and most significant changes occur in the articular cartilage and this chapter will focus on these.

Articular cartilage

Articular cartilage is a specialized form of connective tissue that covers and protects the ends of the bones in synovial joints. For the knee joint this makes up the smooth surfaces covering the femoral and tibial condyles and the under surface of the patella. The surface is smooth and slippery with an extraordinarily low coefficient of friction, while the deeper layer merges with a calcified layer (the tidemark) that interlocks with the subchondral bone (Fig. 6.2).

Interesting facts

Normal articular cartilage is made up of 80% water.

Cartilage is an elastic, resilient structure that acts as a shock absorber to protect the underlying bone. The properties of articular cartilage depend on the composition and structure of the extracellular matrix, and the synthesis and maintenance of this matrix is dependent on the chondrocytes.

Interesting facts

The chondrocyte has a unique role in both the synthesis and degradation of its surrounding extracellular matrix. The chondrocyte can turnover, i.e. divide, but the rate is very slow in adult life and decreases with age.

During skeletal development, the articular cartilage forms from very densely packed mesenchymal cells that differentiate into chondrocytes, which proliferate rapidly and synthesize the large amounts of extracellular matrix. The extracellular matrix is made up predominantly of water (up to 80%), collagen and proteoglycans (discussed below), which are produced and maintained by the relatively sparse cells, the chondrocytes. It is the combination of collagen, proteoglycan and water that gives articular cartilage its unique properties. The collagen forms a network of fibrils that gives the overall framework and shape of the cartilage and provides pockets or compartments that are filled with the water-binding proteoglycan complexes that regulate the compressibility.

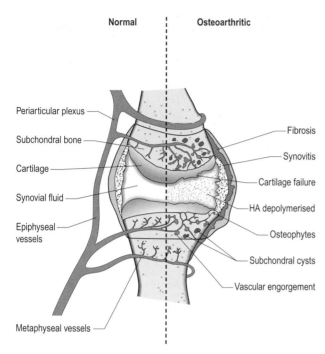

Fig. 6.1 Structures in a normal synovial joint, including articular cartilage, synovial fluid and synovial membrane, together with changes seen in those structures with osteoarthritis. (Based on a drawing by Professor Peter Ghosh, Raymond Purves Laboratory, Institute of Bone and Joint Disease, University of Sydney.)

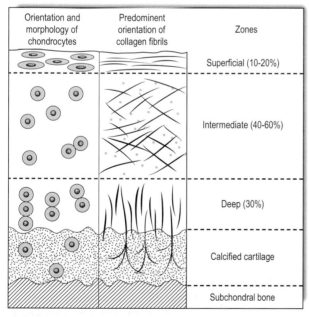

Fig. 6.2 Normal articular cartilage, illustrating the variability in density and orientation of the chondrocytes and collagen network in different layers. (Based on a drawing by Professor Peter Ghosh, Raymond Purves Laboratory, Institute of Bone and Joint Disease, University of Sydney.)

The ability of articular cartilage to resist compressive deformation is largely due to the entrapment of high concentrations of the polyanionic large proteoglycan aggrecan within the collagen fibrillar network. The osmotic pressure provided by the glycosaminoglycan (GAG) chains on the aggregated aggrecan molecules is resisted by and constrained within the insoluble collagenous meshwork. Degradation of cartilage is a central pathological feature of arthropathies such as osteoarthritis and rheumatoid arthritis, and involves proteolytic cleavage of both its major structural elements, namely aggrecan and type II collagen. Proteolysis and subsequent loss of the GAG-rich region of aggrecan from cartilage is an early event in cartilage degeneration, while significant catabolism of the collagen fibrillar structure occurs later and may represent the point of irreversible cartilage damage.

> ### Interesting facts
>
> There are more than 13 different types of collagen throughout the body. The main one in articular cartilage is collagen Type II.

The functional integrity of the articular cartilage in a healthy joint depends on the chondrocyte synthesizing the many different matrix components in the appropriate amounts and in the right sequence. Since cartilage lacks blood and lymphatic vessels, the survival and synthetic activity of the chondrocyte depends on the diffusion and transport of nutrients and metabolites through the matrix. Thus a fine balance exists between anabolism (synthesis) and catabolism (tissue breakdown) with ongoing tissue remodelling part of the normal healthy process.

> ### Interesting facts
>
> Articular cartilage has no blood or neural supply and relies on diffusion of nutrients and waste products through the proteoglycan and collagen matrix.

In 'disease', osteoarthritis, this equilibrium is disturbed with the balance tipped in favour of degenerative changes and the chondrocyte failing to keep up, despite an observed initial increase in chondrocyte numbers and synthetic processes.

The chondrocyte

Chondrocytes play a unique role in regulating both synthetic and catabolic processes in health and disease. They make up less than 5% of the total volume of the cartilage. Each chondrocyte establishes a specialized microenvironment and is responsible for the turnover of extracellular matrix in its immediate vicinity. Cells in different parts of the tissue appear to have metabolic differences, because different components of the matrix are required to maintain structure and function.

Chondrocytes vary in shape, size and number of cells per area depending on their different anatomical locations, even within different regions of the normal knee joint. Close to the surface they are flatter, smaller and generally have a greater density than the cells deeper in the matrix. Each chondrocyte sits within a lacuna (space). Collagen fibres come right up to the edge of the lacunae, which are filled with fine fibrillar material. Unlike the osteocyte in bone, their cytoplasmic processes do not make contact with processes of other chondrocytes i.e. they have little or no cell-cell contact. They have low numbers of mitochondria, which reflects their low oxygen consumption rates. In adult cartilage, the rate of cell division is very low but division does occur in response to injury or disease. Chondrocytes, particularly in the deeper uncalcified zone, have prominent endoplasmic reticulum and Golgi apparatus responsible for protein synthesis and sulphation of the mucopolysaccharides that form the proteoglycan side-chains. Lipid occurs intracellularly and as a diffuse layer around the cells, and probably contributes to cartilage lubrication.

A number of *in vivo* and *in vitro* studies have shown that environmental changes can alter chondrocyte function and thus the surrounding matrix. There appears to be an optimal window of mechanical loading. At low levels of mechanical stress, as would occur with bed rest or disuse, there is increased catabolic activity; at physiological levels there is anabolic activity; while at higher stress levels, as would occur with obesity or carrying heavy loads repeatedly, the chondrocyte is unable to adapt and catabolic processes outstrip the anabolic activity.

Biochemistry

Collagen network

There are at least 13 different types of collagen in the connective tissues throughout the human body. In articular hyaline cartilage, the predominant components are types II, IX and XI with small amounts of others.

Type II collagen is the predominant fibrous component making up 90–95% of the primary collagen and 40–70% of the total dry weight of articular cartilage. It forms a three-dimensional cross-banded network of fibrils that maintain the 'shape' of the cartilage structure. It is secreted by the chondrocytes as procollagen molecules that consist of polypeptide chains organized as a triple helix. These grow and aggregate to form fibrils that then develop strong covalent interfibrillar cross-links. The minor collagens, such as types IX and XI are thought to be important for regulating structure and interactions.

In osteoarthritis, collagen network swelling has been noted as one of the earliest features of the fibrillation process. The chondrocyte is known, when stimulated by inflammatory mediators such as the cytokine interleukin-1 (IL-1), to produce enzymes called metalloproteinases (including stromelysin and collagenases) that degrade the collagen molecules into fragments. This contributes to the loosening of the collagen network and allows the increased water content that is also a feature of early osteoarthritis.

Proteoglycans

Proteoglycans are the predominant molecules trapped in the collagen fibrils and make up 15–40% of the dry weight of articular cartilage. They have many negative charges and thus are highly hydrophilic, which leads to trapping of water which, in turn, contributes to the shock-absorbing capacity.

Interesting facts

Proteoglycans have a very strong negative charge that helps trap the water in the cartilage as well as being able to repel each other when the cartilage is compressed which gives cartilage its resilience and ability to maintain its shape.

Proteoglycans are made up of a core protein with glycosaminoglycan (GAG) side-chains; GAGs are linear polysaccharides made up of many repeating disaccharide units—including keratan sulphate (KS) and chondroitin sulphate (CS)—together with numerous other oligosaccharides.

Most proteoglycans exist in the cartilage matrix as aggregates. As many as 100 proteoglycan monomers will lock onto a central hyaluronic acid (HA) filament, stabilized by link protein (Fig. 6.3). Their aggregate molecular weights are enormous—1 to 2 million daltons (Da).

Proteoglycans play a crucial role in the ability to absorb loading forces in a reversible way. They are responsible for restricting water flow and thus resist deformation during compressive loading. As the tissue is compressed, e.g. in weight bearing, some water is squeezed out, but much is held in by the attractive forces of the proteoglycans; the proteoglycans come into closer contact but are repelled by their strong charges, preventing deformation. As the load is removed, the tissue rapidly regains its form by taking on the water again.

The highly charged state of proteoglycans also stops the flow of large molecules across the tissue but allows the smaller molecules to diffuse through, which is an important mechanism for delivering nutrients to the avascular cartilage.

Pathophysiology of osteoarthritis

When the delicate balance of cartilage matrix synthesis and destruction is upset, the net result is articular cartilage loss and the degenerative process that ensues is osteoarthritis. Despite significant advances in our understanding of cartilage structure, there is still a lot to learn about the mechanisms of cartilage destruction. While it is felt that the initial pathology in osteoarthritis involves the articular cartilage, it is evident from very early stages that there are changes also in the synovial lining, the synovial fluid and the underlying subchondral bone.

Articular cartilage

Macroscopically, the cartilage surface undergoes three phases of degeneration starting with fibrillation and progressing through to erosion and cracking to expose the underlying subchondral bone. Eventually, the bone surface may be denuded of its cartilage cover, a process termed eburnation. In the knee joint, the areas of cartilage damage are most apparent on the surfaces exposed to excessive load bearing and may be quite focal in the early phases.

At the biochemical level, the main changes in osteoarthritis involve an increase in the water content of the articular cartilage, a decrease in the proteoglycan concentration and loss of the collagen network. In the early phases, the articular cartilage will actually thicken and swell because of the increased water and early increased synthesis of proteoglycans. However, these changes leave the cartilage less compressible, more permeable to tissue breakdown products and thus more prone to damage from impact loading. The collagen network also breaks down as enzymes are released from stressed chondrocytes and synovial lining cells. The enzymes belong to a family called metalloproteinases, of which collagenase is a member. The cartilage softens (termed chondromalacia) and progresses to fibrillation of the surface layers.

Microscopically, there is evidence of chondrocyte necrosis as well as focal clumps or clones of increased proliferation. The proliferating cells are attempting repair and have been shown to increase proteoglycan production locally. The 'repaired' cartilage tends to be more cellular and, at points where erosions have occurred and bone has been denuded, it has the properties of fibrocartilage rather than the resilient hyaline cartilage of a normal healthy joint. The main collagen type in fibrocartilage is type I rather than type II and the increased fibrous content offers less protection to the underlying bone.

Pathology occurs in all joint tissues in OA, including bones, menisci, ligaments and synovium but the central

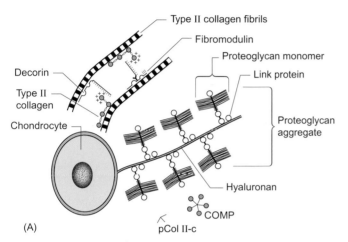

(A)

Aggrecan

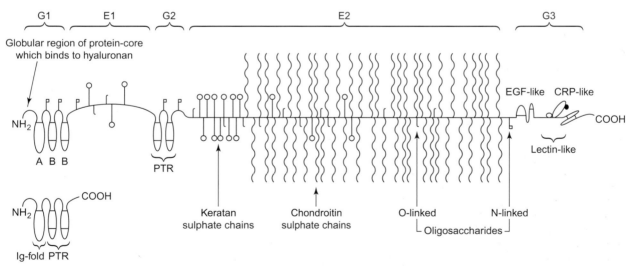

(B)

Link protein
(stabilizes interaction of aggrecan monomer with hyaluronan)

Fig. 6.3 Fine structure of articular cartilage. (A) The chondrocyte in its lacuna; the collagen fibrils, secreted by the chondrocyte, of which type II is the predominant type that bonds via proteins to create the tight mesh; and between the collagen network the aggregates of proteoglycan molecules, linked via the link protein to hyaluronan. (B) A large proteoglycan molecule, aggrecan, made up of a protein core with three globular domains (G1, G2, G3) and two extended segments (E1, E2) to which are bound the glycosaminoglycans, keratan and chondroitin sulphate, and the oligosaccharides. The link protein is attached at the G1 region and binds to hyaluronan to form proteoglycan aggregates. (Based on drawings by Professor Peter Ghosh, Raymond Purves Laboratory, Institute of Bone and Joint Disease, University of Sydney.)

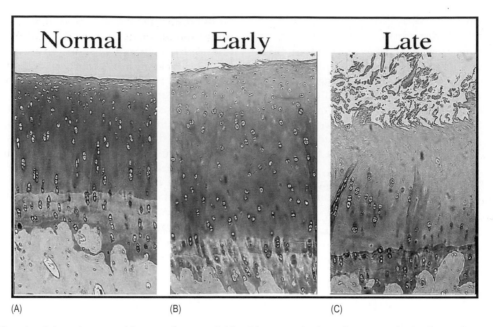

Fig. 6.4 (A–C) Cartilage breakdown is a central feature of osteoarthritis with progressive loss of aggrecan (stained) in early OA and eventual disruption of the collagen network late.

feature is progressive degeneration of the articular cartilage (Fig. 6.4). Articular cartilage has a very poor reparative capacity, and ultimately it is the breakdown and erosion of this tissue that signifies end-stage arthritis necessitating joint replacement surgery.

What mechanisms are important in cartilage breakdown?

Cartilage is aneural, avascular, sparsely populated with cells (chondrocytes) and predominantly comprised of extracellular matrix (Fig. 6.4A). The major matrix proteins are type II collagen which forms a structural scaffold, and aggrecan (the aggregated proteoglycans) which is substituted with negatively charged glycosaminoglycans. The swelling pressure of the aggrecan is balanced by the tension in the collagen network, and together they endow cartilage with its resilience under compression. Progressive breakdown of cartilage in OA involves proteolysis of both aggrecan and type II collagen. Aggrecan breakdown precedes and is independent of collagen degradation, and both *in vitro* and *in vivo* is due to the action of members of the *A Disintegrin And Metalloproteinase with ThromboSpondin motif (ADAMTS)* family of enzymes. In particular ADAMTS-4 and -5 appear to be the physiologically important 'aggrecanases'. Although cartilage has a limited ability to repair, aggrecan can be replenished by the chondrocytes and the mechanical properties of the tissue restored if the destructive insult is removed prior to disruption of the collagen network. Once significant disruption of the collagen network occurs (Fig. 6.4C), cartilage damage is irreparable with further collagen breakdown resulting in progressive cartilage loss.

Interesting facts

The aggrecan is broken down by members of the ADAMTS family (*A Disintegrin And Metalloproteinases* with *ThromboSpondin*) motif, ADAMTS 4 and 5 appear to be the most important.

Fibrillar type II collagen is resistant to degradation by all proteinases at 37°C and neutral pH, except the collagenolytic metalloproteinases (MMPs) (MMP-1, -2, -8, -13 and -14). It has been shown that cytokine-stimulated collagenolysis in articular cartilage is due to the action of MMPs with MMP-13 being the principal enzyme both *in vitro* and *in vivo*.

Interesting facts

A family of enzymes call the metalloproteinases (MMPs) breakdown the collagen and matrix. MMP-13 appears to be the most important.

Activation of MMPs in cartilage

MMPs are secreted as zymogens and must be activated extracellularly where their activity is then controlled by tissue inhibitors of metalloproteinases (TIMPs). Chondrocyte mRNA levels for numerous MMPs including MMP-2, -9 and -13 are significantly increased in OA cartilage in both animals and humans. While OA is often considered a 'non-inflammatory' arthropathy, chondrocyte-derived cytokines such as IL-1 and TNF are known to play a direct role in human cartilage degradation by MMPs. However, the precise regulatory pathway whereby chondrocyte MMP expression is regulated, and therefore the identification of potential therapeutic targets, is still the subject of intensive investigation.

Interesting facts

The inflammatory cytokine IL-1 plays a role in stimulating the chondrocyte to release MMPs.

Subchondral bone

As the articular cartilage is eroded, the underlying bone becomes exposed to wear and tear, causing a polishing effect on the surface and microfractures of the bony trabeculae. In response, there is increased osteoblastic activity and new bone formation. The surface may also undergo focal pressure necrosis. As the overlying cartilage is denuded, subarticular cysts may develop. This is thought to be due to the combination of the focal necrosis and the transmission of intra-articular pressures through to the marrow spaces of the underlying bone. Cysts can collapse or may regress or even disappear if the surface becomes covered with regenerative fibrocartilage. Vascular engorgement, slowing of blood flow and bone marrow oedema in the subchondral bone are all features documented at different stages of the osteoarthritis cycle and are thought to contribute to some of the clinical features of pain.

Synovium

As discussed in Chapter 1, the normal synovium consists of two layers: the lining layer of cells, known as the intima, and the remaining subsynovial tissue or subintima. The normal intima is formed by an interlacing layer, one to three cells (synoviocytes) deep, that merges with the underlying connective tissue. There is no basement membrane between. The lining is generally smooth with few folds and the subintima has connective tissue cells (fibroblasts) only and relatively few blood vessels and endothelial cells.

In osteoarthritis, products released from the breakdown of the cartilage and bone evoke an inflammatory response in the synovium, which becomes both hyperplastic, with increased numbers of synovial lining cells, and hypertrophic, with small villi or folds developing in the membrane, infiltration of lymphocytes and plasma cells and an increase in the vascularity in the subintimal layer. This is in contrast to rheumatoid arthritis where the synovial inflammation is thought to be the primary pathology, leading to secondary cartilage destruction in which the synovial proliferation is much more marked. One of the functions of the synovial membrane is to provide nutrients for the avascular articular cartilage, but if thickened and scarred, it may not function as well and thus may perpetuate the degenerative cycle. The influx of inflammatory cells releases mediators that further contribute to tissue damage.

Synovial fluid

Normal synovial fluid is clear, pale yellow in colour and very sticky or viscous (see Ch. 1). It is a dialysate of plasma combined with hyaluronic acid that is produced by the synovial cells. The molecular weight of HA determines the elasticity and viscosity of the fluid. A normal knee joint contains 0.5–1.5 mL of fluid, which coats the surface of the articular cartilage, providing lubrication for movement, a vehicle for flow of nutrients from the fluid into the articular cartilage matrix and a shock-absorbing cushion on weight bearing. In OA there is often an increased volume of fluid but the hyaluronic acid content and thus the viscosity and other mechanical properties of the fluid are reduced. The fluid is still usually clear and non-inflammatory in OA but if cartilage fragments and/or low-grade inflammation are present, it will have a more turbid appearance.

Normal fluid may produce a 'string' sign, in which the fluid drop can hang from a thread of synovial fluid owing to the high viscosity. The greater the level of inflammation, the more fluid and the less viscous it becomes. Normal synovial fluid has very few white cells ($<100/mm^3$) and fluid from osteoarthritis is also characteristically non-inflammatory. Cell counts may be slightly higher ($100–2000/mm^3$) but cells will be predominantly mononuclear, unlike in rheumatoid arthritis where cell counts are much higher ($>5000/mm^3$) with a higher percentage of polymorphonuclear cells. Higher levels of cells may be associated with inflammation due to calcium pyrophosphate or hydroxyapatite crystals that may be present at sites of tissue damage. Increased white cell numbers may, in turn, be associated with accelerated tissue damage because of the release of inflammatory mediators.

Clinical features of osteoarthritis

Symptoms and signs of osteoarthritis are summarized in Box 6.1.

Symptoms

The key clinical features of OA are joint pain and disability associated with varying degrees of swelling, deformity and decreased range of motion. OA emerges as a clinical syndrome when there is sufficient joint damage to cause impairment of function.

Symptom onset is usually very gradual over a number of years, with pain as the key feature. It is likely that the degenerative changes in the articular cartilage have been progressing for many years before pain develops. The pain is usually deep, aching and poorly localized. In the early phases it is related to activity, being worse at the end of the day. In more advanced stages of joint degeneration there will be pain at rest. OA usually progresses very slowly and symptoms will fluctuate over many years. Not all patients will progress to advanced rest pain and loss of function. Studies of osteoarthritic knee X-rays suggest that only a third will progress significantly over a 10-year period.

Osteoarthritis can affect any joint but most commonly affects the hands, knees, spine (where it is called spondylosis), feet and hips. Involvement of other joints such as

Box 6.1 Symptoms and signs of osteoarthritis

Symptoms
- Joint pain
  - gradual onset
  - deep, aching, poorly localized
  - activity related, worse at end of day
  - later stages, pain at rest
- Joint stiffness
  - early feature
  - usually a few minutes, rarely exceeds 15–30 min
  - after inactivity ('gelling') and when first getting out of bed
- Crepitus
- Limitation of joint motion
- Loss of function
  - difficulty rising from chair, toilet
  - trouble turning taps

Signs
- Tenderness on palpation
- Pain on passive motion
- Crepitus on joint motion
- Joint enlargement—bony spurs and osteophytes, synovitis
- Limitation of range of motion
- Deformity

Box 6.2 Possible sources of pain in osteoarthritis

Intra-articular
- Periosteum, osteophyte formation
- Subchondral bone pressure, micro-fractures, engorgement
- Intra-articular ligament degeneration
- Capsule distension
- Synovitis

Periarticular
- Tendons, fasciae
- Bursitis
- Muscle spasm
- Nerve pressure

Psychosocial

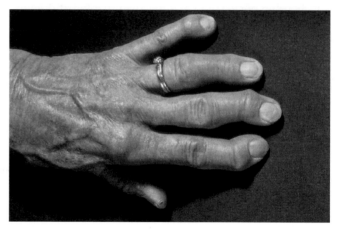

Fig. 6.5 An osteoarthritic hand with bony swelling and deformities at all the distal interphalangeal (DIP) joints (Heberden's nodes) and the third and fourth proximal interphalangeal (PIP) joints (Bouchard's nodes). Deformity is also present at the first carpometacarpal (CMC) joint at the base of the thumb.

shoulders, elbows and wrists does occur but other causes of arthritis should always be considered.

The cause of the pain is usually multifactorial. Interestingly, the cartilage itself, although considered to be the initial site of pathology in the pathogenesis of osteoarthritis, has no nerve supply and therefore is not a source of pain. Pain comes from both intra-articular and periarticular structures (Box 6.2). Intra-articular sources include periosteal stretching and elevation over remodelling bone and osteophyte formation, trabecular microfractures in subchondral bone, pressure on exposed subchondral bone in advanced stages, vascular engorgement of the bone, degenerative changes in intra-articular ligaments, inflammation of the synovial lining, pinching or abrasion of the synovial villi, and distension of the synovial capsule.

Periarticular sources include the tissues, tendons and bursae around the joints, which become stretched and/or inflamed, spasm of the muscles around the joints or pressure on local nerves.

Joint stiffness is localized to the involved joints and usually of short duration, in contrast to the more prolonged and generalized stiffness of the inflammatory rheumatoid arthritis. It rarely lasts more than 15–30 min and is most notable when first mobilizing in the morning after waking, or after inactivity during the day (referred to as gelling), e.g. long car trips, sitting in the waiting room, watching a movie.

Patients will often complain of crepitus or grating that they can feel and hear as they move the joints. Later in the course of the disease, they will notice limitation of joint movement and difficulty carrying out some activities such as turning on taps or opening jars for osteoarthritic hands; getting up from a chair or toilet seat, going up and down stairs, bending and kneeling for osteoarthritic knees and hips. The loss of function may be quite marked early in osteoarthritic hands in the presence of pain due to inflammation and soft tissue swelling. However, this tends to settle over months to years to leave a stiffened joint with bony enlargement (Fig. 6.5) but quite reasonable function. In osteoarthritic knees (Fig. 6.6), degenerative tears in the menisci or loose bodies of broken-off articular cartilage may lodge between other intra-articular structures during joint movement causing locking and catching. Changes in joint alignment and weakness of muscles around the joint may also cause a feeling of the joint 'giving way' in later-stage disease.

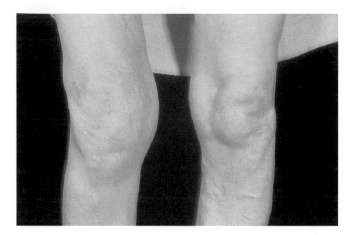

Fig. 6.6 Bilateral osteoarthritic knees with the right knee most affected. Bony swelling and low-grade soft tissue swelling is evident, with probable effusion in the suprapatellar pouch on the right. There is some valgus deformity suggesting loss of articular cartilage from the lateral tibiofemoral joint.

Systemic features with generalized morning stiffness, fevers, weight loss, significant fatigue or anorexia are not features of osteoarthritis, and other causes for the pain should be considered.

Signs

The signs depend on the joints involved and the stage of the degenerative process, which could be at very different stages for different joints in the one patient.

In the early stages there may be very few signs. Later, joints may be tender to palpation along the joint line or surrounding tissues, particularly if synovitis is present. Pain may be present on passive motion, usually at the extremes of the joint range. Later, there is loss of full range of motion that may be due to a number of features, including change in joint surfaces, muscle spasms, and tendon and capsular contractures. Crepitus is often palpable on movement of the joint, and is particularly evident under the patella on flexion and extension of the knee. Crepitus appears to be due to cartilage loss and joint surface irregularity. Swelling may be palpable, both bony swelling as a result of osteophyte formation and soft tissue swelling because of joint effusions and synovitis. In the hand, the hard swelling of the bony osteophytes classically involves the distal interphalangeal joints (called Heberden's nodes), the proximal interphalangeal joints (called Bouchard's nodes) and the first carpometacarpal joint at the base of the thumb. Ongoing joint destruction due to cartilage loss and subchondral bone collapse combined with proliferative bone overgrowth can lead to deformities and joint subluxation. Fusion or ankylosis of the joints is rare, apart from distal interphalangeal joints in the hands. Surrounding muscle atrophy is common, particularly at the knee and thumb.

Essential anatomy of the knee joint

Like the hip joint, the knee joint is a synovial joint. It is formed by three articulations:

- that between the lateral femoral and tibial condyles with its corresponding meniscus

- that between the medial femoral and tibial condyles with its corresponding meniscus

- that between the patella and the femur.

All of these articulations share the same articular (joint) cavity (Fig. 6.7). Functional aspects of the anatomy of the knee will be discussed in more detail in Chapter 10.

The magnetic resonance images (MRIs) of the normal knee in Figure 6.8 outline clearly the structures that would be seen on anatomical dissection. Both menisci and articular cartilage can be visualized, which is not possible with plain radiography.

The knee is predominantly a hinge joint with the main movements being extension and flexion. A small amount of rotation is required to allow the full extension. The knee should normally extend to a straight line (0 degrees) and flex to 130–150°.

Menisci

The medial and lateral menisci are crescent-shaped, fibrocartilaginous disks interposed between the femoral and tibial condyles. They are usually referred to somewhat misleadingly as the knee 'cartilage' and are often injured, requiring surgical debridement or removal. They are unique to the knee joint and should not be confused with the specialized articular cartilage that is hyaline and fused to the ends of the bones in all synovial joints. The outside edge of the menisci is thick and attaches to the joint capsule, while the inside edge is thin and essentially unattached.

Articular ligaments

The bones of the knee are stabilized by the articular ligaments, the main ones being:

- the articular capsule

- the ligamentum patellae (or patellar ligament)

- the medial and lateral collateral ligaments

- the anterior and posterior cruciate ligaments.

The *articular capsule* is a fibrous structure that surrounds the joint and merges with and is strengthened by the other surrounding fascia lata, tendons and ligaments.

The *ligamentum patellae* is the extension of the quadriceps femoris muscle on the anterior thigh and is responsible for extension of the knee. It fans out around the

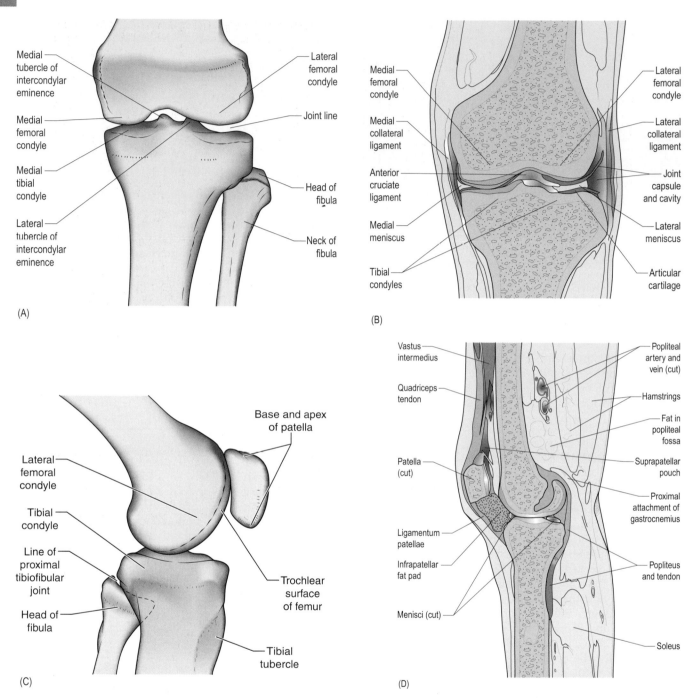

Fig. 6.7 The normal knee: (A) anatomical bony landmarks (anteroposterior view); (B) soft tissue structures, showing articular cartilage, menisci, synovial membrane and main knee ligaments (coronal section); (C) bony landmarks (lateral view); (D) soft tissue structures (sagittal section).

patella and continues distally to insert into the tibial tuberosity. A small infrapatellar fat pad lies beneath the tendon and the underlying synovial membrane.

The *lateral collateral ligament* is a strong fibrous cord that runs from the lateral femoral condyle to the lateral side of the fibular head. The *medial collateral ligament* is a broader more membranous structure that attaches to the medial femoral condyle just below the adductor tubercle and runs to the medial condyle of the tibia and the

medial surface of the tibial shaft. This ligament helps to prevent lateral movements of the femur on the tibia.

The *anterior cruciate ligament*, which keeps the tibia from moving forward on the femur, is attached anteriorly to the intercondylar spine of the tibia and extends posteriorly and superiorly to the lateral femoral condyle, attaching to its medial and posterior portion. The *posterior cruciate ligament*, which keeps the tibia from moving backwards on the femur, is attached to the posterior

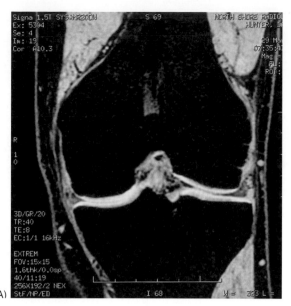

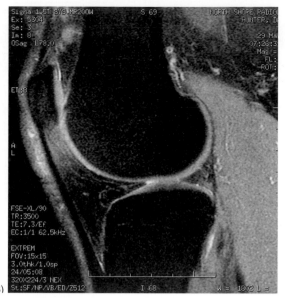

Fig. 6.8 MRI of a normal knee joint: (A) anteroposterior view; (B) lateral view. The epidermal layer, subcutaneous fatty tissue and muscle planes are clearly delineated. No effusion or soft tissue swelling is evident. The underlying bone shows no cysts or oedema. It is covered by a layer of articular cartilage (appears white on these films) of normal thickness without any evidence of thinning. The menisci appear as wedge shapes between the joint surfaces.

Case 6.1 Osteoarthritis: 2

Case note: Examination

When examining any joint, remember to *look*, *feel* and *move*.

On examination, with Mrs Campbell first standing up with lower limbs exposed, *look* for:

- difficulty rising from a seated position
- deformity
- malalignment
- swelling (anteriorly and posteriorly because Baker's cysts are seen best from behind while the patient is standing)
- muscle wasting
- scars.

Mrs Campbell has mild genu varum (bow-leggedness), which she says has been lifelong but has been more obvious in the right knee in recent years. This would be due to thinning of the articular cartilage in the medial tibiofemoral compartment. Her genu varum would have predisposed her to degenerative change initially and now would be increasing the wear and tear with increased weight bearing through the damaged compartment of the knee.

She had some difficulty rising from the chair and there was some wasting of the quadriceps muscle at the front of the thigh. This would also be associated with her loss of confidence on weight bearing, particularly when walking down stairs or slopes. The tendency is then to 'favour' the knee and not use it as much, thus contributing to further atrophy. Epidemiological studies suggest that quadriceps weakness predicts further deterioration or progression of the arthritis.

This is manifested by more osteophytes and more joint space narrowing seen on X-ray, because of loss of articular cartilage. Management should include attention to building back the quadriceps strength.

When Mrs Campbell turns around, a small 2-cm swelling is evident in her popliteal fossa.

With Mrs Campbell lying on a couch *feel* for:

- increased warmth
- effusion (patellar tap, bulge sign)
- bony swelling
- local tenderness.

Mrs Campbell has some medial joint line tenderness in the right knee, suggestive of local periosteal reaction due to osteophyte formation, low-grade synovitis and/or local bursitis. There is a small positive bulge sign when fluid is 'milked' out of the suprapatellar pouch, consistent with a slight increase in synovial fluid but there is no increased warmth to suggest inflammation. The small swelling in the popliteal fossa is non-pulsatile and soft, consistent with a fluid-filled Baker's cyst.

Move for:

- crepitus
- pain
- restriction
- ligament instability
- locking, catching or meniscal tears.

Osteoarthritis: 2 (continued)

Mrs Campbell has retropatellar crepitus of both knees that is more marked on the right, reduced bulk on contraction of her quadriceps muscles on the right side compared with the left, particularly in the medial band, tightness in her hamstring muscles but no ligamentous instability, and McMurray's sign (discussed in Ch. 10) of meniscal damage is negative.

General examination shows that she has some asymptomatic bony osteophytic swelling of the distal and proximal interphalangeal joints in her hands consistent with Heberden's and Bouchard's nodes, respectively. Other joint and spinal movements are within normal limits. She weighs 70 kg and is 160 cm tall. Her body mass index (BMI = weight (kg)/height (m)^2) is 27.3, which puts her in the moderately overweight range.

In order to focus on what is happening in Mrs Campbell's knee and what might be causing the pain, an understanding of the anatomy of the knee joint is required.

intercondylar notch of the tibia and to the posterior part of the lateral meniscus. It passes superiorly and anteriorly to attach to the lateral and anterior portion of the medial femoral condyle. The cruciate ligaments also help to control rotation of the knee.

Interesting facts

The bones of the knee are stabilized by the articular capsule, the ligamentum patellae, the medial and collateral ligaments and the anterior and posterior cruciate ligaments. The overlying quadriceps femoris muscle is another essential element for maintaining stability.

Synovial membrane and adjacent bursae

As these structures are often the source of pain in OA, they are briefly introduced here. The synovial membrane of the knee is the largest in any of the synovial joints and has numerous reflections and extensions that can form pockets of fluid. There are also multiple bursae surrounding the knee at sites where tendons and ligaments are required to glide over bony prominences. The knee cavity extends superiorly beneath the quadriceps muscle for as much as 6 cm above the superior pole of the patella. In pathological states when there is excess fluid, swelling will often first be noted in the suprapatellar pouch. In some instances when there has been a chronic excess of synovial fluid, the synovial cavity will 'blow-out' at sites of weakness in the capsule forming cysts that may or may not remain in communication with the joint cavity. The popliteal fossa in the posterior aspect of the knee is a common site for this and the swelling has been called a Baker's cyst.

Some of the more prominent bursae around the knee include:

- The prepatellar bursa, which lies on the anterior aspect of the knee between the skin and the patella

- The infrapatellar bursa, which has two components, a small superficial infrapatellar bursa between the skin and the proximal part of the ligamentum patellae (patella tendon) and a deep infrapatellar bursa that lies beneath the distal part between the tendon and the infrapatellar fat pad

- The semimembranosus bursa, which is located posteriorly on the medial aspect of the knee and lies between the semimembranosus muscle and the medial head of the gastrocnemius muscle. It will usually communicate with the medial gastrocnemius bursa, which lies deep to it between the medial head of the gastrocnemius and the articular capsule and communicates, in turn, with the knee joint cavity

- Posteriorly on the lateral aspect lies the subpopliteal recess of the synovial cavity between the popliteus tendon and the lateral femoral condyle. In this region also lies the other gastrocnemius bursa between the lateral head of the muscle and the articular capsule

- The anserine bursa, so named for its 'goose-neck' shape, lies on the medial aspect of the knee between the medial collateral ligament and the common tendon insertions of the sartorius, gracilis, and semitendinosus muscles as they attach to the medial tibial condyle and shaft. It is felt to be the source of pain in many patients with early medial tibiofemoral joint involvement.

Muscles

Quadriceps femoris covers the anterior and lateral aspects of the thigh and is responsible for extension. The lateral portion is the vastus lateralis, the medial portion the vastus medialis, and between these lies a double layer with rectus femoris superficially and vastus intermedius beneath. The four muscle bellies merge into a common tendon that encloses the patella and merges with the ligamentum patellae, which inserts into the tibial tuberosity. The quadriceps femoris is essential for maintaining stability of the knee joint on weight bearing. The vastus medialis is often the first to waste in painful conditions of the knee and because this portion is responsible for the final 10° of extension it is critical for normal weight bearing.

The hamstring muscles make up the bulk of the posterior aspect of the thigh and are the main muscles responsible for knee flexion. They are formed by the biceps femoris, semitendinosus and semimembranosus.

The gastrocnemius muscle forms the bulk of the calf muscle and helps to limit hyperextension of the knee.

Nerves

Flexion The hamstrings are supplied by the sciatic nerve and its tibial and peroneal branches (L4,5, S1,2,3 nerve roots).

Extension The quadriceps is predominantly supplied by the femoral nerve (L2,3,4 nerve roots).

Epidemiology of osteoarthritis

Osteoarthritis, also referred to as osteoarthrosis and degenerative joint disease, is the most common form of arthritis. It is a heterogeneous group of conditions with different parts of the skeleton being involved at different rates and having variability in risk factors for development and progression of the disorder.

Classification

Classically, the diagnosis of osteoarthritis in epidemiological and clinical studies has been taken from the characteristic radiographic changes described in the *Atlas of Individual Radiographic Features in Osteoarthritis* (Altman et al 1995). These features include (Fig. 6.9):

- formation of osteophytes on the joint margins or in ligamentous attachments

- narrowing of the joint space

- sclerosis and/or cysts in the subchondral bone

- altered shape of the bone ends.

Prevalence estimates will vary depending on which criteria have been used to classify osteoarthritis. Prevalence of knee osteoarthritis is low before age 40 years (<5%), and then increases with age, with females having greater frequency than males at each age group and at each joint site. Among 45- to 65-year-old women (Mrs Campbell's age range), clinically symptomatic osteoarthritis would be expected with approximately 5% prevalence, while X-ray changes consistent with knee osteoarthritis may be present in up to 20%. Radiological estimates are higher than self-reported clinical osteoarthritis and the two are not always well correlated. It is likely that MRI will take over as the gold standard for assessing structural changes of OA, as changes can be seen in the articular cartilage long before radiological changes are evident on plain X-ray. Although MRI is a highly sensitive tool, further evaluation is required to determine correlations with clinical symptoms.

Box 6.3 Risk factors for development of knee osteoarthritis

Unalterable
- Age
- Female sex
- Race
- Genetics, family history

Potentially alterable
- Obesity
- Injury
- Occupational overuse
- Malalignment
- Past inflammatory process

Risk factors for the development of osteoarthritis (Box 6.3)

Racial differences

Some racial differences have been shown in the distribution of the joints affected by osteoarthritis. For example, African-American females appear to have higher rates of knee osteoarthritis than Caucasian females but are less likely to have the Heberden's nodes; African-Blacks, Chinese and Asian-Indians have all been shown to have lower prevalence of hip osteoarthritis compared with European Caucasians.

Age

There is a dramatic increase in the incidence and thus prevalence of osteoarthritis with age. There is an exponential rise from around age 55 years, which then appears to plateau around 75–80 years. By the time our skeletons reach 80+ years, radiological changes of osteoarthritis are almost universal in joints so far examined in large population-based studies, including hands, cervical and lumbar spines and knees.

Symptomatic and radiographic knee osteoarthritis is very uncommon before the age of 40 years.

Family history: genetic factors

Genetic factors appear to be the most important in generalized nodal (that is, accompanied by Heberden's nodes) osteoarthritis. Early studies found at least a two-fold increase in Heberden's nodes among mothers of OA subjects and a three-fold increase among sisters. There appears to be an autosomal dominant inheritance among females and a recessive inheritance in males.

More recently, twin studies have shown a clear genetic predisposition with a heritability of 65% for OA hand, 50% for OA hip and 45% for OA knee when radiographs were compared between identical and non-identical twins, and a 70% heritability of degenerative disc changes seen in the cervical and lumbar spine on MRI.

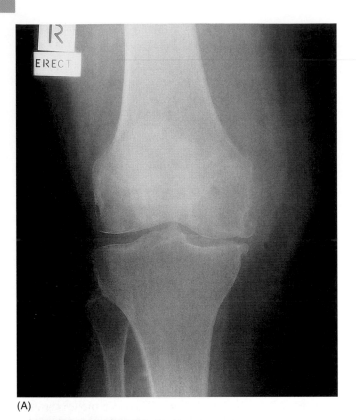

(A)

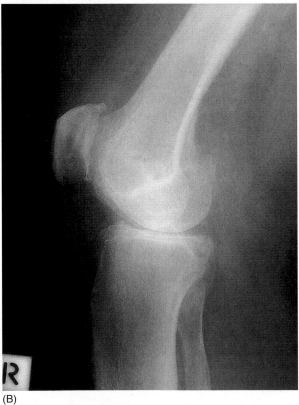

(B)

Studies among rare clusters of multi-case families with early-onset, aggressive osteoarthritis have identified a number of different abnormalities/mutations in the gene for type II collagen, *COL2A1*. However, studies among larger groups of osteoarthritic patients, including those with generalized nodal osteoarthritis, have not found an increase in these mutations when compared with control groups. More recent genetic epidemiology studies have demonstrated a major genetic component to osteoarthritis (OA), with heritability estimates of over 50% for most joint sites. These studies have also highlighted differences in the degree of OA heritability between joint sites and between the sexes, implying a high level of heterogeneity.

Several new arthritis susceptibility genes have been identified including *GDF5* (growth differentiation factor 5), *FRZB* (frizzle-related protein). Common variants at these genes affect either the structural properties of the protein (*FRZB* and *IL4R*) or the transcription of the gene (*BMP5* and *COL9A1*). The variants are particularly relevant to the development of hip OA in females.

Interesting facts

New arthritis susceptibility genes have been identified including *GDF5* (growth differentiation factor 5) and *FRZB* (frizzle-related protein).

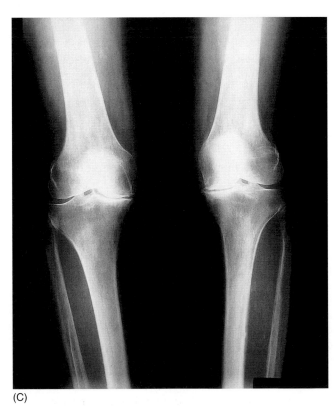

(C)

Fig. 6.9 Radiographic changes in osteoarthritis. (A) AP weight-bearing X-ray of a right knee showing moderate changes of OA with joint space narrowing and osteophytes most marked at the medial tibiofemoral joint, and early joint space narrowing in the lateral compartment. (B) Lateral view of the same knee showing osteophytes representing moderate patellofemoral compartment OA. (C) AP weight-bearing X-ray showing typical advanced bilateral OA most marked in the medial tibiofemoral compartments, with advanced joint space narrowing, subchondral sclerosis and varus deformity.

Trauma/injury

Joint injury is a well-documented risk factor for subsequent osteoarthritis development. This is shown for major ligamentous damage around a joint or damage to the bones and growth plates within joints. Injury is particularly apparent as a risk factor for knee osteoarthritis in the setting of a damaged or removed meniscus, or derangement of the supportive anterior cruciate or collateral ligaments. The time lag between significant injury and subsequent osteoarthritis is in the order of 10–15 years in human studies. In experimental animal models of osteoarthritis, however, the articular cartilage damage occurs very early following anterior cruciate ligament disruption or removal of the medial meniscus.

Occupational 'overuse'

Certain occupations that involve repeated heavy use of particular joints over long periods of time have been associated with the development of osteoarthritis. Occupations that require repeated knee bending, heavy lifting, climbing and carrying have shown an increase in knee osteoarthritis, particularly for males, while farmers appear to be at particular risk for hip osteoarthritis.

Obesity

Obesity is associated with the development of knee osteoarthritis in both sexes but the association is strongest for women. Initial epidemiological evidence was cross-sectional but the association has now been confirmed in a number of prospective studies. Mean body mass index is significantly higher among those with knee osteoarthritis than those without. The risk of osteoarthritis is increased at least two-fold when those in the heaviest groups are compared with individuals in the lightest groups. In addition, obesity is a predictor of disability related to radiographic changes and appears to be related to the radiological progression of osteoarthritis once identified. At a population level obesity represents one of the most important potentially modifiable risk factors for osteoarthritis of the knee. The association is not as clear cut with osteoarthritis of hips or hands.

Interesting facts

Obesity is a major modifiable risk factor for osteoarthritis of the knee, particularly in women.

Sport and recreational activities

There is consensus that extreme levels of physical activity among elite competitive sportsmen and women may lead to greater risk of osteoarthritis of the knees and hips. However, although epidemiological studies have shown conflicting results, a moderate level of activity, in the absence of joint injury or anatomical malalignment, is unlikely to be a risk factor for development of osteoarthritis.

These factors and other secondary causes of osteoarthritis may predispose to the development of osteoarthritis as shown in Figure 6.10.

Risk factors for progression

Epidemiological studies have identified female gender, obesity, quadriceps strength and having nodal hand osteoarthritis as strong predictors of radiological progression of knee osteoarthritis. In addition, some preliminary reports have shown associations with other factors that warrant further study. These include a raised C-reactive protein and positive technetium bone scan suggestive of inflammation, a diet low in vitamin C and other antioxidants, and low vitamin D.

Management of osteoarthritis

Management of osteoarthritis has focused on symptom modification, predominantly characterized by pain relief. As the mechanisms surrounding cartilage failure are likely to be multivariate in nature, it is likely that strategies to repair the 'failing' articular cartilage will also need to target multiple mechanisms. Despite many promising *in vitro* and *in vivo* animal experiments, to date no disease or structure-modifying drug for osteoarthritis has been confirmed in long-term human studies. The main candidates that have shown some promise in trials to slow the rate of cartilage degeneration include glucosamine, diacerein and doxycycline (the latter two perhaps through their ability to reduce the cytokine interleukin 1 (IL-1) activity).

Nevertheless, there is now considerable scientific evidence about what can be done to help prevent osteoarthritis from getting worse. The myths that 'nothing can

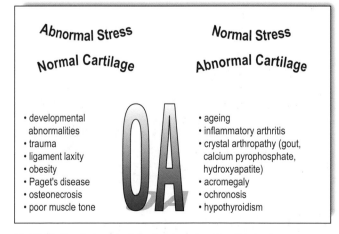

Fig. 6.10 The factors contributing to secondary OA. Factors are divided into two groups: those that place abnormal stress on baseline normal cartilage; and those that have abnormalities in biochemistry or structure of the articular cartilage but are not subject to abnormal stresses. It is recognized that some individuals will have contribution from multiple factors covering both groupings.

Case 6.1 Osteoarthritis: 3

Case note: Risk factors and approach to management

We can see from the details that Mrs Campbell has nodal osteoarthritis and numerous risk factors for osteoarthritis of the knee, including a strong family history, obesity, a history of trauma, anatomical malalignment and the finding of more generalized joint involvement.

The main features of management of Mrs Campbell's knee osteoarthritis include:

- pain reduction
- reduction and prevention of disability
- modification of risk factors
- prevention of progression

Box 6.4 Treatments with randomized controlled trial evidence for symptomatic benefit in knee osteoarthritis

Non-pharmacological

- Patient education and self-management
- Exercise—aerobic, muscle strengthening, range of motion, tai chi
- Physiotherapy—active therapies
- Lateral heel wedges for medial tibio-femoral OA
- Knee braces for varus or valgus instability
- Weight loss—reduced kilojoule intake and exercise
- TENs
- Acupuncture
- Regular telephone contact

Topical/injectable

- Capsaicin
- Anti-inflammatory gels
- Intra-articular hyaluronan
- Intra-/periarticular corticosteroids

Oral

- Analgesics (paracetamol, ibuprofen)
- Non-steroidal anti-inflammatory drugs
- COX-2 selective NSAIDs
- Glucosamine and chondroitin sulphate (only select products found to be better than placebo)
- Weak opioids, e.g. tramadol for chronic pain not responsive to other measures

be done about it' and that 'it is just something to be put up with' need to be dispelled. The knowledge that the disease progresses only *very* slowly over 10 years in the majority of knee osteoarthritis patients and that most will not need joint replacement surgery can make a big difference to the patient's outlook.

All patients presenting with symptomatic osteoarthritis of the knee should be given education, an exercise prescription and suggestions for pain relief. Management should start with these principles and continue with them throughout. Thus, at whatever stage in the disease process a patient is seen, education and discussion about the disease and non-pharmacological measures should be undertaken. Treatments supported by randomized controlled trial evidence are listed in Box 6.4.

The typical management approach to symptomatic osteoarthritis of the knee is shown in Box 6.5 and discussed further below.

Patient education and support

Patient education and self-help courses have been shown in randomized trials to be cost-effective and associated with reduced pain, increased wellbeing, increased knowledge, reduced use of healthcare services and increased compliance with exercises. The effect sizes are small for these types of interventions, however, all osteoarthritis guidelines and chronic disease management programmes strongly recommend education about the disease and active self-management strategies to explain the importance of exercise and weight-loss in particular. Clinical status and symptoms have also been shown in small randomized trials to be improved if patients are contacted regularly by telephone.

Exercise

Exercise is also important at all stages of knee osteoarthritis. The vastus medialis muscle wastes early and

quickly when there is pain and even more so when there is swelling as well. Maintaining quadriceps strength, which is the main support mechanism for the knee, may help prevent radiological progression and disability. Regular aerobic exercises have been shown in elderly men and women with established osteoarthritis to be safe and effective in reducing pain and improving wellbeing. Exercises to improve aerobic fitness, muscle strength and range of motion are all highly recommended for OA management at all stages of the disease. The psychosocial benefits of exercise should also not be underestimated. Exercise and increased physical activity when combined with weight-loss strategies have the greatest chance of reducing the pain and disability associated with knee OA in those who are overweight. Referral to a physiotherapist may aid the process and encourage ongoing adherence to exercise recommendations as well as providing any manual therapy.

Weight reduction

Many patients, particularly women, are overweight. Sound epidemiological evidence has shown that being overweight is strongly associated with radiological progression and disability of knee osteoarthritis. Recent

Box 6.5 Key steps in management

Step 1

Education, reassurance, exercises, intermittent or regular analgesics, topical preparations

- *Non-pharmacological intervention*: patient education, reassurance, strengthening exercises, weight reduction counselling, orthotics, walking aid and consider trial of glucosamine
- *Analgesics*: oral paracetamol/acetaminophen either as required, 500–1000 mg before and/or after activity, building up to 1000 mg twice to three times daily (avoid narcotic-containing preparations for long-term use). Consider new slow release paracetamol preparations for more persistent pain
- *Topical treatment*: anti-inflammatory (e.g. diclofenac, ketoprofen, piroxicam, methylsalicylate) or analgesic capsaicin-based creams (which act by depleting substance P in nociceptors) used up to four times daily

Step 2

Step 1 + trial of NSAIDs, ±intra-articular viscosupplementation or steroids

- Lowest dose of least toxic NSAIDs, e.g. ibuprofen 400–800 mg b.d. or diclofenac 50 mg b.d.
- Consider intermittent use—use with paracetamol/acetaminophen
- In high-risk patients (elderly, previous ulcer history) consider prophylaxis with misoprostol or proton pump inhibitors (e.g. omeprazole, lansoprazole) or use of the COX-2 selective NSAIDs (celecoxib)
- Consider course of intra-articular hyaluronan for activity-related pain
- Consider intra-articular or periarticular corticosteroids if there are elements of inflammation clinically

Step 3

Consider surgery

randomized trials combining weight loss and exercise strategies have resulted in improvement in symptoms with a reduction in pain and an increase in mobility and physical function. It has yet to be proven in prospective randomized studies whether weight reduction can help prevent progression of the arthritis.

TENS and acupuncture

Both TENS (transcutaneous electrical nerve stimulation) machines and acupuncture have been shown in randomized placebo-controlled trials to reduce pain associated with OA knee.

Other non-pharmacological Interventions

Walking aids, knee braces in the presence of varus or valgus instability, insoles with lateral heel wedges for medial-tibiofemoral compartment involvement and thermotherapy (both hot and cold) have been shown to provide small improvements in symptomatic OA knee.

Analgesics

Many patients with osteoarthritis of the knee will get adequate symptom relief—control of pain—with regular oral paracetamol/acetaminophen use. Intermittent use is also beneficial for activity-related pain. There is not much to be gained by using combination codeine-containing analgesics chronically. They are more expensive and may contribute to unwanted side-effects of drowsiness, increased risk of falling in the elderly, constipation and even addiction, with minimal or no improvement in pain relief.

Non-steroidal anti-inflammatory drugs

These agents have been discussed in Chapter 1. Individual patient variability in response to both efficacy and toxicity has been documented and it may be worth trying several different NSAID regimens. One systematic review was unable to detect a significant difference in efficacy between different NSAIDs for OA of the knee, whilst another meta-analysis observed a hierarchy for toxicity, with ibuprofen and diclofenac consistently showing the lowest peptic ulcer risk and longer-acting NSAIDs such as piroxicam and ketoprofen the highest risk. The combination of paracetamol in conjunction with NSAIDs has been shown to give added pain relief and may also lower the overall use of the NSAID. NSAIDs are often preferred over paracetamol for short-term symptom relief but side-effects from NSAIDs are common, particularly in the elderly, in patients with reduced renal function or in those who are taking antihypertensives so their long-term use is not recommended. All guidelines suggest these agents should be used at the lowest dose for the shortest duration possible to provide symptom relief.

Several NSAID compounds (celecoxib, meloxicam) have been developed that have selectivity for blocking the cyclooxygenase 2 (COX-2) enzyme responsible for production of prostaglandins at sites of inflammation, without blocking cyclooxygenase 1 (COX-1), which is expressed constitutively and is responsible for the production of prostaglandins in the gastric mucosa where it has a protective effect. These NSAIDs appear to have equivalent efficacy to available NSAIDs but with reduced propensity to cause gastric irritation. They appear not to have any effect on thromboxane and platelet activity, so do not confer any anticoagulant or antiplatelet risk or benefit. They still have the potential to exacerbate fluid retention, renal insufficiency, hypertension and congestive cardiac failure and must be used with caution in patients with these co-morbidities.

Topical therapies

Topical anti-inflammatory gels and creams can provide small improvements in pain and stiffness.

Interesting facts

Management of OA should include a combination of non-pharmacological and pharmacological interventions.

Corticosteroids

Oral corticosteroids should never be used for the treatment of osteoarthritis. Topical steroids do not have a role either. Soft-tissue and intra-articular injections of corticosteroids are widely used but have not been well tested in placebo-controlled trials. In early knee osteoarthritis, some of the pain may be due to anserine bursitis and infiltration of this region with steroids and local anaesthetic may improve symptoms. Peripatellar injection of steroid and anaesthetic may also provide pain relief. Intra-articular steroids for knees, first CMC joints and inflamed PIP joints can offer temporary relief in many patients, usually of 6–8 weeks' duration. However, the response appears to wane with repeated injections. Once marked joint space narrowing has developed, corticosteroid injections are unlikely to be of any value.

Viscosupplementation

Hyaluronan is the main component of normal synovial fluid. In osteoarthritis the elasticity and viscosity of the fluid is reduced owing to degradation of the hyaluronan polymers. A number of randomized controlled trials suggest that intra-articular injections of a cross-linked polymer derived from hyaluronan can reduce pain and stiffness and improve physical disability and poor quality of life associated with OA of the knee for an average duration of 6 months after a series of 3–5, weekly intra-articular injections. However they have not been shown to slow the progression of arthritis and the logistics and cost associated with repeated intra-articular administration has tended to limit their uptake.

Glucosamine and chondroitin sulphate

A number of trials have shown that these compounds, produced from marine fish and mammalian cartilage, may offer symptom relief for osteoarthritis, equivalent to NSAIDs but with greatly reduced potential for adverse effects. Doses of 1500 mg glucosamine and/or 1200 mg chondroitin are recommended daily. They take 3–6 weeks to provide benefit but can also have a sustained effect following cessation of treatment. More recent overviews of all published trials have suggested that the effect on symptoms is no better than placebo. In theses studies however, some 50–60% of placebo patients reported symptom improvement. Most guidelines suggest giving them a trial for 4–6 weeks and discontinuing if no significant improvement in symptoms is felt. Preliminary studies suggest they may be associated with slowing of the cartilage degeneration if taken long term (2–3 years) but more work is required before they can be considered a proven disease- or structure-modifying agent for osteoarthritis.

Interesting facts

No cure exists but several products show some promise of slowing disease progression including glucosamine, diacerein and doxycycline.

Surgery

The main principles of surgical treatment for osteoarthritis are:

- to improve pain
- to correct deformity.

For knee osteoarthritis, the types of surgery available include arthroscopy, osteotomy, arthroplasty and arthrodesis.

Arthroscopy This is useful in the setting of a joint that is locking or catching frequently because this may be due to a degenerative meniscal tear or loose body. Lavage and debridement in this setting can help. In the absence of these pathologies there is little evidence that arthroscopy will benefit the diffusely arthritic knee.

Osteotomy This involves the cutting of a wedge of bone and pinning to realign the weight-bearing surfaces of the knee. It is most useful in younger patients (under 55 years) in whom the osteoarthritis is limited to the medial tibiofemoral compartment and significant genu varum has developed. It does not alter the joint surfaces but redistributes the weight bearing more evenly through the medial and lateral compartments. It has a modest success rate.

Arthroplasty Joint replacement involves the cutting away of the diseased surfaces of the joint and its replacement with artificial components of metal and special plastic. This usually involves a complete resurfacing of the femoral and tibial condyles, with or without a button on the back of the patella. Pain relief is usually dramatic but range of motion rarely goes back to normal. Recently, partial or hemi-arthroplasty has had a revival in which just one compartment of the joint is replaced (usually the medial tibiofemoral compartment). This is only successful in the setting of osteoarthritis limited to that one compartment and in the absence of significant malalignment.

Arthrodesis Joint fusion is considered, rarely, for knee osteoarthritis in the setting of a joint that has failed because of repeated infection. Although it achieves pain relief, it is very disabling to live with a stiff leg.

When to have surgery

The choice of surgical management is dependent on a number of patient-related factors including age, anatomical

Case 6.1 Osteoarthritis: 4

Case note: Management

Mrs Campbell was referred to a self-management programme, given advice on weight reduction and an exercise programme that included daily quadriceps straight-leg raising exercises, walking 2–3 times a week for 20 min and attending a weekly Tai-chi class. She uses paracetamol/acetaminophen before and after activities, massages her knee with a topical anti-inflammatory gel when needed and also takes regular glucosamine. Her symptoms are reasonably controlled with this and to date she does not require NSAIDs and is unlikely to require surgery for many years.

reduction in pain and disability and improvement in quality of life in the majority, with benefits being sustained for up to 10 years in more than 80% of patients.

Further reading

Altman Jr, R.D., Hochberg, M., Murphy, W.A., et al., 1995. Atlas of individual radiographic features in osteoarthritis. Osteoarthritis and Cartilage 33 (Suppl A), 3–70.

March, L.M., 1997. Osteoarthritis. In: Brooks, P.M. (Ed.), MJA Practice Essentials in Rheumatology. AMPCo, North Sydney, pp. 28–33.

Moore, K.L., Dalley, A.F., 1999. Clinically Oriented Anatomy, fourth ed. Williams & Wilkins, Baltimore.

Zhang, W., Moskowitz, N., Nuki, G., et al., 2008. OARSI recommendations for the management of hip and knee osteoarthritis, Part II: OARSI evidence-based, expert consensus guidelines. Osteoarthritis and Cartilage 16, 137–162.

alignment and mechanical stability of the knee, and the level of pain and disability. Total knee joint replacement is a highly cost-effective operation resulting in a significant

CRYSTAL ARTHROPATHIES AND THE ANKLE

Neil McGill

Chapter objectives

After studying this chapter you should be able to:

1. Understand the possible causes of acute arthritis in a single joint and the approach to diagnosis.

2. Understand normal uric acid handling in the body, factors resulting in a high serum uric acid (hyperuricaemia) and how drug therapy can influence the production or excretion of uric acid.

3. Understand the principles of treatment of acute arthritis (a) when crystal arthritis is known to be the diagnosis and (b) when the diagnosis is unclear.

4. Appreciate joint aspiration technique using the ankle as an example.

5. Appreciate the indications and strategies for long-term prevention of gout, including avoidance of adverse drug interactions.

6. Be aware of the associations of gout and calcium pyrophosphate dihydrate deposition, with particular emphasis on those conditions that pose a threat to future health and are preventable/treatable.

7. Understand the principles of treatment of calcium crystal associated arthritis.

Introduction

Gout is the commonest inflammatory arthropathy in men over the age of 40 years and is a cause of severe joint pain. Clinicians in all areas of medicine can expect to be confronted with a patient with acute gout who requires prompt effective therapy. Septic arthritis can present in the same manner and needs prompt but very different, therapy. The correct approach to assessment and diagnosis should allow the disorders that cause acute monarthritis to be differentiated promptly so that the correct therapy is used. Gout is often accompanied by a range of other health problems such as obesity, hypertension, hyperlipidaemia (elevated serum lipids) and alcohol excess. Although it may have been gout that led to the patient–doctor interaction, recognition and effective management of these other health problems may bring rewards greater than simply controlling gout.

Effective management for gout is available in the vast majority of cases. Achieving good compliance in the long term is the major practical problem and success in that aspect is based on the patient obtaining sufficient information to understand the need for lifelong therapy.

The calcium crystal associated arthropathies that occur with sufficient frequency to warrant consideration in this text can be divided into calcium pyrophosphate dihydrate (CPPD) and basic calcium phosphate (BCP) associated arthropathies. The presence of CPPD deposition in a person less than 55 years of age should prompt consideration of underlying causes such as haemochromatosis. Calcium crystal associated arthropathies can masquerade as other disorders and thus the correct identification is helpful in avoiding unnecessary treatment.

This chapter will review the principles of investigation of acute monarthritis, joint aspiration technique (using the ankle as an example), risks of hyperuricaemia, production and handling of uric acid in normal and disordered circumstances, and principles of the treatment of gout. Calcium crystal associated disorders will also be briefly reviewed with an emphasis on aspects with direct clinical relevance.

Differential diagnosis of acute monarthritis of the ankle

As discussed in Chapter 1, an acutely painful swollen joint can be explained by bacterial infection, crystal-induced inflammation (gout or pseudogout), trauma, haemarthrosis (bleeding into the joint) and occasionally by disorders such as rheumatoid arthritis, psoriatic arthritis or reactive arthritis. The postoperative period is a time of increased risk for acute crystal-induced arthritis, particularly gout. Invasive procedures also have the potential to cause bacteraemia that could lead to septic arthritis, although the risk of that occurring at the time of a sterile procedure such as arthroscopy is very low. One could consider the possibility of trauma (e.g. while

---

Gout: 1

Case history

Mr Taufaao, a 43-year-old Tongan man, awoke at 0400 h with pain in the left ankle. By 0800 h his ankle was swollen, red and warm. The previous day he had had an arthroscopy of his right knee because of a meniscal tear, suffered while playing touch football 2 months earlier. He had suffered several sprains of both ankles in the past as a result of rugby and he had one previous episode of right knee pain and swelling, also associated with a rugby injury. He had not previously experienced spontaneous joint pain. He worked as a security guard, enjoyed eating and would usually drink about four small bottles of full-strength beer each day.

He had not been aware of any other prior health problem. His elder brother and father had both had joint problems that he thought might have been gout. His father died at the age of 54 years of a heart attack and his mother remained well at the age of 68 years, although she was overweight.

On examination, he was overweight (120 kg, height 182 cm), afebrile and was barely able to walk owing to the combined effect of pain in the left ankle and post-arthroscopy discomfort in his right knee. The arthroscopic wounds were clean and there was no inflammation in that region. His left ankle was swollen, warm, tender and slightly red. His blood pressure was 180/95, there was no sign of liver disease, and urinalysis was normal.

---

anaesthetized) but for trauma to produce a red, swollen, warm joint, the injury needs to be substantial. Thus, the most likely diagnoses are crystal-induced arthritis or sepsis. They both typically produce an abrupt onset of marked joint inflammation.

Joint aspiration to allow examination of the synovial fluid is the best way of establishing the diagnosis. It should be performed promptly using correct aseptic technique and the fluid obtained should be promptly examined and processed for culture. Aspiration will require knowledge of the anatomy of the ankle region.

Essential anatomy

The ankle joints

The ankle region comprises three joints:

1. the true ankle (tibiotalar) joint between the tibia and the talus

2. the subtalar joint between the talus and calcaneus

3. the talonavicular joint between the talus and the navicular (Fig. 7.1A).

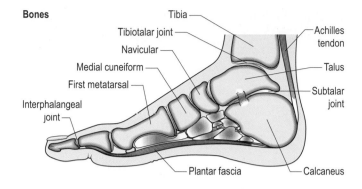

Bones

Tibia

Tibiotalar joint

Navicular

Medial cuneiform

First metatarsal

Interphalangeal joint

Achilles tendon

Talus

Subtalar joint

Plantar fascia

Calcaneus

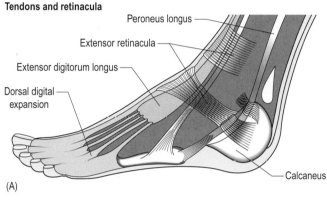

Tendons and retinacula

Peroneus longus

Extensor retinacula

Extensor digitorum longus

Dorsal digital expansion

Calcaneus

(A)

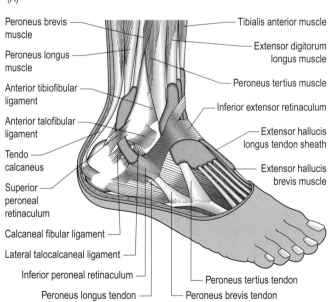

Peroneus brevis muscle

Peroneus longus muscle

Anterior tibiofibular ligament

Anterior talofibular ligament

Tendo calcaneus

Superior peroneal retinaculum

Calcaneal fibular ligament

Lateral talocalcaneal ligament

Inferior peroneal retinaculum

Peroneus longus tendon

Tibialis anterior muscle

Extensor digitorum longus muscle

Peroneus tertius muscle

Inferior extensor retinaculum

Extensor hallucis longus tendon sheath

Extensor hallucis brevis muscle

Peroneus tertius tendon

Peroneus brevis tendon

(C)

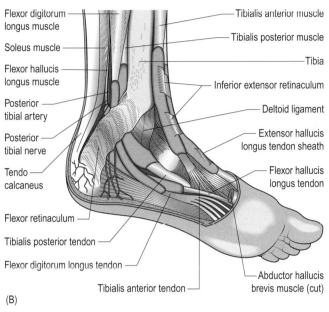

Flexor digitorum longus muscle

Soleus muscle

Flexor hallucis longus muscle

Posterior tibial artery

Posterior tibial nerve

Tendo calcaneus

Flexor retinaculum

Tibialis posterior tendon

Flexor digitorum longus tendon

Tibialis anterior tendon

Tibialis anterior muscle

Tibialis posterior muscle

Tibia

Inferior extensor retinaculum

Deltoid ligament

Extensor hallucis longus tendon sheath

Flexor hallucis longus tendon

Abductor hallucis brevis muscle (cut)

(B)

Fig. 7.1 Basic anatomy of the ankle. The relationships of (A) bones (upper; medial view), and tendons and retinacula (lower; lateral view); (B) tendons, ligaments and blood vessels (medial view); and (C) tendons and ligaments (lateral view).

Involvement of any of these three joints will cause 'ankle' pain. The tibiotalar joint is a true hinge joint whose movement is almost entirely limited to plantar flexion (downwards) and dorsiflexion (upwards). The fibula articulates on the lateral side of the tibia but does not bear weight. The subtalar joint allows the foot to be inverted or everted. The midtarsal joints, including the talonavicular joint, allow forefoot supination and pronation.

Articular capsule, ligaments and tendons

The articular capsule is lax on the anterior aspect but tightly bound on both sides by strong medial and lateral ligaments. All the tendons crossing the ankle joint lie superficial to the articular capsule and are partly enclosed in synovial sheaths (Fig. 7.1B). Disorders of the peroneal tendons (inferoposterior to the lateral malleolus), the tibialis posterior tendon (inferoposterior to the medial malleolus), the tendons that run anterior to the ankle joint (such as tibialis anterior, extensor hallucis longus and extensor digitorum longus) or the Achilles tendon also cause 'ankle' pain. Which structure is responsible for the patient's pain can often be determined by testing specific movements and the patient's ability to resist movement in specific directions. The tibialis posterior muscle helps to maintain the ankle in a position of inversion, and the peroneal muscles help to maintain eversion.

Blood vessels and nerves

The major neurovascular bundles of the foot and ankle are the dorsalis pedis artery and anterior tibial (deep peroneal) nerve, which run longitudinally anterior to the ankle and over the dorsum of foot, and the posterior tibial artery and nerve, which course behind the medial malleolus.

Investigations and diagnosis

Aspiration and synovial fluid analysis

An anterior approach to the ankle is usually used. The joint line should be carefully palpated with the help of passive movement of the joint (if the patient actively moves the ankle, then tendon movement obscures the joint line). The point at which the needle enters the skin is approximately 1 cm proximal to the tip of the medial malleolus. The needle is directed posteriorly.

Joint aspiration is usually performed as a clean (not sterile) procedure. Thus, palpation of the joint line and marking the site with an indentation of the skin needs to be performed prior to cleaning the skin. The solution used to clean the skin (e.g. iodine) should be allowed to dry. Gloves are worn to protect the person performing the aspiration against blood-borne viral infection. Unless the person performing the aspiration is very experienced and can confidently place the needle in the joint space at the first attempt, local anaesthetic should be used to anaesthetize the skin and periarticular structures. The needle route should avoid the major tendons anterior to the ankle and the dorsalis pedis artery. If joint fluid is not obtained on the first attempt, then the needle should be slightly repositioned.

The synovial fluid obtained should be examined promptly; including macroscopic appearance, cell count, Gram stain, culture and microscopic examination for crystals. In Chapter 1 we described the characteristics of synovial fluid in normal and abnormal joints. Here, we will consider only those aspects of synovial fluid analysis that apply to crystal identification. Examination for crystals requires only a tiny amount of synovial fluid (even an apparently 'dry' tap may yield enough) but the examination should be performed immediately. Polarized microscopy allows the identification of urate crystals (strongly negatively birefringent needle-shaped crystals) and CPPD crystals (weakly positively birefringent rod-shaped or

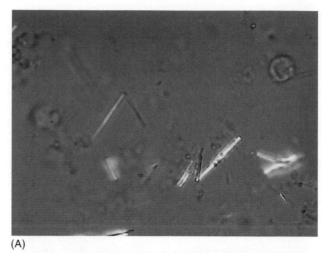

(A)

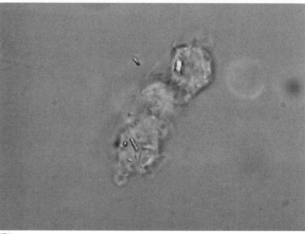

(B)

Fig. 7.2 Crystals in synovial fluid: (A) monosodium urate monohydrate; (B) calcium pyrophosphate dihydrate.

rhomboidal crystals) as shown in Fig. 7.2. The technique is not difficult but the experience of the observer and the adequacy of the microscope (e.g. rotating stage) can make a major difference to accuracy. CPPD crystals are often missed, and thus a repeat examination of a fresh specimen may be appropriate if the diagnosis appears likely, but no crystals are seen initially.

Other investigations

Other investigations can provide useful supplementary information but cannot replace synovial fluid examination. X-rays can detect or help to exclude pre-existing joint or bone disorders, chondrocalcinosis (CPPD deposition in cartilage) and bone trauma. It is sensible to assess laboratory parameters of inflammation, such as white cell count and ESR, for comparison with future results but they assist little in the differentiation of septic from gouty arthritis. The serum uric acid level is of little help in the setting of possible acute gout. A normal level does not exclude gout and an elevated level does not confirm

<table>
<tr><td>Case 7.1</td><td>Gout: 2</td></tr>
</table>

Investigations

Mr Taufaao's synovial fluid was opaque, creamy-yellow in colour and had reduced viscosity. The cell count was 23×10^9/L, almost all neutrophils. Numerous urate crystals, both extracellular and within neutrophils, were identified using a polarizing microscope. Gram staining and subsequent culture were negative. The diagnosis of acute gout was thus established with certainty. Although, as far as Mr Taufaao was aware, his gout started abruptly, the factors that led to the episode of acute joint inflammation had been operating for years.

gout. However, the uric acid level is very important in the long-term management of gout.

Pathophysiology of gouty arthritis

Acute gout is caused by the interaction between the inflammatory system (particularly neutrophils) and crystals of monosodium urate monohydrate (urate). Urate crystals form in and around joints and have a predilection for the cooler areas of peripheral joints (because of the decreased solubility of urate at lower temperatures). Although the inflammatory episode comes on abruptly, the formation of urate crystals probably occurs slowly over weeks to months (there remains some doubt as to the maximum speed of urate crystal formation *in vivo*). Urate crystals can only form in a supersaturated solution of sodium urate, which approximately equates to a uric acid concentration above 0.42 mmol/L (7.0 mg/dL). Thus the attack of acute gout is the culmination of a sequence of events:

1. chronic hyperuricaemia

2. urate crystal formation

3. interaction between the inflammatory system and the urate crystals (Fig. 7.3).

We will explore these three stages further.

Uric acid metabolism and hyperuricaemia

Persistent hyperuricaemia is necessary for urate crystal formation. Hyperuricaemia, however, is not sufficient in itself to cause urate crystal formation, as reflected by the finding that only about 20% of subjects with uric acid levels in excess of saturation (0.42 mmol/L) ever develop gout. Nevertheless, there is a strong correlation between the degree of hyperuricaemia and the risk of developing gout, and hyperuricaemia is the only proven independent risk factor for the development of gout. For subjects

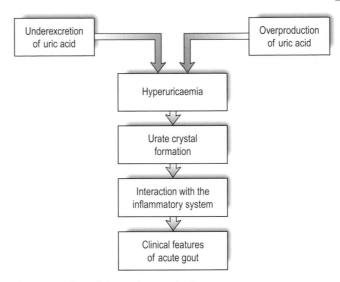

Fig. 7.3 Outline of the pathogenesis of gout.

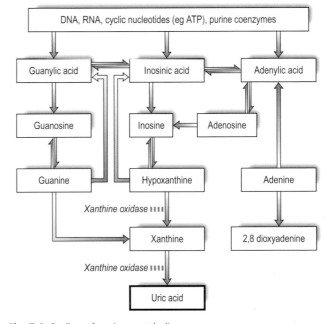

Fig. 7.4 Outline of purine metabolism.

previously free of gout with a uric acid level of 0.42–0.47 mmol/L, 2% will have experienced an attack of gout after 5 years, compared with 30% of those with a uric acid level of >0.60 mmol/L.

Uric acid is a final breakdown product of purine nucleotide turnover (Fig. 7.4). Of uric acid in the body, approximately two-thirds comes from endogenous sources and approximately one-third from food purines, but there is marked variability between individuals (Fig. 7.5). Excretion of uric acid from the body normally occurs mainly via the kidney (accounting for about two-thirds) with the remainder being excreted by the bowel. Uric acid is almost completely filtered at the glomerulus, and then 99% is reabsorbed in the proximal tubule.

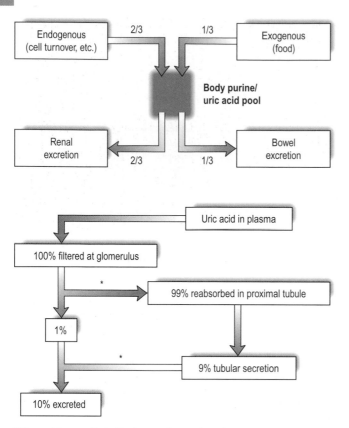

* These steps are affected by drugs such as cyclosporin, diuretics, probenecid, sulfinpyrazone and aspirin.

Fig. 7.5 Overview of uric acid handling.

of nucleic acids, such as myeloproliferative and lympho-proliferative disorders, multiple myeloma, secondary polycythaemia and chronic haemolytic anaemias (e.g. haemoglobinopathies or thalassaemia). Rare enzyme abnormalities (hypoxanthine guanine phosphoribosyl transferase (HGPRT) deficiency, phosphoribosyl pyro-phosphate (PRPP) synthetase overactivity, glucose-6-phosphatase deficiency or fructose-1-phosphate aldolase deficiency) can result in marked uric acid overproduction and familial premature gout.

More than 90% of gouty subjects have impaired renal urate clearance, usually in the absence of any other evidence of renal dysfunction.

Urate crystal formation

Although hyperuricaemia is necessary for urate crystal formation to occur, and the likelihood of urate crystal formation increases with increasing uric acid levels, in the majority of hyperuricaemic subjects, urate crystal formation and gout never occur. When urate crystal formation does occur, it preferentially involves peripheral joints, particularly in the lower limbs, subcutaneous tissue, skin, bone and tendon. Various biological substances have been shown to influence the nucleation and growth of urate crystals (e.g. the immunoglobulin IgG) and it is likely that the balance of biological inhibitors and promoters of crystal formation plays a substantial role in determining whether urate crystal formation occurs and where it occurs. The process of urate crystal formation is slow (weeks to months) and does not produce symptoms.

Crystal-induced inflammation

Most of the time, the body's inflammatory system largely, although not completely, ignores the urate crystals, but eventually the crystals incite an inflammatory response that results in acute gout. Acute attacks of gout can be precipitated by any cause of a rapid fall in the serum uric acid level, acute illness, trauma, surgery, alcohol and food binges. The mechanism by which these insults precipitate acute gout has not been clarified but alteration of the protein coating of the urate crystals is a plausible explanation. Subsequently, usually after many years, chronic inflammatory responses to the crystals and the physical presence of lumps of crystals (tophi) can lead to joint and bone damage. In male-pattern gout, tophi do not usually develop until many years after the initial attack. In postmenopausal women, however, tophi, particularly in osteoarthritic distal interphalangeal joints, occur early and may be seen at initial presentation. Multiple components of the inflammatory system are involved in the production of acute gouty inflammation (Fig. 7.6). *In vivo*, urate crystals are coated by proteins that markedly influence their ability to induce an inflammatory response. Most crystal surface proteins (especially apolipoprotein B) inhibit the production of inflammation. In contrast,

It then undergoes tubular secretion back into the urine such that about 10% of the filtered uric acid is excreted. The extensive handling of uric acid by the renal tubule accounts for the alterations in blood uric acid level that result from drugs and diseases which interfere with tubular function. Low-dose aspirin, diuretics (thiazide and loop), cyclosporine, pyrazinamide, ethambutol, niacin and nicotinic acid influence tubular transport to cause a fall in uric acid clearance, whereas probenecid, sulfin-pyrazone, benzbromarone, losartan and fenofibrate all influence tubular transport such that uric acid clearance is increased. Certain racial groups (e.g. Polynesians) have reduced renal clearance of uric acid despite otherwise normal renal function. Oestrogen increases renal uric acid clearance, whereas alcohol, fructose (soft drinks) and obesity decrease it.

Renal insufficiency due to all causes results in reduced uric acid clearance and hence an increased prevalence of hyperuricaemia and gout. Those renal diseases with predominant tubular involvement result in hyperuricaemia disproportionate to the reduction in glomerular filtration rate (e.g. lead poisoning, medullary cystic disease, poly-cystic disease, cystinuria and analgesic nephropathy).

Less than 10% of gouty subjects demonstrate uric acid overproduction (measured by 24-h urine collection). In this group, one can find diseases with increased turnover

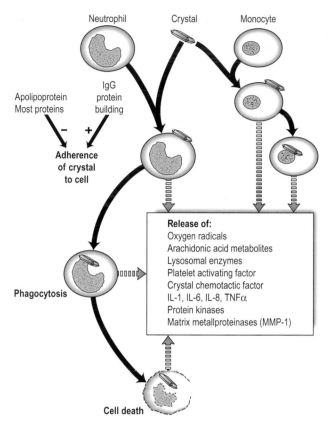

Fig. 7.6 Urate crystal-induced inflammation.

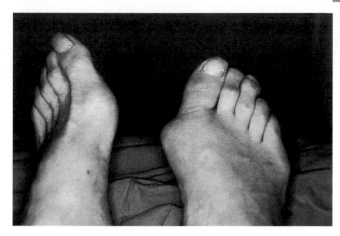

Fig. 7.7 Acute gouty arthritis, here involving the most frequently affected joint—the first metatarsophalangeal joint.

IgG on the crystal surface promotes interaction with the inflammatory system. Urate crystal-induced phosphorylation and activation of the tyrosine kinase Tec leading to release of IL-1 from monocytes, and hence to migration of neutrophil leukocytes into the joint, are important steps in urate crystal-induced inflammation. During the inflammatory response, many mediators are released (chemotactic factors, lysosomal enzymes, eicosanoids (e.g. prostaglandins), interleukin-1 (IL-1), tumour necrosis factor (TNF), IL-6, IL-8, reactive oxygen species and collagenase) and adhesion molecule expression (E selectin) on synovial endothelial cells is increased. Attacks of gout resolve even without treatment, and resolution appears to be mainly due to the switching off of the inflammatory reaction rather than removal of the urate crystals.

Treatment of acute gout

Acute gout is extremely painful (Fig. 7.7) and demands prompt effective therapy. Minimizing the delay between the onset of the acute attack and the commencement of therapy is more important than which form of therapy is used. For patients who are otherwise well, oral non-steroidal anti-inflammatory (NSAID) medication is usually used. Which NSAID is chosen is not so important

and the usual full dose (not higher) should be used. Intra-articular corticosteroid is also very effective and is a particularly good choice in patients with a contraindication to NSAID therapy (such as a history of peptic ulceration, heart failure, renal insufficiency, unstable haemodynamic situation such as following major surgery, anticoagulant therapy, or in situations where interference with platelet function could cause problems, such as in the early postoperative period).

Systemic corticosteroid therapy (synthetic ACTH intramuscularly, triamcinolone intramuscularly, or prednisone orally 20–50 mg daily rapidly reducing to zero over 7–10 days) is also effective and acceptably safe. Traditional high-dose colchicine therapy (1 mg initially then 0.5 mg every 2 h until relief) is poorly tolerated, unpleasant and rarely appropriate, although it is effective, particularly if commenced quickly after the onset of an attack. Low-dose colchicine (0.5 mg twice daily, if renal function is normal) is a useful adjunct to other therapies in acute gout and is effective at preventing recurrence after one-off treatments, such as synthetic ACTH, intramuscular triamcinolone or intra-articular corticosteroid.

If the diagnosis of gout appears likely but synovial fluid cannot be aspirated and thus the diagnosis remains in doubt, the above therapies remain appropriate. It is essential not to use oral antibiotic therapy in this situation because, if the correct diagnosis is septic arthritis, oral antibiotics may suppress the disease and further delay diagnosis. Oral antibiotic therapy is not sufficient treatment for septic arthritis, as discussed in Chapter 11. If what is thought to be acute gout does not respond promptly to the above therapies, then the diagnosis should be reconsidered and further efforts made to obtain synovial fluid from the joint.

Hyperuricaemia can be associated with obesity, hypertension, hyperlipidaemia, insulin resistance, coronary heart disease, excess alcohol ingestion, medication use, renal disease and renal calculi. Many of these conditions warrant intervention in their own right. The risk of gout occurring increases with increasing uric acid levels but is never so high as to warrant drug treatment on that basis prior to an attack of gout. Studies of the effect of hyperuricaemia (in the absence of gout or renal calculi) on renal function and coronary artery disease are limited but have indicated that any effect is small. Hence, asymptomatic hyperuricaemia should not be treated with drug therapy except when there is a possibility of tumour lysis syndrome leading to acute uric acid nephropathy or in the rare patient with a familial cause of uric acid overproduction or familial juvenile hyperuricaemic nephropathy.

Interesting facts

Restriction of dietary purines, within the range that is feasible for a palatable long-term diet, makes relatively little difference to the serum uric acid concentration. Dietary efforts to reduce uric acid should focus on weight reduction and avoidance of excessive alcohol and/or fructose (soft drinks).

Case 7.1 | Gout: 3

Management in relation to risk factors

Although Mr Taufaao was most concerned about his painful ankle, his general practitioner noted that he was Polynesian, overweight, hypertensive, consumed excess alcohol and had a family history of premature vascular disease. This was no coincidence. Hypertension, obesity, insulin resistance, hyperlipidaemia (particularly hypertriglyceridaemia), alcohol excess and Polynesian/Maori race are all associated with hyperuricaemia and gout. Hypothyroidism, renal calculi (uric acid and calcium oxalate) and renal impairment are also associated with gout. Recognition of these other problems in a patient presenting with acute gout can allow intervention to avoid serious consequences in the future. Correction of obesity and alcohol excess will also help management of the gout.

Primarily to reduce his risk of coronary artery disease, Mr Taufaao should modify his diet and lifestyle and reduce his alcohol intake. Obesity and alcohol intake are the most important dietary influences on the uric acid level, although regular consumption of high-purine foods (offal, sardines and similar, meat and yeast extracts), excess fructose (soft drinks) or urinary output less than 1500 mL/day will also have an adverse effect. Unfortunately, in many people, dietary and lifestyle modification is either insufficient to normalize the uric acid level or is not maintained long term. The importance of dietary modification with respect to control of gout (as opposed to beneficial effects on cardiac and other problems) depends on the degree of hyperuricaemia and the magnitude of correctable factors. The reduction in uric acid level that could be achieved by Mr Taufaao is likely to be considerable and of clear clinical importance. On the other hand, a slim non-drinker who has a normal diet and a uric acid level of 0.53 mmol/L has almost no chance of achieving a healthy uric acid level through dietary modification.

Treatment of chronic gout

The indications for hypouricaemic drug therapy for gout are:

- features or complications of chronic gout such as tophi, erosions on X-ray, renal calculi, or failure of symptoms to resolve completely between attacks
- the presence of disorders that make the treatment of acute gout hazardous, such as contraindications to NSAIDs
- renal insufficiency (because of the increased difficulty achieving normouricaemia and overall control of gout if the total body load of urate crystals is high)
- recurrent attacks that have been sufficiently frequent and inconvenient for the patient to prefer to use lifelong daily prophylactic therapy rather than treat the acute attacks as they occur.

The diagnosis of gout should have been established with 'certainty', preferably via the detection of urate crystals in synovial fluid. In many patients with probable gout, the diagnosis has not been confirmed. Although it is appropriate to treat probable acute gout without confirmation of the diagnosis, committing a patient to lifelong prophylactic therapy without a high degree of certainty of the diagnosis is inappropriate. Prophylactic therapy for gout is never urgent and, in the long run, it is better to defer it until the diagnosis has been established with, at least, near certainty. The most common reason for failure of long-term gout therapy is poor compliance. It is essential that the patient plays an active role in the decision to use hypouricaemic therapy and that the patient fully understands the need to continue that therapy lifelong (with rare exceptions). Unless the uric acid level is markedly elevated, it is not usually appropriate to commence long-term hypouricaemic drug therapy after only a single attack of gout.

Interesting facts

Drug therapy options for lowering the serum uric acid level have changed in recent years. The uricosuric agents, sulfinpyrazone and benzbromarone are no longer available in many countries. Febuxostat, a non-purine xanthine oxidase inhibitor, suitable for many patients including those with allopurinol allergy, has become available. Allopurinol remains the most commonly used hypouricaemic drug and the uricosuric agents probenecid, losartan and fenofibrate all continue to provide benefit in selected circumstances.

Hypouricaemic therapy

In most gouty patients, adequate control of the uric acid level can be achieved either with the use of allopurinol, which inhibits xanthine oxidase and hence reduces uric acid production, or with the use of probenecid,

Case 7.1	Gout: 4

Management of chronic gout

Mr Taufaao, in conjunction with his physician, elected not to use long-term prophylactic drug therapy, but he did reduce his alcohol consumption and he managed to lose a small amount of weight. His uric acid level fell from an average of about 0.50 mmol/L to about 0.45 mmol/L. Over the subsequent 2 years, he suffered four further attacks of gout with the last two attacks in close succession. He also noted that his most recent two attacks, although less severe at their peak, were slower to resolve and they caused him to lose days from work. After further consultation, Mr Taufaao elected to commence drug therapy with the understanding that he would need to continue the treatment lifelong.

which increases uric acid clearance through the kidney. Allopurinol is most commonly chosen because of ease of use, fewer tablets in the long term, and suitability for both under-excreters and over-producers. Febuxostat, a non-purine xanthine oxidase inhibitor, is also very effective, although its availability throughout the world is currently limited. Hypouricaemic therapy is best introduced at a low dose so that a gentle fall in the serum uric acid is achieved. The dose is then increased to achieve a uric acid level preferably below 0.36 mmol/L and ideally below 0.30 mmol/L. The starting and maximal doses of hypouricaemic therapy are: allopurinol 100 mg daily, increasing up to 600 mg daily (the maximal dose needs to be reduced in the presence of impaired renal function); probenecid 500 mg daily, increasing up to 2 g daily; febuxostat 80 mg daily, increasing up to 240 mg daily.

Uricosuric therapy is ineffective in patients with significantly impaired renal function and requires a large urine volume and urine alkalinization to reduce the risk of urinary uric acid calculi, particularly in the first few weeks. Aspirin antagonizes the effect of probenecid and, if the two drugs must be used in the same patient, the interval between consumption of the two medications should be at least 6 h.

Any rapid reduction in the serum uric acid level increases the risk of acute gout, and the introduction of hypouricaemic drug therapy is the commonest example. Patients are unlikely to be impressed by their doctor if they suffer their worst ever attack of gout soon after commencing medication which has been promised to rid them of gout in the long term. Low-dose colchicine (0.5 mg b.d., if adequate renal function) is an effective means of preventing acute gout during the introduction of hypouricaemic therapy.

The risk of an acute attack should be discussed in advance and the patient should know what action to take should an acute attack occur. Unless there is a contra-indication, the advice is usually to continue the hypouricaemic drug and low-dose colchicine, and to introduce an NSAID promptly. If a patient suffers a severe attack of gout soon after commencing hypouricaemic drug therapy, it may be necessary to cease the hypouricaemic drug to gain control of the acute attack but, in general, hypouricaemic therapy should not be altered during an acute attack. The duration of colchicine cover is usually between 6 weeks and 6 months, depending on the total urate load. Non-tophaceous patients who have had less than 10 attacks may require only 6 weeks of colchicine, whereas patients with multiple tophi often benefit from remaining on low-dose colchicine for at least 6 months. If a patient suffers an attack of gout soon after ceasing colchicine, it should usually be recommenced and continued for a further 3 months.

Provided an ideal uric acid level (<0.30 mmol/L) has been achieved, there is no reason to alter the hypouricaemic drug therapy just because the patient continues to suffer attacks of gout during the first few months of therapy. The urate crystals that have formed slowly in the body over months and years can continue to cause attacks of gout until they have dissolved, even if the uric acid level has been brought down into the ideal range.

Patients who have a need for non-steroidal anti-inflammatory medication for reasons other than to cover the introduction of hypouricaemic therapy can usually continue their anti-inflammatory in place of colchicine.

Interesting facts

Uric acid excretion is primarily dependent on renal tubular function. Drugs and diseases that affect tubular function have a greater effect on uric acid levels than those which mainly affect glomerular function.

Patients with renal impairment

The presence of renal failure markedly reduces uric acid clearance, and uricosuric therapy is not effective. The active metabolite of allopurinol, oxypurinol, is excreted by the kidney, and the dose of allopurinol thus needs to be reduced. The allopurinol hypersensitivity syndrome (skin rash, hepatitis, interstitial nephritis, substantial mortality) occurs with increased frequency in patients with renal impairment, particularly in association with advanced age and diuretic treatment. It may be impossible to achieve an ideal uric acid level in the face of renal failure. Although chronic colchicine toxicity is more likely to occur in patients with renal failure than in other situations, low-dose colchicine (0.5 mg daily) is often helpful in minimizing the severity of acute gouty episodes, even although the drug does not reduce uric acid levels nor retard chronic gouty joint and bone damage.

Organ transplant recipients frequently receive cyclosporine (which inhibits renal uric acid clearance) or azathioprine (which can be lethal in combination with allopurinol because allopurinol inhibits the metabolism of the active metabolite of azathioprine, 6-mercaptopurine).

Case 7.2 Chondrocalcinosis: 1

Case history

Mr Steele, a 41-year-old carpenter, sought medical advice because of a gradual onset of discomfort and brief morning stiffness in both hands. On specific questioning, he also admitted to right groin pain at the end of the day's work over the last 6 months. He had noted fatigue for several months but had attributed that symptom to his work.

He had no significant past history and he was not aware of any illness in his family. He did not smoke and he drank only a small amount of alcohol.

On examination he had hard enlargement of the index and middle metacarpophalangeal (MCP) joints of both hands. There was thickening of the skin of both palms in keeping with regular physical work as a carpenter. There was no definite evidence of arthritis of the other small joints of the hands and his other upper limb joints were clinically normal. There was mild restriction of internal rotation of the right hip, but otherwise his lower limb joints were normal.

X-rays demonstrated osteoarthritic change in the index and middle MCP joints of both hands and in the right hip. Chondrocalcinosis was present in the triangular fibrocartilage of both wrists, both hips, the pubic symphysis and the menisci of both knees.

Case 7.2 Chondrocalcinosis: 2

Investigations and management

The distribution of joint involvement suffered by Mr Steele (index and middle MCP joints, hip joint) is characteristic of the arthropathy of haemochromatosis and that diagnosis was confirmed, initially by the finding of elevated transferrin saturation and elevated ferritin, and subsequently by genetic testing. He was found to have abnormal liver function tests and mild hepatic fibrosis on liver biopsy, and he was referred for endocrinological assessment, which fortunately excluded diabetes, testicular failure and pituitary disease, all of which can occur as a consequence of excessive iron deposition in haemochromatosis. He commenced regular venesection and his liver function tests returned to normal. His arthritis, however, continued to deteriorate and he subsequently required a right hip replacement. The arthropathy of haemochromatosis, once it is established, does not respond to venesection.

Allopurinol allergy is potentially life threatening. Although allopurinol desensitization is sometimes appropriate, if the uric acid level can be controlled using some other medication, then that option should be used. Gout therapy can produce several important drug interactions. Azathioprine and allopurinol in combination are potentially lethal. In those rare circumstances when the two drugs need to be used concurrently, the dose of azathioprine needs to be reduced markedly. Probenecid interferes with the excretion of methotrexate and can result in increased toxicity. Concurrent aspirin therapy inhibits the uricosuric effect of probenecid. Allopurinol and ampicillin in combination lead to skin rash in about 20% of cases.

Chondrocalcinosis

Chondrocalcinosis (literally calcification of the cartilage) is a term used to describe the radiological appearance of calcium pyrophosphate dihydrate crystal deposition within either fibrocartilage (e.g. menisci) or hyaline cartilage. Chondrocalcinosis becomes increasingly frequent with advancing age such that it can be found in 20% of the population aged in excess of 60 years. At less than 50 years of age, however, it is uncommon and, in this group, the possibility of an underlying cause should be considered. Haemochromatosis, hypomagnesaemia, hypophosphatasia and hypercalcaemia (usually due to primary hyperparathyroidism) are all associated with chondrocalcinosis.

Diagnosis

CPPD deposition can present as a chronic arthropathy, as occurred in Mr Steele's case. It can also result in acute crystal-induced inflammation, 'pseudogout'. This usually involves the knee or the wrist and the patient is usually elderly. Although the diagnosis can be suspected by the finding of chondrocalcinosis on X-ray of the involved joint, the definitive diagnostic investigation is synovial fluid examination to confirm the presence of CPPD crystals (weakly positively birefringent rod-shaped or rhomboidal crystals) and to exclude infection. Rarely, CPPD deposition can produce a pseudorheumatoid appearance. If the clinical features suggest the presence of both osteoarthritis and rheumatoid arthritis, the possibility that all of the manifestations are due to CPPD-associated arthropathy should be considered. CPPD deposition can also be associated with rapidly destructive arthritis resembling neuropathic arthropathy.

Basic calcium phosphates (mainly hydroxyapatite) are found in association with tendon and bursal inflammation (e.g. supraspinatus tendonitis) and the crystals are commonly found in fluid removed from osteoarthritic joints. The role the crystals play in osteoarthritis remains unclear and, at this stage, the finding of BCP crystals in an osteoarthritic joint does not alter clinical management.

Treatment of calcium crystal associated arthritis

Acute joint inflammation in association with CPPD crystals or acute tendon or periarticular inflammation in association with BCP crystals should be treated in a similar manner to acute gout. Prompt institution of treatment with an oral NSAID or intra-articular/intrabursal corticosteroid is most commonly used. The management of chronic arthropathy associated with calcium crystal deposition is the same as the management of chronic osteoarthritis. There is no safe and effective means of dissolving or removing calcium crystals from joints or periarticular sites. Magnesium supplementation has been shown to be of benefit in retarding the progression of CPPD deposition in some patients with hypomagnesaemia.

Further reading

Hochberg, M.C., Silman, A.J., Smolen, J.S., et al. (Eds.), 2008. Rheumatology, fourth ed. Mosby, St Louis.

Moore, K.L., Dalley, A.F., 2006. Clinically Oriented Anatomy, fifth ed. Williams & Wilkins, Baltimore.

DISORDERS OF SKELETAL MUSCLE

8

Rodger Laurent

Chapter objectives

After studying this chapter you should be able to:

1. Understand the structure and function of skeletal muscle.

2. Describe the pathological changes that occur in inflammatory myopathies.

3. Appreciate what investigations are appropriate in a patient with primary muscle disease.

4. Understand the common endocrine and metabolic muscle disorders.

5. Describe the use of various drugs in the treatment of muscle disorders.

6. Understand the basic clinical features of the common inherited muscle disorders.

7. Appreciate the clinical features of fibromyalgia.

Introduction

Skeletal muscle is one of the major tissue components of the human body. Its main function is to convert chemical energy into mechanical work. It is usually under the voluntary control of the central nervous system.

Skeletal muscle also has other functions; it contains about 80% of the body's content of water and is a reservoir for intracellular ions such as potassium. It also functions as a source of energy-rich compounds and is an important producer of body heat.

A myopathy is a primary disorder of the muscle. The acquired myopathies include polymyositis, and endocrine and drug-induced myopathies. The inherited myopathies are rare but need to be considered in someone presenting with weakness because they often have a poor prognosis.

This chapter will discuss the primary muscle disorders. It will not discuss muscle disorders secondary to nerve or motor endplate disorders.

Anatomy of skeletal muscle

The muscle fibre

Muscles are made up of a collection of individual muscle fibres (Figs 8.1, 8.2). Each fibre is a multinucleated cell, which can be up to 10 cm in length with a diameter ranging from 10–100 μm. Normal muscles have the nuclei arranged around the periphery of the cells.

The muscle cell membrane is called the sarcolemma and the cytoplasm, the sarcoplasm. The sarcolemma has the property of excitability and can conduct the electrical impulses that occur during depolarization. A system of tubules, the transverse tubules or T-tubules, begins at the sarcolemma and extends into the sarcoplasm. They allow rapid distribution of the signal to contract throughout the muscle fibre.

The muscle fibre contains numerous myofibrils, which are 1–2 μm in diameter and the length of the cell (Fig. 8.1A). Myofibrils shorten and are the structures responsible for muscle contraction. They shorten the fibre because they are attached to the sarcolemma at each of its ends. Mitochondria and glycogen granules are situated between the myofibrils.

The myofibrils consist of bundles of filaments, which are made up of the proteins actin and myosin, and are organized in repeating functional units called sarcomeres. Sarcomeres are the smallest functional units of the muscle fibre (Fig. 8.1C). The actin filaments are thin and the myosin filaments are thick. The thick filaments lie at the centre of the sarcomere with the thin filaments at either end. On either side of the centre, there is an area of overlap between the thin and thick filaments in which each myosin filament is surrounded by a hexagonal array of actin filaments. The arrangement of the myosin and actin filaments gives a banded appearance to the muscle and is the reason it is called striated muscle. The sarcomeres are separated by a dense area called the Z line. The M line is at the middle of the sarcomere and consists of proteins that bind the thick myosin filaments. The actin and myosin filaments are joined by molecular cross-bridges and, during contraction, these cross-bridges repeatedly disengage and engage at successive sites, with the result that the actin and myosin filaments slide upon one another and the myofibrils shorten.

The myofibril is surrounded by a sheath of membranes called the sarcoplasmic reticulum. At the zone of overlap between the thick and thin filaments, the tubules of the sarcoplasmic reticulum enlarge and form chambers called terminal cisternae. A transverse tubule is situated between two terminal cisternae and the resulting complex is called a triad. The cisternae contain large stores of calcium ions. Release of calcium from these structures initiates the muscle contraction.

The size of the muscle varies in proportion to the size of the fibres with larger fibres being present in larger muscles. Consistent physical exercise can increase the muscle fibre diameter in both sexes.

Skeletal muscle structure

Each fibre is surrounded by a thin layer of collagen, called the endomysium. The fibres are then joined together in bundles to form fascicles, which are surrounded by a further layer of connective tissue called the perimysium (Fig. 8.1A). Groups of fascicles form the whole muscle, which is surrounded by a strong layer of collagen, called the epimysium. The epimysium merges with the peritenon of the tendon and the periosteum.

The arrangement of the fascicles is variable and depends on the task of that specific muscle. Factors such as the amount and direction of the force required or the amount of muscle shortening determine the muscle

---

Case 8.1 Myopathy: 1

Case history

Mr Colin Brown is a 47-year-old man who presents to his general practitioner complaining of weakness in both legs when getting out of a chair. He first noticed muscle weakness about 6 months earlier, when he had difficulty walking up and down the stairs at work. He also noticed that his arm and leg muscles were often painful after exercise and occasionally his thigh muscles would be tender. Over the last 2 months, he has noticed increased tiredness.

The history raises the possibility of a disorder of skeletal muscle. It would be important to consider what other clinical information is required and what should be specifically looked for on physical examination.

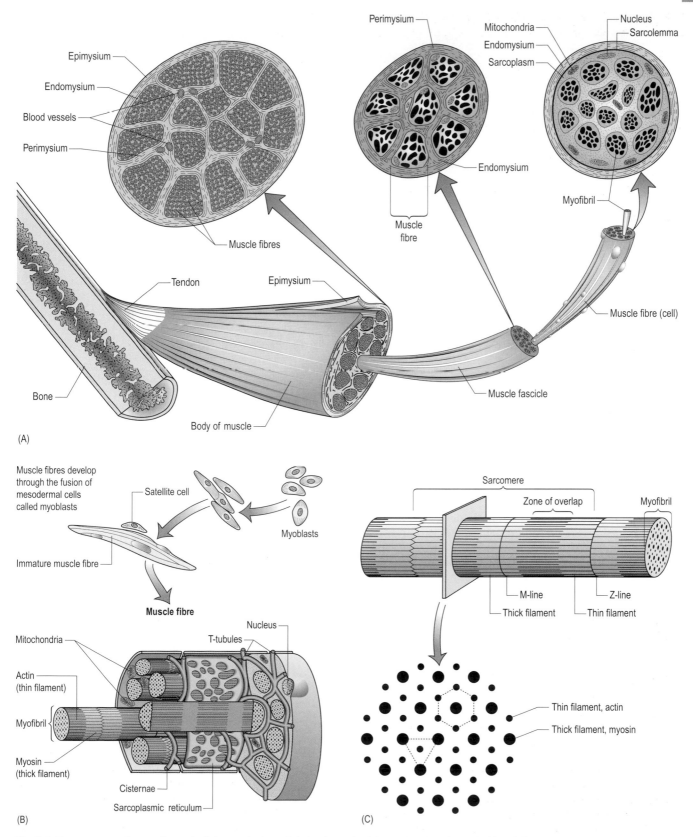

Fig. 8.1 The structure of normal muscle: (A) organization of skeletal muscle; (B) organization of muscle fibre; (C) sarcomere structure. Skeletal muscle consists of fascicles enclosed by the epimysium. Bundles are separated by the connective tissue fibres of the perimysium and, within each bundle, the muscle fibres are surrounded by the endomysium. Each myofibril consists of a linear series of sarcomeres.

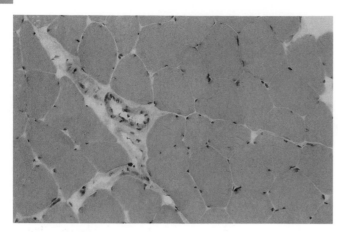

Fig. 8.2 Histological appearance of normal muscle.

Table 8.1 Characteristics of the major muscle fibre types

	Fibre type		
	1	2A	2B
Speed of conduction	Slow	Fast	Fast
Resistance to fatigue	High	Intermediate	Low
Type of metabolism	Oxidative	Oxidative/ glycolytic	Glycolytic
Mitochondria	Many	Intermediate	Few

architecture. Two examples are an arrangement of the fascicles parallel to the long axis of the muscle, as in the gastrocnemius (calf) muscle, or a convergent arrangement where the origin covers a wide area and the fascicles converge to a common attachment site, as in the pectoralis major muscle. The pectoralis major muscle has its origin covering a wide number of ribs, converging to a tendon that attaches to the upper humerus.

Types of muscle fibres

Muscle fibres (Table 8.1) are divided on the basis of their morphology and physicochemical characteristics into two major groups: type 1 and type 2 fibres. Each type has different functions. The type 1 muscle fibres, slow oxidative, have a slow speed of contraction and a high resistance to fatigue. Their metabolism is oxidative and they have an increased concentration of myoglobin, which has an increased capacity to transport oxygen. They also have numerous mitochondria. Type 1 fibres generally have a greater capillary blood supply than type 2 fibres.

The type 2 muscle fibres have anaerobic metabolism and use glycogen as their source of energy. They have higher levels of the enzymes that are associated with anaerobic metabolism. These fibres contract at a much faster rate and have a low resistance to fatigue. They also have fewer mitochondria than type 1 fibres. Type 2 fibres can be subdivided into types 2A, fast oxidative-glycolytic, and 2B, fast glycolytic. Type 2A fibres have a mixture of oxidative and glycolytic metabolism. They have a slightly slower contraction rate than type 2B fibres, but are more resistant to fatigue.

Fibre types are determined by innervation, with all muscle fibres supplied by a single neuron being of the same histological type. The cranial muscles, for example the masseter muscle, are an exception to this rule. The percentages of the different fibre types within a muscle can be affected by exercise or inactivity. Therefore, there is considerable variation between individuals.

The distribution of these muscle fibres is related to their function. The type 1 fibres lie in deeper planes nearer to the trunk or limb axes. They usually span a single joint and their actions are predominantly to maintain posture. Type 2B are more common in the lower limbs and type 1 in the upper limbs.

Neuromuscular junction

The neuromuscular junction is the structure that transmits the nerve impulse to the muscle to initiate muscle contraction. As the axon approaches the muscle it divides into a fine network of terminal branches. Each muscle fibre has a single neuromuscular junction where the axon of the neuron joins the fibre. The terminal end of the axon is adjacent to the motor endplate, a region of the sarcolemma or muscle cell membrane. The nerve and motor end plate are not in direct contact but are separated by a space, the synaptic cleft. Activation of the muscle is then by chemical transmission. The axon contains the transmitter acetylcholine, which, when released, binds to receptors on the motor endplate.

This depolarizes the sarcolemma and the action potential spreads across the sarcolemma and down the transverse tubules into the interior of the cell to the triads. The action potential stimulates the release of calcium and subsequent muscle contraction. The effect of the acetylcholine is short-lived because the area is rich in the enzyme acetylcholinesterase, which rapidly destroys the acetylcholine. Certain drugs act at the neuromuscular junction to affect these processes, e.g. curare competes with acetylcholine for endplate receptors and suxamethonium produces a depolarization block.

Muscle and tendon receptors

The position of the joints and the amount of contraction required by a muscle are obtained by sensors called receptors. They provide information that determines how we move and are important for neuromuscular coordination. The main receptors that affect muscles are the muscle spindles and Golgi tendon organs. Receptors in the ligaments and joint capsule are important for joint position sense.

A muscle spindle is a spindle-shaped stretch receptor found in most muscles but especially concentrated in muscles that exert fine motor control, such as the small muscles of the hand. The muscle spindle is about $100\,\mu m$ in diameter and up to $10\,mm$ in length. Muscle spindles receive a sensory innervation from groups Ia and II afferent nerve fibres and a motor supply from dynamic γ and static δ motor axons (see Ch. 3 for revision of nerve fibre types).

Another type of stretch receptor is the Golgi tendon organ formed by the terminals of a group Ib afferent nerve fibre. Golgi tendon organs are arranged in series within the tendon adjacent to the musculo-tendinous junction. They can be activated by either stretch or muscle contraction. Golgi tendon organs signal the force that develops in the tendon on muscle contraction, whereas muscle spindles provide feedback about the amount and rate of muscle stretch.

Interesting facts

The position of the joints and the amount of contraction required by a muscle are obtained by sensors called proprioceptors. They provide information that determines how we move. The main proprioceptors that affect muscles are the muscle spindles and Golgi tendon organs. Proprioceptors in the ligaments and joint capsule are important for joint position sense.

Muscle metabolism

Muscle requires a large amount of energy to function adequately. Muscle contains large energy reserves, these being adenosine triphosphate (ATP) and other high-energy compounds, especially creatine phosphate and glycogen.

Resting muscle generates ATP, which is stored among the myofilaments. The cell produces more ATP than can be stored, and excess is stored as creatine phosphate. ATP and creatine are converted to adenosine diphosphate and creatine phosphate, which is stored in the muscle. When energy is required, the reverse occurs, releasing ATP and creatine. This reaction is facilitated by the enzyme creatine kinase. At rest, the muscle contains six times as much creatine phosphate as ATP. When the ATP and creatine phosphate supplies are exhausted, glycogen becomes the energy source. Glycogen is broken down into glucose, which is metabolized to ATP. This can be done by aerobic or anaerobic respiration, depending on the supply of oxygen. Mitochondria produce ATP from glucose by aerobic respiration.

At low levels of muscle activity, aerobic respiration is sufficient to provide energy for the muscle. At maximum muscle activity, mitochondria produce about one-third of the required ATP, and the rest is produced by anaerobic glycolysis. Anaerobic glycolysis as a method of energy production has some disadvantages. It is relatively inefficient, requiring 18 molecules of glucose to provide the same amount of energy as from one glucose molecule by aerobic metabolism.

Muscle contraction

Muscle contraction is due to the actin and myosin filaments sliding alongside each other. There are chemical bonds between actin and myosin, and contraction involves changes in these bonds that alter the relative positions of the filaments. At rest, the interaction between actin and myosin is prevented by the proteins tropomyosin and troponin. Calcium ions prevent troponin and tropomyosin from blocking contraction, and calcium levels in the resting muscle are low. The calcium level rises rapidly at time of contraction, which stops the troponin and tropomyosin from blocking contraction. Contraction is stopped by active removal of the calcium from the cell.

Muscle contraction can be divided into three stages: latent phase, contraction phase and relaxation phase. The latent phase begins from the time of stimulation and consists of the action potential sweeping across the sarcolemma releasing calcium ions. In the contraction phase, there is interaction between the actin and myosin filaments. This is followed by the relaxation phase where calcium levels fall and the filaments no longer interact.

There is a certain range over which muscles contract efficiently. A muscle contracts efficiently until it has shortened by about 30%. If the muscle is overstretched or significantly contracted, then it is less efficient.

Muscles work in groups and, on the basis of their actions, can be described as agonists, synergists or antagonists. The agonist is the muscle primarily responsible for producing a particular movement, for example the hamstring muscles producing knee flexion. A synergist assists the prime mover or stabilizes the joint, for example supraspinatus muscle assisting the deltoid in early shoulder abduction. The antagonist is a muscle whose action is the opposite of the agonist. It does not relax but maintains tension to ensure a smoother movement of the joint. For example, the hamstring muscles are antagonists to the quadriceps muscle, the agonist, when it is contracting and flexing the knee.

There are two main types of muscle contraction, isotonic and isometric. In isotonic contraction, as the muscle shortens, the muscle tension remains constant at a level sufficient to do the required amount of work. In isometric contraction, the length of the muscle remains constant with increasing muscle tension. Isometric contraction is the type of contraction in muscles used to maintain posture.

Control of muscle function

Each fibre has a motor endplate on which the nerve fibre terminates. The functional unit of activity is a motor unit, which combines numerous fibres that are supplied by a single anterior horn cell and its axon. The individual muscle fibres that make up the motor unit are scattered throughout the muscle but contract together under the influence of the anterior horn cell. All muscles fibres supplied by a single motor neuron are of the same histochemical type, either type 1 or type 2.

All of the muscle fibres controlled by a single motor neuron form a motor unit. Small motor units where a motor neuron may control two or three muscle fibres are found in muscles where fine control is required. The converse is found in muscles that do not need fine control, for example the gastrocnemius or gluteus maximus. The amount of tension produced in a contracting muscle depends on the frequency of stimulation and the number of muscle units involved.

The nervous system controls the force of the contracting muscle by varying the number of motor neurons activated at any one time. For each movement, there is a progressive increase in the number of motor units contracting to provide an even increase in tension. Maximum tension in a muscle occurs when all the motor units are contracting.

Muscle tone is the resting tension in a skeletal muscle. It occurs because there are always a few motor units contracting in a resting muscle. These contractions do not cause enough tension to produce movement. Muscle tone is maintained by a normal reflex arc, whereby a signal is sent from the muscle spindles to a lower motor neuron in the posterior root ganglion which then sends a signal to the appropriate muscles to adjust the extent of their contraction. Changes in tension in a muscle result in activation of the muscle spindles so that the contraction of other muscles is altered to correct the tension in that muscle. This reflex arc is also under the control of the central nervous system.

Resting muscle tone is important for maintaining normal posture, and provides support for the joints to stabilize their position and help prevent sudden changes in the position. Muscle tone is increased in upper motor neuron lesions, for example in cerebral cortical damage that occurs in cerebrovascular accident. This is thought to be due to loss of cortical control of motor neurons, which increase their activity. There is no muscle wasting. A reduction in muscle tone, hypotonia, occurs in lower motor neuron disorders. These occur in spinal and/or peripheral nerve damage. This results in muscle atrophy. Examination of muscle tone provides important clues to the cause of muscle weakness.

Interesting facts

Myotonia is delayed relaxation of the muscle after contraction. It is an important feature of dystrophia myotonica but can be due to other causes, where it is less severe, which include hypothyroidism, prolonged cold exposure, extreme physical exercise and medication, e.g. propranolol.

Muscle fatigue

Muscle fatigue is a transient and recoverable reduction in the force of muscle contraction which occurs during exercise. There are numerous causes for fatigue and their role and interactions are not clearly understood. Fatigue can be influenced by local muscle factors, the central nervous system and general fitness. The type of exercise also influences fatigue, with the factors that cause fatigue during high-intensity exercise, for example sprinting, being different to those during low-intensity endurance exercise, for example long-distance running. Muscle fatigue can occur earlier than expected depending on various factors that include reduced blood flow or low energy reserves because of poor diet, illness or metabolic disorders. The recovery period after exercise can take from several hours to about a week, depending on the exercise.

Cramp is a prolonged, painful muscle contraction, which can occur following severe exercise. During cramp, the muscle fibre membrane conducts action potentials at abnormally high frequencies in the absence of nerve stimulation. This is due to changes in membrane permeability brought about by changes in ion concentration in the tissue fluids secondary to dehydration and loss of sodium ions.

Ageing and the muscular system

There are several changes in muscle with ageing that result in a reduction of anaerobic and aerobic performance by 30–50% at the age of 65 years. These include selective type 2 fibre atrophy, a reduction in the number of myofibrils and reduced mitochondria and glycogen reserves. There is also an increase in fibrous tissue throughout the muscle, which reduces its flexibility. The number of motor units also falls with age due to a sporadic death of motor units, which cannot regenerate. There is a sprouting from the surviving axons to reinnervate the denervated muscle which increases the size of the surviving motor units. However, the surviving motor units reach a stage where they can no longer support the remaining denervated muscle fibres and muscle fibres are lost. This also contributes to the loss of strength and fine motor control. Conduction velocity in the motor nerves slows with age in adults. The reduction in muscle strength and endurance associated with ageing can be slowed by regular exercise.

Investigations

General investigations

In patients presenting with 'muscle' disease, a number of general investigations are usually performed to exclude other causes of 'weakness' and these usually include measurement of haemoglobin, white cell count, platelets, ESR and, depending on the history and examination, urea and creatinine, liver function tests and autoantibodies.

Muscle-specific investigation

Creatine kinase

This enzyme is important in muscle metabolism and appears in blood when muscle damage occurs, making it

Myopathy: 2

Case note: Clinical examination

We can now answer the question of what other clinical information is required in Mr Brown's case. Muscle disorders usually present with a limited number of symptoms. Pain and weakness are the most common presenting symptoms. Tenderness, twitching and cramps are less common. Muscle wasting and contractures usually occur late in the illness. However, the clinical history is still important, as it is essential to try to determine the cause of the muscle symptoms as well as the appropriate investigations required to make the diagnosis.

It is important to determine whether there are any other neurological symptoms, e.g. numbness, 'pins and needles', dysaesthesia or cranial nerve symptoms, to help determine whether it is a primary muscle disorder or secondary to peripheral nervous system involvement. Enquire about symptoms of connective tissue disease, e.g. photosensitivity, skin rash, Raynaud's phenomenon, arthritis, pleurisy or pericarditis. Family history is important to exclude a congenital problem, e.g. muscular dystrophy. Congenital conditions, however, are usually manifest in childhood or the early 20s. It is also important to take a history of current drug exposure, as a variety of drugs have been associated with muscle disease, as discussed below. Tiredness and fatigue are features of many diseases but can occur in some endocrine disorders, so it is important to determine whether there are other symptoms relevant to an endocrine disorder such as hyper/hypothyroidism.

With regard to the physical examination, it is important to try to determine whether the muscle pain and weakness are due to a primary muscle disorder or secondary to involvement of the nervous system. Neurological abnormalities, in particular lesions of the spinal cord or peripheral nerves, may have associated sensory symptoms and signs. This indicates that the problem is not a primary muscle disorder.

The clinical examination should carefully evaluate all muscle groups both proximally and distally, including the trunk and cervical muscles. This will give you information about the muscle groups involved; whether they are proximal or distal, symmetrical or unilateral, diffuse or related to a particular nerve root distribution. A full neurological examination should be performed to determine whether there is any other neurological abnormality.

The examination of muscle strength involves general functions as well as testing of specific muscles or muscle groups. The patient should be observed walking, getting out of a chair, using a step(s), sitting up from a supine position and holding arms above the head.

Specific muscle testing involves isometric contraction against resistance. The grading system for power is that described in the Medical Research Council Memorandum of 1943 (*Aids to the investigation of peripheral nerve injuries,* War Memorandum No. 7). This is:

- Grade 0, no contraction
- Grade 1, flicker or trace of contraction
- Grade 2, active movement with gravity eliminated
- Grade 3, active movement against gravity
- Grade 4, active movement against gravity and resistance—this can be subdivided into 4−, 4 and 4+ to indicate slight, moderate and strong resistance
- Grade 5, normal power.

This is a subjective scale but is the most appropriate for routine clinical use. There are numerous devices for accurately measuring muscle power, but size or cost precludes their use in the clinical setting.

A general physical examination is also required. Sometimes muscle disorders can be part of a more diffuse disorder, e.g. systemic lupus erythematosus, and there may be other clinical signs, such as a skin rash or arthritis (see Ch. 9). Hyperthyroidism and hypothyroidism can also be associated with muscle disorders and once again, examination should be able to determine whether the patient is clinically euthyroid.

---

the most useful serum enzyme marker of muscle pathology. Damage to the muscle cell membrane, e.g. from inflammation or ischaemia, allows creatine kinase and other enzymes to leak from the muscle cell into the circulation. There are other enzymes that are also elevated with muscle damage, but the creatine kinase has the best correlation with disease activity and is the best measure of muscle damage and response to treatment. It is relatively specific for muscle and usually elevated in myositis. However, there are other causes of an increased level of creatine kinase, which always need to be considered. The more common of these are severe exercise, muscle trauma, drugs and hypothyroidism.

Electromyography

Electromyography and nerve conduction studies are useful in determining if the problem is due to a primary myopathy or neuropathy. Some myopathies have a characteristic pattern, e.g. dystrophia myotonica, but usually the changes are non-diagnostic.

Muscle biopsy

When the diagnosis is uncertain, a muscle biopsy is the most useful investigation. Not all muscle disorders have abnormal histology but it is usually helpful in the more serious conditions.

Atrophy is the commonest abnormality of muscles and there are varying patterns of atrophy. If there is denervation of the muscle, then there is atrophy of both type 1 and type 2 fibres. This is non-selective atrophy and indicates an abnormality in the nerve supplying the muscle.

Selective type 1 atrophy is very rare. It has been described in myotonic dystrophy and rheumatoid arthritis. In contrast, selective type 2 fibre atrophy is common and non-specific and it is not associated with any special disease. Type 2 fibre atrophy can occur with corticosteroid use, Cushing's syndrome (a condition of excess endogenous production of corticosteroids) and inactivity.

Genetic studies

There are an increasing number of identifiable genetic abnormalities that are associated with the inherited muscle disorders. They are usually identified with a muscle biopsy, and should be considered if the history and examination is consistent with an inherited disorder. These patients and families will also require genetic counseling.

Muscle diseases

Muscle disease can be divided into two broad groups, acquired and inherited. The term muscular dystrophy usually applies to a muscle disease that is inherited. The genetic defect associated with inherited muscle diseases has been identified in an increasing number of diseases over recent years. This trend will continue with constant changes in the classification of inherited muscle diseases.

Acquired muscle diseases

Idiopathic inflammatory myopathies

This group of muscle disorders consists of polymyositis, dermatomyositis and inclusion body myositis. Clinical features and histology are helpful in distinguishing between the three types.

Polymyositis and dermatomyositis

Polymyositis and dermatomyositis both have inflammation in the muscle with dermatomyositis also having characteristic skin changes.

The incidence of polymyositis and dermatomyositis is 5–10 per million per year. Polymyositis is slightly more common than dermatomyositis and more common in females by a ratio of 2:1. The peak age of onset is between 40–60 years.

Clinical features

The major clinical feature is proximal muscle weakness and increased muscle fatigue with exercise. The pattern is similar for polymyositis and dermatomyositis, although dermatomyositis may be more rapidly progressive than polymyositis, which usually has a slower more insidious onset. Polymyositis is slowly progressive, whereas the muscle weakness in dermatomyositis may have a fluctuating course. There is symmetrical involvement of the large proximal muscles of the shoulders, arms and thighs. There may also be weakness of the trunk and neck muscles and the muscles of swallowing. Distal muscle involvement is rare. Muscle pain (myalgia) and tenderness is usually mild and occurs in about 50%. It is more likely to occur in those who have rapidly progressive weakness. Muscle wasting occurs late in the disease and can lead to muscle contractures.

Systemic features These include fever, weight loss, fatigue and malaise. Raynaud's phenomenon occurs in about 20–30% of patients.

Lung involvement The lungs can be affected in both polymyositis and dermatomyositis, either due to interstitial lung disease or as a direct result of muscle weakness.

The most frequent lung complication is interstitial lung disease. It occurs in about 30–40% of patients. The lung disease can precede the onset of the myositis in about 40%, and it is clinically indistinguishable from idiopathic pulmonary fibrosis. The main abnormalities in the respiratory function tests are a reduction in total lung capacity, vital capacity and diffusing capacity. Interstitial lung disease in polymyositis and dermatomyositis is associated with the antibody to the Jo-1 antigen. The association is less significant for dermatomyositis. Jo-1 antibody is present in about 5% of polymyositis patients without interstitial lung disease and 60–70% of those with interstitial lung disease.

Involvement of the respiratory muscles may lead to respiratory failure, and involvement of the pharyngeal muscles may also make these patients at increased risk of aspiration pneumonia. This only occurs in patients with severe disease.

Heart involvement Cardiac abnormalities may be present in about 70% of patients but are usually asymptomatic. The major abnormalities are conduction disturbances, arrhythmias and myocarditis. The commonest conduction disturbances on electrocardiogram are left anterior fascicular block and right bundle branch block. Congestive cardiac failure due to myocarditis is rare.

Gastrointestinal involvement The predominant gastrointestinal feature is dysphagia, which occurs in about 12% of patients. Weakness of the pharyngeal muscles or the muscles of the proximal oesophagus can result in difficulties in swallowing, or regurgitation of liquids when attempting to swallow. These abnormalities occur in those with severe disease.

Association with malignancy There is no increased risk of malignancy in patients with polymyositis. The prevalence is about 10%, which is similar to an age-matched population. However, there is an increased risk of malignancy in dermatomyositis with about 25% having a malignancy. This group is unlikely to have features of a connective tissue disorder or myositis-specific antibodies. Therefore, in patients with dermatomyositis, care must be taken in the history and examination to detect symptoms and signs of malignancy.

Overlap with other connective tissue diseases Polymyositis or dermatomyositis may be associated with systemic sclerosis, systemic lupus erythematosus, rheumatoid arthritis or Sjögren's syndrome. This association is more common with polymyositis. This group is less likely to have an increased risk of malignancy.

Investigations

Creatine kinase Serum levels of creatine kinase usually correlate with the disease activity. Most patients with polymyositis and dermatomyositis have elevation of creatine kinase and its level is a useful guide for monitoring the effects of treatment.

Electromyography Electromyography can detect abnormalities in about 90% of patients with active polymyositis, although they are not diagnostic.

Muscle biopsy This is the most definitive test, and in patients suspected of polymyositis or dermatomyositis, a muscle biopsy is mandatory. There are some differences in the histopathology between polymyositis and dermatomyositis. In polymyositis the inflammatory cell infiltrate is in the region of the endomysium and is predominantly CD8+ T lymphocytes and macrophages. In dermatomyositis the inflammatory cell infiltrate is predominantly perivascular and consists of CD4+ T lymphocytes, macrophages and some B lymphocytes. Muscle cells show variation in size, central nuclei, necrosis and regeneration in both types of myositis.

Autoantibodies There is an association between polymyositis and antibodies to the enzymes aminoacyl-transfer RNA synthetases. The reason for this association is unknown. Jo-1, an autoantibody against histidyl-tRNA synthetase, is the commonest antisynthetase antibody. It occurs in 5% of those with polymyositis without lung disease and 60–70% of those with lung involvement.

Treatment

Corticosteroids are the most effective treatment and are usually commenced at a high dose, typically 1 mg/kg of prednisone per day. This dose is maintained until the serum level of creatine kinase is normal and muscle power has almost returned to normal. If the corticosteroids are reduced before there has been adequate control of the myositis, then there are more likely to be flares in the disease and it becomes difficult to control.

High-dose corticosteroids are associated with side-effects, and other agents, including azathioprine, methotrexate and ciclosporin, are often used to control the myositis. This allows a lower maintenance dose of prednisone. The 5-year survival is about 80%, with the 8-year

---

Case 8.1 Myopathy: 3

Case note: diagnosis

Further history taking revealed that Mr Brown had had asthma for 6 years, requiring oral corticosteroids for the past 3 years. There was no other significant past history or symptoms. His family history does not include muscle disorders. Physical examination showed symmetrical proximal muscle weakness, more marked in the legs than the arms. The remainder of the neurological examination was normal; in particular there was no evidence of sensory impairment. He did not have any rash. The remainder of the physical examination was normal.

The most likely diagnosis is polymyositis or its variants, e.g. inclusion body myositis. Steroid myopathy should be considered. The absence of other features made an associated connective tissue disorder or endocrine disorder unlikely. Specific tests include measurement of serum creatine kinase, which was elevated at 2500 IU/L (normal 40–300 IU/L).

Mr Brown was subsequently referred to a rheumatologist for further investigation. Chest X-ray was normal and respiratory function tests showed a mild impairment of diffusing capacity but were otherwise normal. There was an antibody to Jo-1. A muscle biopsy showed irregularity in the size and shape of muscle fibres, including necrotic fibres, regenerative fibres and a variable inflammatory infiltrate. These changes were consistent with polymyositis (Fig. 8.3).

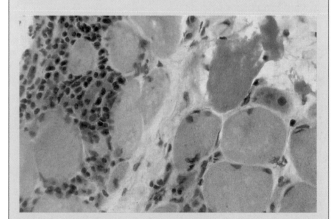

Fig. 8.3 Histological appearance with polymyositis.

---

survival being about 73%. The major causes of death are malignancy, infection and pulmonary involvement. Early treatment improves the prognosis.

Inclusion body myositis

Inclusion body myositis is more common than polymyositis and dermatomyositis and has a poorer prognosis. It usually affects people over the age of 50 years and is more common in males. It has a slower, more insidious onset than polymyositis and the clinical pattern is usually different. The predominant weakness is in the proximal muscles, particularly the quadriceps, but there may also be distal muscle involvement, particularly weakness of the finger flexor and the foot extensor muscles. Rarely, there can be an associated polyneuropathy. Compared with polymyositis, dysphagia, due to involvement of the swallowing muscles, is more common. They can also develop mild facial weakness which is not found in polymyositis or dermatomyositis.

The creatine kinase is elevated but levels are much lower than in polymyositis. Inclusion body myositis is less likely than polymyositis or dermatomyositis to be associated with a connective tissue disorder or have autoantibodies. A muscle biopsy is essential to make the diagnosis. The histology is similar to polymyositis with the addition of rimmed vacuoles and cytoplasmic inclusions. There is the accumulation of β-amyloid and tau proteins in the muscle.

The electromyogram is similar to that of polymyositis.

Treatment is the same as for polymyositis, but inclusion body myositis responds poorly to treatment and is usually slowly progressive.

Infections and muscles

Myalgia is the commonest muscle symptom associated with infections, and occurs with most viral infections. It resolves with the illness, there is no weakness and the creatine kinase is normal.

Myositis may be associated with microbial agents and has been described with numerous viruses, particularly influenza and Coxsackie A and B viruses. It presents with muscle pain, mild weakness and there may be a high creatine kinase level, which rapidly returns to normal without treatment after about 1 week. Pyomyositis is a bacterial infection of muscle that is rare and serious. Parasite infections are most likely to be toxoplasmosis and trichinosis. They usually give diffuse muscle pain and are often diagnosed by muscle biopsy.

Endocrine myopathies

Muscle weakness occurs with several endocrine disorders, where it can occasionally be the presenting symptom. If any of these endocrine disorders is suspected, then the appropriate additional endocrine investigations are also required. With all these endocrine disorders, correction of the endocrine abnormality results in the return of muscle function to normal.

Thyroid disease

Hyperthyroidism produces generalized weakness and occasionally there may be associated paralysis of the extraocular muscles. Proximal muscle weakness is usually the presenting symptom, although there is usually less obvious distal muscle weakness. The creatine kinase level is normal or only slightly elevated. Muscle biopsy shows only occasional non-selective fibre atrophy.

In hypothyroidism there will be proximal muscle weakness and patients are more likely to have myalgia. There is often slowness of contraction and delayed relaxation of the reflexes. In contrast to hyperthyroidism, the creatine kinase level is elevated.

Cushing's syndrome

Cushing's syndrome is associated with proximal muscle weakness, which is due to the effect of cortisol on muscle cell metabolism. The pattern of muscle involvement is similar to that associated with excess exogenous cortisol. The creatine kinase level is normal and histology shows type 2 fibre atrophy.

Acromegaly

Acromegaly is associated with proximal weakness. The muscle histology is unusual, with type 1 fibre hypertrophy and type 2 fibre atrophy.

Disorders of calcium metabolism

Hyper- and hypocalcaemia can be associated with muscle weakness with or without pain. Creatine kinase level is usually normal and the histological changes consist of type 2 fibre atrophy.

Drug-induced muscle disease

A wide range of drugs can affect muscle function because of a direct effect on the muscle. It is important to remember that drugs can also affect the nerves or neuromuscular junction, and this will have a secondary effect on muscle function. The true frequency of drug-induced muscle involvement is not known. The clinical features are usually muscle pain, tenderness and weakness. The weakness is usually proximal and the creatine kinase level may be elevated.

Because a wide range of drugs have been described as causing muscle disease, any history of a patient with muscle disease should include a detailed history of medications. A temporal association between first taking the drug and the onset of muscle symptoms is important. Sometimes the only way to determine if the drug is the cause is to stop it. Most of the drug associations are based on case reports, which may not always be reliable. The drugs more commonly associated with muscle disease are shown in Box 8.1.

Cholesterol-lowering drugs are probably the commonest cause of drug-induced myopathy. Statin-induced

Box 8.1 Drugs commonly associated with muscle disease

- Cholesterol-lowering drugs:
  - clofibrate
  - HMG-CoA enzyme inhibitors
- Alcohol
- Zidovudine
- Vincristine
- Lithium
- Cimetidine
- Ciclosporin

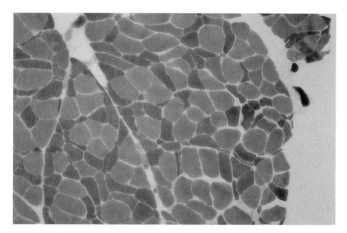

Fig. 8.4 Muscle biopsy showing type 2 fibre atrophy. The type 2 fibres are darker.

muscle involvement can include myalgia, elevated creatine kinase, myositis and rhabdomyolysis. It is more common in the first few months after starting the statin but can occur at any time. Stopping the drug usually results in resolution of the muscle disorder.

Diuretics can produce widespread muscle weakness with or without pain and associated elevation in creatine kinase level. This is essentially a hypokalaemic myopathy and it also occurs with the excessive use of laxatives.

Corticosteroid-associated myopathy is associated with proximal weakness with a normal level of creatine kinase. The effect of the corticosteroid on the muscle is dose dependent. Myopathy is more common with the fluorinated steroids, particularly triamcinolone and betamethasone. It can also occur with prednisone and reports vary as to the dosage required to produce a myopathy. The histological changes are a type 2 fibre atrophy (Fig. 8.4).

Alcoholic myopathies are of two major types. Chronic alcoholics may develop slowly progressive proximal muscle weakness. There may be a neuropathic component to the weakness. Acute alcoholic myopathy can occur after an episode of heavy drinking. There is pain, cramps, and muscle swelling that can lead to rhabdomyolysis with very high serum creatine kinase levels.

The alcoholic myopathies improve when alcohol consumption is stopped.

Inherited muscle disorders

Dystrophinopathies

The dystrophinopathies are associated with a defect in the dystrophin gene which is on the X chromosome. As a consequence, they usually involve males. The gene mutation results in a deficiency of the protein dystrophin, which is in the cell membrane and important for reducing myofibril plasma membrane contraction-induced injury. There are varying levels of deficiency depending on the genetic defect. However, they all present with proximal muscle weakness and an elevated creatine kinase. The two most common dystrophinopathies are Duchenne muscular dystrophy and Becker muscular dystrophy. There is no known treatment for these disorders.

Duchenne muscular dystrophy

This is a severe progressive disease of males. The incidence is 20–30/100 000 males per year. It usually presents with proximal muscle weakness during the first 2 years of life. There is a continuous slow decline in muscle strength and most are unable to walk by 7–12 years. Enlargement of the calf and occasionally the quadriceps muscles occurs at some stage of the illness, although it subsequently disappears. There is a severe deficiency of dystrophin with levels in the muscle being less than three percent. A muscle biopsy is required for diagnosis. The creatine kinase level is elevated, particularly in the early stages.

Becker muscular dystrophy

Becker muscular dystrophy is associated with a partial deficiency of dystrophin. The clinical pattern is similar, but less severe than that of Duchenne muscular dystrophy. Its onset is usually between the ages of 5–15 years and it has an incidence of 2–5/100 000 males per year.

Myotonic dystrophy

This is a rare disorder where there is a delay in muscle relaxation after a contraction. It is clinically detected by a delay in relaxation of hand grip. It is inherited, usually by autosomal dominant inheritance with a wide spectrum of clinical manifestations. There is mutation in the gene encoding for dystrophia myotonica protein kinase which results in a defect in the RNA product of the mutant gene. This results in defective RNA splicing which affects a variety of cell functions and is considered to be the reason for the clinical heterogeneity of the disease.

Dystrophia myotonica is a systemic disorder that involves other systems in addition to the muscles. The prevalence is about 15/100 000 per year. The features include myotonia, facial myopathy, distal muscular atrophy, cataracts, frontal baldness in males, gonadal atrophy, cardiomyopathy, reduced lung function, impaired thyroid activity and impaired glucose metabolism, hyperostosis of the skull vault and impaired mental function, especially cognitive defects.

It usually presents with difficulty in walking and weakness of the hands, between the ages of 20–50 years. EMG shows myotonic changes and the creatine kinase level is elevated. Muscle biopsy shows an increase in the number of nuclei, which are arranged in long rows in the centre of the fibre, a variation in the fibre size and necrosis of sections of the muscle fibre. The condition is slowly progressive and patients are unable to walk after about 20 years of disease. Death is due to cardiac failure or respiratory infection. However, there is considerable variation in the age of onset and rate of progression. There is no treatment for this condition.

Facioscapulohumeral muscular dystrophy

Facioscapulohumeral muscular dystrophy initially involves the facial muscles and may present with difficulty in closing the eyes. Subsequently, there is weakness of the shoulder girdle muscles and there may also be weakness of the abdominal muscles and lower limb muscles. In the leg the tibialis anterior is involved and the gastrocnemius is normal. The incidence is 1–3/100 000 per year. It is an autosomal dominant disorder and the genetic defect is a deletion at the subtelomeric region of chromosome 4q. How this gene abnormality affects muscle function is unknown. The level of creatine kinase is normal or only mildly elevated. There are non-specific changes on muscle histology. The rate of progression is variable but most of those affected have a normal life expectancy.

Metabolic myopathies

These are inherited disorders of metabolism of glycogen and lipids that can cause impaired muscle function. They are usually due to an enzyme defect, most frequently a deficiency, which affects normal muscle metabolism. There may be involvement of other organs, which include the liver. There is a different clinical pattern for different enzymes.

Many of these metabolic myopathies have symptoms only with exercise. Those associated with glycogen metabolism usually produce pain and weakness early in exercise, whereas those associated with lipid metabolism develop these symptoms late in exercise. The extent of exercise and severity of symptoms varies for each enzyme. They can also produce progressive weakness. There is often an increase in serum creatine kinase levels.

Muscle histochemistry or enzyme studies are required to make the diagnosis.

Ion channel disorders of muscle

Inherited ion channel disorders are a diverse group of conditions due to a mutation in genes encoding ion channels which results in dysfunction of these channels. Most affect the nervous system or muscle. The main muscle disorders are hyperkalaemic and hypokalaemic periodic paralysis.

Hyperkalaemic periodic paralysis is caused by a mutation in the gene that affects the sodium channel. It usually develops in the second decade, improves in the third and is slightly more common in males.

There are intermittent attacks, which usually present with symmetrical proximal muscle weakness. It can progress to involve distal muscles, but there are no changes in sensation or higher function. Precipitating factors include rest following intensive exercise, cold, carbohydrate-rich meals and alcohol.

Hypokalaemic periodic paralysis is caused by mutations affecting a component of the calcium entry channel. It usually begins at an earlier age but is similar to and milder than the muscle involvement in hyperkalaemia.

Mitochondrial myopathy

Mitochondrial myopathies are a heterogeneous group of inherited myopathies due to abnormalities in the structure and/or function of the skeletal muscle mitochondria. Most have clinical features affecting other systems and the clinical picture can be quite varied.

Patients present with a proximal muscle weakness but may also have distal muscle weakness early in their illness. Many present in childhood and the condition is first evident only after intense exercise. There are subgroups that have cerebral dysfunction or are associated with chronic progressive external ophthalmoplegia. These additional features are helpful in the diagnosis and differentiate the condition from polymyositis. The diagnosis is made on muscle biopsy, which shows a pattern of 'ragged-red' fibres owing to increased mitochondria around the cell periphery. There is no effective treatment for these myopathies.

Muscle disorders in which pain is the main feature

Myofascial pain syndromes

Myofascial pain refers to a localized area of pain within a muscle. It is usually caused by acute overload of a muscle, fatigue due to chronic overuse or direct trauma. Any muscle group can be involved and there is a characteristic pain pattern for each muscle. The pain is usually over the involved muscle but there is also a referred pain pattern that is specific for each muscle.

Case 8.1 Myopathy: 4

Case note: Treatment

You will recall that investigations in Mr Brown were consistent with a diagnosis of idiopathic polymyositis. Steroid myopathy was unlikely because of the high creatine kinase level and the absence of type 2 fibre atrophy on muscle biopsy. However, Mr Brown may develop type 2 fibre atrophy secondary to the increased prednisone required for the polymyositis.

Mr Brown was instructed by his rheumatologist to increase his prednisone to 50 mg/day and start taking azathioprine at 100 mg/day. After 6 weeks, his muscle power had returned to normal and his creatine kinase was 145 IU/mL. The prednisone was reduced over the next month to 10 mg/day and the over the next 3 months to 5 mg/day. Mr Brown's muscle power and creatine kinase level remain normal. Lung function tests remain unchanged.

Box 8.2 Fibromyalgia

- **Occiput.** At the insertion of the suboccipital muscles.
- *Low cervical.* Under the sternomastoid muscle at the anterior aspect of the intra-transverse spaces at C5–C7.
- *Trapezius.* At the midpoint of the upper border of the trapezius muscle.
- *Supraspinatus.* At the origin of the supraspinatus muscle above the scapular spine, near the medial border.
- *Second rib.* At the second costochondral junction.
- *Lateral epicondyle.* 2 cm distal to the epicondyle.
- *Gluteal.* At the upper outer quadrant of the buttock in the anterior fold of the muscle.
- *Greater trochanter.* Posterior to the trochanteric prominence.
- *Knee.* At the medial fat pad, proximal to the joint line.

The other feature of myofascial pain is a localized tender area, often called the 'trigger point', within the involved muscle. Sometimes bands of tight muscle fibres can be palpated within the muscle.

There is restriction of movement on stretching the involved muscle group and there may be weakness on isometric contraction. Myofascial pain is distinguished from other causes of muscle pain and weakness because it is usually restricted to one or two muscle groups. A careful clinical examination is required to identify the involved muscle. A correct diagnosis is important, because therapy has to be directed at the involved muscle.

Levator scapulae myofascial pain The levator scapulae muscle is one of the more common muscles that has myofascial pain symptoms. The muscle extends from the upper medial border of the scapula to the transverse processes of the first four cervical vertebrae. The levator scapulae muscle, in conjunction with the other shoulder muscles, has an important action in stabilizing and moving the scapula and is associated with movement of the shoulder.

Levator scapulae pain is at the angle of the neck and may radiate down the medial border of the scapula or out to the posterior aspect of the shoulder joint. Associated with this will be some restriction of neck movements and pain on stretching the levator scapulae muscle. Tenderness is maximal over the angle of the neck along the line of the muscle. Levator scapulae myofascial pain is often precipitated by using a keyboard in an abnormal position with the neck rotated but can occur in sports, e.g. swimming, where frequent neck rotation is required. Treatment consists of stretching and strengthening exercises for the individual muscle and correction of the precipitating cause.

Fibromyalgia

Fibromyalgia is a condition characterized by widespread muscle pain, in combination with tenderness at 11 or more of 18 specific tender point sites (Box 8.2). There is usually associated sleep disturbance and fatigue. It occurs most frequently in the 30–60 year age group, and 80–90% of patients are women. Fibromyalgia may occur on its own or be associated with other rheumatic disorders. Fibromyalgia that is associated with other rheumatic disorders, e.g. rheumatoid arthritis, is clinically identical to fibromyalgia occurring on its own.

Clinical features

The pain most commonly involves muscles of the axial skeleton, including the shoulder and pelvic girdles. There is no diurnal variation in symptoms.

The pain is poorly localized but there are specific areas of tenderness, tender or trigger points, which are specific and consistent from patient to patient. Figure 8.5 shows the 18 tender points, of which 11 must be tender on digital palpation to make a diagnosis of fibromyalgia.

Other features of fibromyalgia include irritable bowel syndrome, headaches, paraesthesia, urinary urgency and anxiety.

The disturbed sleep pattern is an important feature of fibromyalgia. The electroencephalographic changes during sleep in patients with fibromyalgia have shown a disturbance of Stage IV, non-rapid eye movement sleep. This disturbance is due to the rapid alpha rhythm normally found in REM sleep intruding into the slow delta rhythm of Stage IV or deep sleep. It is associated with non-restorative sleep and waking unrefreshed in the morning. Induction of this type of sleep pattern has been shown to produce symptoms and signs of fibromyalgia.

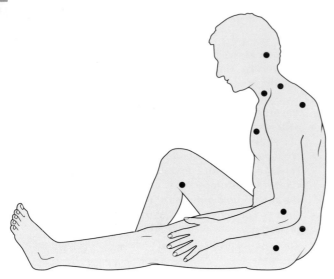

Fig. 8.5 Tender points in fibromyalgia. There are nine tender points on each side, making a total of 18 tender points.

All investigations are normal, including erythrocyte sedimentation rate, C-reactive protein and creatine kinase levels. If any of the laboratory tests are abnormal, then causes other than fibromyalgia need to be considered for the myalgia.

Management

Numerous treatments have been tried but the only ones that have been shown to be of any value are exercise and tricyclic antidepressants. This latter group of drugs is usually taken at night and corrects the abnormal sleep pattern.

Prognosis

The condition is chronic and it is difficult to treat. It tends to remain stable without any significant deterioration and about 60% of patients still have moderate symptoms 3 years after diagnosis. An understanding of the illness helps the patients' anxiety and improves their ability to cope with the disease.

Further reading

Hochberg, M.C., Silman, A.J., Smolen, J.S., et al. (Eds.), 2003. Rheumatology, third ed. Mosby, Philadelphia.

Karpati, G., Hilton-Jones, D., Griggs, R.C., 2001. Disorders of Voluntary Muscle, seventh ed. Cambridge University Press, Cambridge.

Moore, K.L., Dalley, A.F., 1999. Clinically Oriented Anatomy, fourth ed. Williams & Wilkins, Baltimore.

Tortora, G.J., Derrickson, B., 2006. Principles of Anatomy and Physiology, eleventh ed. Wiley, Hoboken.

AUTOIMMUNITY AND THE MUSCULOSKELETAL SYSTEM

9

Nicholas Manolios

Chapter objectives

After studying this chapter you should be able to:

1. Understand the features of autoimmune disease in the musculoskeletal system.

2. Understand the basis of immune complex disease pathogenesis.

3. Understand the use and interpretation of autoantibodies.

4. Understand the clinical features of systemic lupus erythematosus (SLE).

5. Understand the clinico-pathological correlation of symptoms and signs in SLE.

6. Understand the treatment of SLE.

Introduction

Systemic lupus erythematosus (SLE) is the prototypic autoimmune disease, characterized by excessive auto-antibody production, immune complex formation and immunologically-mediated tissue injury at multiple sites. It is a clinically heterogeneous disorder with a broad spectrum of presentations. Although the immune mechanism/s responsible for the breakdown of tolerance against self-antigens is unknown, a genetic influence in disease predisposition has been clearly demonstrated. Like most other connective tissue disorders, auto-antibody testing can be of value in making the diagnosis. These results must always be correlated with the patient's symptoms and signs for correct interpretation. Treatment is symptomatic and aimed at suppressing an altered immune system that causes end-organ damage. In Chapter 1 we dealt with another autoimmune disease—rheumatoid arthritis. This chapter will be illustrated by a case of SLE that tracks its course over several years to illustrate its clinical and immunological features.

Interesting facts

Lupus with its characteristic butterfly rash was long considered a skin disease. Kaposi in 1870 recognized that lupus had other extra-cutaneous manifestations such as arthritis and at the turn of the century, Osler recognized the systemic nature of the disease. In the 1920s Libman and Sacks differentiated the effects of lupus on the heart from that of rheumatic fever and, in 1938, Hargraves noted the LE-cell phenomenon, which later became the test for lupus. Steroids revolutionized the treatment of lupus in the 1950s; anti-nuclear antibodies were introduced for the identification and diagnosis of lupus in the 1960s. The survival of lupus patients has dramatically increased over the last 50 years. In 1953, 4 years after diagnosis 50% of patients had died. Nowadays, the majority of cases can be controlled with proper treatment.

Immunology

Autoimmunity

Despite the heterogeneity of clinical features of SLE discussed later in this chapter, one characteristic laboratory finding is the presence of antibodies generated by the person's own immune system against a wide range of 'self' antigens, such as deoxyribonucleic acids (DNA) and ribonucleoproteins. Since these antibodies are directed against 'self' antigens they are called 'autoantibodies'. A schematic representation of an antigen–antibody (immune) complex is shown in Figure 9.1. The exact reason for this breakdown of immune tolerance is still unclear. The consequence of immune complex deposition in many vascular beds throughout the body results in a wide variety of clinical presentations. These manifestations are dictated

Case 9.1 SLE: 1

Case history

Melanie, an 18-year-old woman initially presented to her GP complaining of joint pain in both hands. On specific questioning it was noted that she had felt unwell over the preceding several months and was experiencing increasing lethargy which was disproportionate to her daily activities. Other features noted in her history were the presence of facial rash, alopecia (hair loss) and mouth ulcers. There was no history of drug ingestion, overseas travel, diarrhoea, urinary tract symptoms or recent upper respiratory infection. The patient had a twin sister and two other siblings who were well. There was no family history of arthritis.

Physical examination revealed an ill-looking woman with a malar rash in a butterfly distribution over the face. The hair was sparse and there were mouth ulcers in the buccal cavity. Examination of the musculoskeletal system revealed tenderness in the proximal interphalangeal and metacarpophalangeal joints of both hands consistent with a symmetrical polyarthritis. There were small effusions present in both knees. There were no nodules or psoriatic skin changes. Heart sounds were dual with no murmurs and breath sounds were normal.

A presumptive diagnosis of SLE was made. To confirm the clinical suspicion and to assess the extent of disease activity, she underwent a variety of serum and urine tests including testing for various autoantibodies. The serum tests showed a mild anaemia, elevated ESR, a positive antinuclear antibody (ANA) at a titre of 1:640 with a homogeneous pattern and positive antibody to the Sm antigen. Biochemistry and urinalysis were normal. The patient was started on prednisone and hydroxychloroquine.

by the site and extent of the inflammatory process, triggered by the antibody–antigen complex.

Immunopathology

An autoimmune disease like SLE is characterized by the production of many autoantibodies. Their exact role in disease aetiopathogenesis remains unclear. Some autoantibodies have been shown to contribute directly to the clinical picture by causing cell death. For example, anti-erythrocyte antibodies result in haemolysis (red cell lysis) and lymphocytotoxic antibodies are responsible for the reduced lymphocyte count (lymphopenia) that occurs in active lupus. An alternative mechanism of tissue injury is deposition of antigen–antibody complexes with complement activation. This is seen particularly in the kidney and skin. Complement and pro-inflammatory cytokine production result in polymorph trafficking into the area in question. Further release of pro-inflammatory mediators from mast cells, basophils and polymorphs

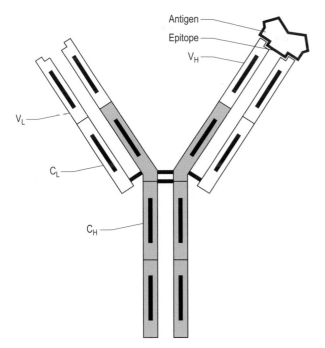

Fig. 9.1 Interaction of an antibody with antigen. Key for abbreviations: V_L = variable region of the light chain, V_H = variable region of the heavy chain, C_L = constant region of the light chain and C_H = constant region of the heavy chain. The epitope refers to the component of the antigen that binds to the antibody.

perpetuate the inflammatory cascade. Platelet aggregation and clot formation result in microthrombi formation and tissue ischaemia. This is compounded by the release of proteases, hydrolytic enzymes and free radicals. Complement activation may also lead both directly (via complement components C5–9) and indirectly to cell lysis. Resultant end-organ damage in various tissues such as the kidney, skin and brain are responsible for the clinical manifestations of the disease. Under normal circumstances, antigen–antibody complexes are rapidly and efficiently cleared by phagocytes. However, defective mechanisms of immune complex clearance may perpetuate the inflammatory response.

Complement receptors (CR) bind different complement fragments produced during complement activation. They are found on erythrocytes (CR1), B cells (CR2), macrophages and polymorphonuclear cells (CR3, CR4). Deficiency in these receptors may lead to continued inflammation and immune complex deposition. Immune complexes may also be cleared via the immunoglobulin portion of Fc receptors expressed on monocytes, polymorphonuclear cells and other immune cells. The Fc receptors are encoded by genes on chromosome 1 and have different forms (alleles) that may influence immune complex handling.

Cutaneous immunopathology

In skin, the three key features are immune complex deposition, vascular inflammation and mononuclear cell infiltration. Immunoglobulin and complement deposition occurs at the dermo–epidermal junction, presumably because this is highly vascular. This can be detected in a skin biopsy by immunofluorescence and is called the 'lupus band test'. Immunofluorescence involves staining with specific antibody preparations labelled with fluorescent compounds and examining for fluorescence by microscopy. It is not completely specific for SLE, being seen in other autoimmune conditions such as rheumatoid arthritis.

Renal immunopathology

Immune complex deposition in the glomeruli is the main immunopathogenic mechanism that results in tissue injury. Immunofluorescence often reveals the deposition of IgG, IgM, IgA, C3, C4 and C1q. This will be discussed again later.

Central nervous system immunopathology

The pathogenesis of central nervous system lupus is uncertain, but immune deposition and activation in the cerebral vasculature may result in microvascular and macrovascular thromboses (clots) with resultant cerebral oedema and ischaemia. Other possible mechanisms include a direct effect of autoantibodies on neuronal tissue with resultant dysfunction. Anti-ribosomal P antibodies have been associated with psychosis in SLE. It is important to exclude other diagnoses such as infection, renal failure, malignant hypertension and drug-related effects in an often immunosuppressed patient.

Serological manifestations of autoimmunity

Complement

In autoimmune disease, activation and deposition of complement components induced by antigen–antibody complexes cause tissue damage such as glomerulonephritis (glomerular inflammation) in the kidney. Low serum levels of complement (C3, C4) reflect consumption and are useful in assessing disease activity. Contrary to what may be expected, complement factor deficiency is associated with a predisposition to SLE, possibly due to a decrease in the ability to solubilize immune complexes leading to tissue deposition and inflammation. C1q/r/s and C4 deficiencies show the strongest association with SLE, whereas C2 deficiency may manifest a lupus-like disease with cutaneous manifestations. C3 deficiency is rare.

Antinuclear antibodies

The most typical serologic abnormality in SLE is the presence of ANA antibodies. These antibodies are usually directed against intra-nuclear proteins involved in DNA packaging, RNA splicing or RNA translation. The two important features of an ANA are: (1) the titre (extent of serum dilution that still gives a detectable pattern) and (2) the pattern of immunofluorescence.

Titre

The titre does not always correlate with activity, since it is the avidity of antibody binding that is important and not the amount. More than 95% of patients with SLE have a positive ANA. ANA-negative SLE is very uncommon and may be due to the presence of anti-cytoplasmic antibodies, the commonest being SS-A (also known as

Ro). Our patient had a moderately positive ANA at a titre of 1/640. It is important to remember that a positive ANA is not diagnostic of SLE and can occur with other illnesses, for example bacterial and viral infection, drug therapy and other inflammatory disorders. About 5% of the normal population have a positive ANA at a titre of ≥1:160.

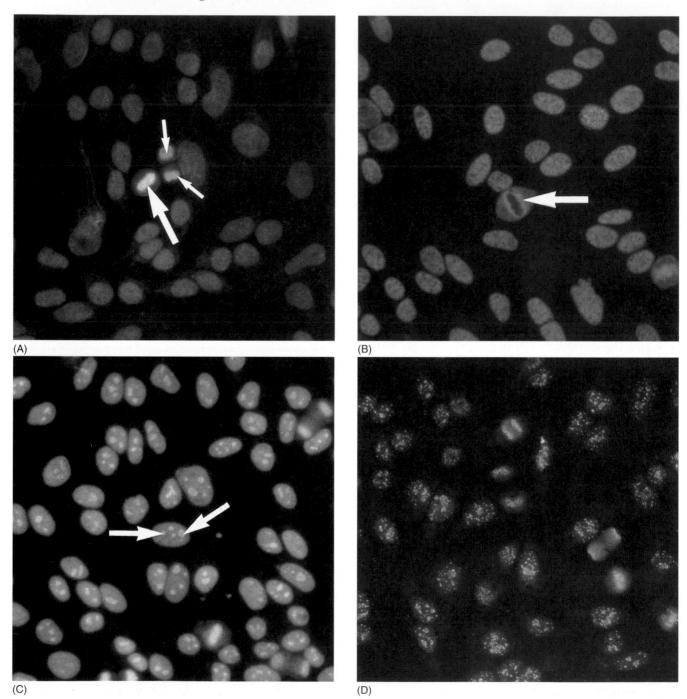

(A)

(B)

(C)

(D)

Fig. 9.2 Fluorescence micrographs of ANA staining patterns. (A) Homogeneous: the arrows indicate staining of DNA inside the nucleus. (B) Speckled: the arrow indicates staining of non-DNA fragments. Compare it with (A), where there is clearly staining of DNA. (C) Nucleolar: this indicates staining of the nucleolus (arrows). (D) Centromere: as the antigen is the centromere, there are exactly 46 nuclear speckles (courtesy of the Immunology Laboratory, Institute of Clinical Pathology and Medical Research, Westmead Hospital).

Table 9.1 ANA patterns and disease associations

Pattern	Antigen	Association
Homogeneous	Deoxyribonucleic acid, histones	SLE; Drug-induced lupus
Speckled	SS-A, SS-B, Sm, RNP	SLE; Sjögren's syndrome; MCTD
Nucleolar	–	Scleroderma; Polymyositis
Centromere	Centromere	Limited Scleroderma (CREST)
Speckled and nucleolar (mixed)	SS-A, SS-B, Sm, RNP	Raynaud's; Overlap syndromes; Myositis; Lupus; Sjögren's

ANA, antinuclear antibody; MCTD, mixed connective tissue disease.

Table 9.2 Specific autoantibodies and their disease association

Antibody	Disease association
dsDNA	SLE
Sm	SLE
SS-A/Ro with SS-B/La	Primary Sjögren's syndrome
SS-A/Ro without SS-B/La	SLE, Sjögren's syndrome
Jo-1	Polymyositis/dermatomyositis
RNP	Mixed connective tissue disease
Scl-70	Diffuse scleroderma
Anti-centromere	Limited scleroderma (CREST)

Staining patterns

Different staining patterns (Fig. 9.2) reflect the nature of the antigen and its distribution. Their disease associations are summarized in Table 9.1. Different patterns include:

Homogenous pattern This pattern is most common in SLE and drug-induced lupus erythematosus. The antigen is usually DNA, histones or deoxyribonucleoprotein.

Rim pattern This pattern is also associated predominantly with SLE. It is thought that rim and homogenous are essentially the same pattern, but appear slightly differently due to sectioning of cells.

Speckled pattern This is the most frequent staining pattern and the pattern that usually occurs in other illnesses and normal people with low titres of ANA.

Anti-centromere pattern This specific speckled pattern is due to antibodies to the centromere and results in exactly 46 nuclear speckles. Anti-centromere antibodies are associated with the CREST syndrome, a limited variant of the disease scleroderma. The latter is also known as systemic sclerosis. CREST comprises C for calcinosis (calcium hydroxyapatite deposition in soft tissues), R for Raynaud's phenomenon (abnormal vascular sensitivity of the digits on exposure to cold, characterized by a classical three-phase colour change of white, then blue, then red), E for esophageal dysfunction (usually manifest initially as difficulty swallowing), S for sclerodactyly (thickening of the skin of the digits) and T for telangiectasia (localized capillary dilatation and tortuosity in the skin). Anti-centromere antibody is uncommon in the more diffuse form of systemic sclerosis and is only rarely found in other connective tissue disorders.

Nucleolar pattern This pattern is suggestive of systemic sclerosis or polymyositis.

Specific antibodies

Once an ANA is detected, the next step is to define the antigen. This is important because specific autoantibodies are usually associated with a particular autoimmune disease.

Antibodies to dsDNA

Antibodies to double-stranded DNA (dsDNA) are specific for SLE, being present in 40% of patients. Elevated levels are usually associated with active disease, but patients can have elevated DNA antibodies and be clinically quiescent. Rapid rises or falls in DNA antibody levels with doubling or halving time of 4 weeks or less, may precede flares in the disease. Levels may fall with successful treatment. The presence of dsDNA correlates well with the probability of development of lupus nephritis (kidney disease). Many normal people have IgM antibodies to single-stranded DNA (ssDNA). However, IgG antibodies to dsDNA are less prevalent in normal controls and are highly suggestive of SLE. They have a pathogenic role by complexing with DNA trapped in glomeruli or by direct attachment to glomerular structures. Their complement-fixing ability then results in tissue damage.

Serum complement levels of C3 and C4 are useful in monitoring disease activity in conjunction with dsDNA levels. A rapid rise or fall of dsDNA levels in association with a fall in complement C3 and/or C4, is more likely to be significant than when the complement levels remain normal.

Antibodies to extractable nuclear antigens

The extractable nuclear antigens (ENA) consist of a number of antigens which include ribonucleoprotein (RNP), Smith antigen (Sm), SS-A/Ro, SS-B/La, Jo-1, ribosomal-p, and Scl-70. Their disease associations are summarized in Table 9.2. Autoantibodies can also be useful in helping with the diagnosis of connective tissue disorders (Table 9.2). The clinical findings are the most important factor in determining which autoantibody to measure.

Anti-RNP Antibodies to RNP are present in about one-third of patients with SLE and are the only autoantibodies present in patients with so-called 'mixed connective tissue disease'.

Anti-Sm Anti-Sm antibody is highly specific for SLE but is present in only about 20% of patients. Therefore, although it is very specific, it is not particularly sensitive. Our patient had a positive anti-Sm antibody.

Anti-SS-A/Ro Anti-SS-A/Ro is a relatively common antibody found in about 30% of people with SLE and 75% of patients with primary Sjögren's syndrome (indeed SS is an abbreviation of Sjögren's syndrome). Sjögren's syndrome is characterized by chronic inflammation of the lacrimal and salivary glands, causing dryness of the eyes and mouth respectively, and is frequently associated with rheumatoid arthritis. People with SLE who have anti-Ro are more likely to have cutaneous involvement. Women with this antibody, when pregnant, are more likely to have children with congenital heart block. This applies particularly if they also have antibodies to SS-B/La.

Anti-SS-B/La Antibodies to SS-B/La are less common and usually occur in conjunction with anti-SS-A/Ro. They are present in only about 10% of people with SLE and in about 50% of primary Sjögren's syndrome. Their presence may indicate a milder course of disease in SLE. The presence of both SS-A/Ro and SS-B/La is more commonly associated with primary Sjögren's syndrome.

Antibodies to Scl-70/Topoisomerase-1 Antibodies to Scl-70 are highly specific for diffuse scleroderma. They occur in about 50% of patients with diffuse scleroderma.

Antibodies to Jo-1 Antibodies to Jo-1 are present in 30% of people with polymyositis, particularly in those who also have pulmonary fibrosis as discussed in Chapter 8.

Antibodies to ribosomal-p These antibodies are present in about 15% of SLE, and may be associated with psychiatric manifestations of SLE. However, the association is not strong enough to make them of diagnostic value.

Anti-phospholipid/anti-cardiolipin antibodies

These consist of a number of antibodies that bind to different negatively charged phospholipids of the cell membrane. They include lupus anticoagulant and anti-cardiolipin (ACA) antibodies which can be independently positive. Lupus anticoagulant may prolong the clotting time of various bleeding tests such as the activated partial thromboplastin time (APTT). However, despite the prolonged APTT, the patient is actually at increased risk of thrombosis. How these antibodies induce thrombosis is unknown.

Clinical features and epidemiology

SLE is traditionally considered to be present in women of child-bearing age, with a peak incidence between 15 and 40 years of age. However, the onset can range outside of these age groups to involve infants and the elderly.

Some 90% of patients with SLE are female. This strong correlation suggests that hormonal factors may be involved in disease development. The female-to-male ratio of incidence ranges from 5:1 at teenage to its peak (9:1) in the 30s. The ratio then declines (2:1) as age increases to over 60 years, and in infants. It has been postulated that sex hormones play an important role in disease predisposition and may modulate the immune system, either by oestrogens inhibiting and androgens accelerating clearance of circulating immune complexes; oestrogens stimulating antibody production by B cells; and/or androgens stimulating T suppressor/cytotoxic cell activity. Females may develop full-blown SLE after receiving high-dose oestrogens for oral contraception.

SLE has no geographic limitation and a worldwide prevalence that varies from 15–207/100 000 per head of population. The incidence (number of new cases per head of population per year) rates also vary between studies and range from 1.8–7.6/100 000 per year. In general the prevalence is approximately 1 in 2000, although this may vary depending on geographical (racial) differences, ethnicity and socioeconomic status.

SLE is commoner in Afro-Caribbeans (prevalence rate of 207/100 000) and Asians (49/100 000) compared with Caucasians (20/100 000). Interestingly, despite the high incidence and prevalence of SLE in Blacks in the UK and USA, lupus is thought to be almost non-existent in West and Central Africa where most of these people originated. These results suggest that there may be more than genetic influences determining susceptibility and that environmental factors are likely to be important.

Pathology

The pathologic findings of SLE are widely distributed throughout the human body and reflect tissue damage due to immune complex deposition and primary or secondary infiltration of tissue with mononuclear cells. The pathology is characterized by inflammation, blood vessel abnormalities secondary to immune complex deposition and/or cellular infiltrate. Pathological findings in the kidney are described below.

The kidney in SLE

The WHO classification of lupus nephritis is shown in Table 9.3. Light microscopic examination of the kidney reveals increases in mesangial cells and matrix, an inflammatory cellular infiltrate and basement membrane damage. Mesangial proliferative nephritis has the best prognosis and is characterized by immune complex and complement deposition predominantly in the mesangium with an increase in mesangial cellularity and matrix. Focal and segmental proliferative nephritis has involvement of some parts (segmental) of some glomeruli (focal) only. This is manifested by an increase in the resident glomerular endothelial and mesangial cells as well as infiltrating inflammatory cells.

Case 9.1 SLE: 2

Case progress

Melanie remained stable for 2 years. At the end of this period, she again became unwell and developed a malar rash, polyarthritis, chest pain, shortness of breath and vasculitic lesions on her hands. An abnormal urinary sediment with haematuria and proteinuria was noted on urinalysis. Proteinuria usually indicates excessive leakiness of the glomerular basement membrane which, in combination with haematuria, almost certainly

indicates glomerular inflammation. Accordingly, a renal biopsy was performed and confirmed acute glomerulonephritis (Fig. 9.3). The results of laboratory tests revealed she was anaemic, had an elevated ESR and C-reactive protein, normal creatinine, low C3 and C4 and her dsDNA was markedly elevated. The patient was commenced on high-dose prednisone and azathioprine. Her clinical picture stabilized with the institution of the above therapy.

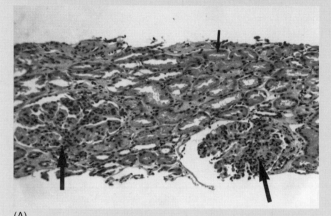

(A)

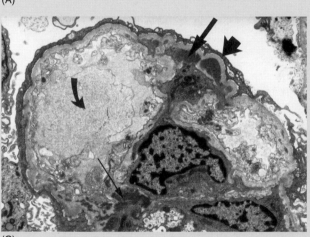

(C)

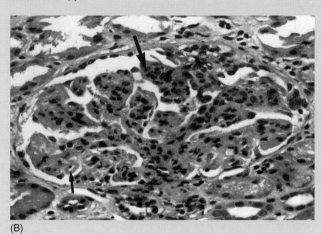

(B)

Fig. 9.3 (A) Low power photomicrograph of a renal biopsy showing two glomeruli (large arrows) and normal tubules (small arrow). (B) High power photomicrograph of a glomerulus showing features of a diffuse proliferative glomerulonephritis. There is an increase in mesangial cellularity (large arrow) and lobulation as well as thickened capillary loops (small arrow). (C) Electron micrograph of a capillary loop showing fusion of foot processes (short wide arrow) in diffuse proliferative glomerulonephritis (Type IV). Other notable features are subendothelial electron-dense deposits (straight large arrow) and focal mesangial deposits (straight thin arrow). The curved arrow indicates the capillary lumen (courtesy of Dr Thomas Ng, Institute of Clinical Pathology and Medical Research, Westmead Hospital).

This form of nephritis has a variable prognosis. Diffuse proliferative nephritis is the most concerning form of lupus nephritis. There are usually significant increases in glomerular cellularity, fibrin deposition and necrosis resulting in crescent formation. On electron microscopic examination, the immune deposits reside in the mesangium and on the subepithelial and subendothelial sides of the glomerular basement membrane. Another form of nephritis is membranous nephritis. This has diffusely thickened capillary loops with marked proteinuria. Advanced sclerosing nephritis is characterized by glomerular fibrosis and sclerosis.

Other clinicopathologic correlations

Constitutional symptoms of lethargy, malaise, and feeling unwell are common features of active SLE and may herald the onset of a flare. Cytokines produced as a result of inflammation are believed to be responsible for the lethargy and fatigue. Serum levels of tumour necrosis factor alpha (TNF-α), IFN-α, IFN-γ and IL-6 are elevated in SLE while TNF-α levels have been shown to correlate with disease activity in SLE. These symptoms are non-specific and one should be cautious

Table 9.3 World Health Organization classification of lupus nephritis

	Type	Approximate prevalence (%)
I	Normal glomeruli	<10
II	Mesangial proliferative	10
III	Focal and segmental proliferative	15
IV	Diffuse proliferative	50
V	Membranous	15
VI	Advanced sclerosing	<10

Adapted from Becker G J, Whitworth J A, Kincaid-Smith P 1992 Clinical nephrology in medical practice. Blackwell, Victoria.

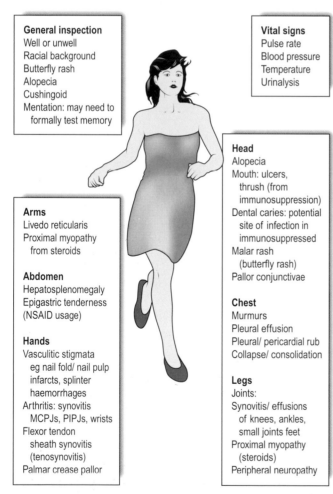

General inspection
Well or unwell
Racial background
Butterfly rash
Alopecia
Cushingoid
Mentation: may need to
   formally test memory

Vital signs
Pulse rate
Blood pressure
Temperature
Urinalysis

Head
Alopecia
Mouth: ulcers,
   thrush (from
   immunosuppression)
Dental caries: potential
   site of infection in
   immunosuppressed
Malar rash
   (butterfly rash)
Pallor conjunctivae

Chest
Murmurs
Pleural effusion
Pleural/ pericardial rub
Collapse/ consolidation

Legs
Joints:
Synovitis/ effusions
   of knees, ankles,
   small joints feet
Proximal myopathy
   (steroids)
Peripheral neuropathy

Arms
Livedo reticularis
Proximal myopathy
   from steroids

Abdomen
Hepatosplenomegaly
Epigastric tenderness
(NSAID usage)

Hands
Vasculitic stigmata
   eg nail fold/ nail pulp
   infarcts, splinter
   haemorrhages
Arthritis: synovitis
   MCPJs, PIPJs, wrists
Flexor tendon
   sheath synovitis
   (tenosynovitis)
Palmar crease pallor

Fig. 9.4 Clinical manifestations of SLE. This is a multi-system disease.

of underlying infection. The major clinical features to examine for are depicted pictorially in Figure 9.4. The common clinicopathological features are discussed below.

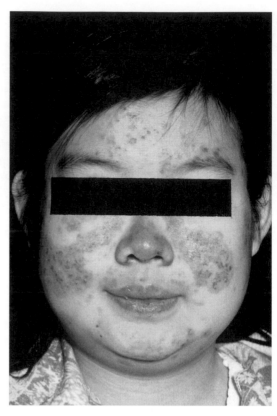

Fig. 9.5 The malar (butterfly) rash of SLE (courtesy of Professor Les Schrieber, Department of Rheumatology, Royal North Shore Hospital).

Skin

Skin lesions in SLE patients are classified as either acute (butterfly rash, photosensitivity), sub-acute (sub-acute cutaneous lupus erythematosus or SCLE) or chronic (discoid). The characteristic acute malar butterfly rash seen in acute flares presents as an erythematous, elevated, and painful photosensitive lesion (Fig. 9.5) that spares the nasolabial fold. The malar rash is the commonest recognized skin manifestation of SLE. Conditions such as cellulitis of the face or rosacea do not spare the nasolabial fold. Other acute lesions include erythema in sun-exposed areas (photosensitivity) or blistering lesions in dark-skinned individuals. It has been found that lymphocytes from SLE patients are activated by light in the near ultraviolet (360–400 nm) wavelength. This heightened activity may result in tissue damage and exposure of an autoantigen which further stimulates the immune-mediated process occurring in skin. Localized fixed lesions may also be seen and are termed discoid lupus. These are erythematous plaques or papules with a hypopigmented central area that may occur in the presence or absence of systemic manifestations of SLE.

Other non-specific dermatological manifestations of SLE are protean and may include panniculitis, urticaria and vasculitic lesions such as palpable purpura. Histologic examination of the skin reveals non-specific inflammation

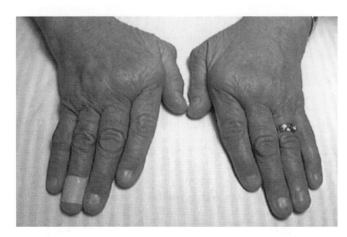

Fig. 9.6 A lupus patient with Jaccoud's arthritis. The features include a symmetric deforming hand arthritis with ulnar deviation at the metacarpophalangeal joints. Unlike rheumatoid arthritis, the deformities are reducible and there are no signs of joint erosion on X-ray.

with abundant immune deposits on immunofluorescence at the dermo–epidermal junction.

Musculoskeletal

Arthralgia and/or arthritis are the commonest clinical manifestations of SLE. Synovitis is due to inflammation induced by deposition of antigen–antibody immune complexes with complement activation and release of inflammatory cytokines, of which TNF-α and interleukin-1 and -6 (IL-1, IL-6) feature prominently. The arthritis seen in SLE usually affects the small joints of the hand, wrists and knees. Although most cases of SLE arthritis are symmetric, asymmetric presentations can occur. It may be distinguished from rheumatoid arthritis (RA) because it is non-erosive. Although nodules are more common in RA, they may also occur in SLE. Tenosynovitis is frequently seen in SLE. Significant joint deformity may occur in SLE. This pattern of non-erosive but deforming disease is termed 'Jaccoud's arthritis' and may be confused with RA. In these patients, the hand deformities include subluxation with ulnar deviation at the metacarpophalangeal joints (Fig. 9.6). This is a non-erosive arthritis and the deformities are reducible—unlike the fixed deformities seen in RA. Radiological examination of the hands reveals only peri-articular osteoporosis due to disuse and soft tissue swelling, but no erosions or joint destruction. This is often surprising given that significant deformity may be present clinically.

Avascular necrosis of bone may be seen in SLE, particularly in the presence of a positive anti-cardiolipin antibody. It is more commonly seen in the context of corticosteroid usage, however, this diagnosis should always be considered in a patient with SLE who presents with acute onset severe bony pain, regardless of whether or not they are being treated with corticosteroids. The underlying mechanism is presumed to be thrombotic in aetiology.

Renal

This is one of the major determinants of morbidity and mortality in lupus. Patients do not usually volunteer symptoms pertaining to this system until late in the course of renal failure. Symptoms may include shortness of breath, headache, oliguria (reduced urine output) and ankle oedema. Lupus nephritis may often be clinically silent. It is worth remembering that urinalysis should be considered as part of the physical examination. It provides an immense amount of clinical information. In this case, it identified the onset of lupus nephritis. Although renal involvement is suggested by an elevated creatinine, proteinuria, haematuria and presence of casts, the only way to accurately determine the type and extent of renal involvement is by renal biopsy and histologic examination. However, given that a renal biopsy may be complicated by significant morbidity, for example bleeding, it is usually only indicated if an abnormality is detected in one or more of the above parameters.

Once performed, histologic and immunologic examination of the tissue obtained is useful in both diagnosis and prognosis. The presence of acute inflammatory changes such as cellular proliferation, cellular crescents and leukocyte infiltration, necessitates the institution of potent immunosuppressive therapy in an attempt to reverse the inflammatory changes and prevent further renal damage. On the other hand, while the presence of chronic changes such as sclerotic glomeruli and fibrosis may augur poorly for the patient's renal function, it does not require the commencement of immunosuppressive therapy.

Neuropsychiatric

SLE may affect the central and peripheral nervous systems and cause abnormal (psychiatric) behaviour. Central nervous system (CNS) involvement may be sub-divided into: (a) organic brain syndrome, manifested by focal signs, seizures, strokes or chorea; or (b) psychosis, often with depression, dementia, hallucinations, and delusions. The diagnosis of neuropsychiatric lupus is difficult and a large number of imaging techniques (e.g. MRI, CT scan, PET) are not specific in making the diagnosis. However, the presence of multiple high-signal lesions on MRI in a young person with appropriate autoimmune serology is highly suggestive of cerebral lupus. These imaging modalities are useful in excluding other causes of CNS dysfunction such as infection in SLE patients. The diagnosis of neuropsychiatric lupus is predominantly a clinical one.

Pulmonary

Lung involvement in SLE may include pleurisy, pneumonitis, pulmonary haemorrhage, pulmonary hypertension and pulmonary embolism. Pneumonitis may simulate pneumonia with clinical features of fever, cough and haemoptysis. Serositis is a generic term for inflammation of serosal membranes lining visceral and thoracic organs. Pleurisy and pericarditis are two examples and may manifest as inflammation or effusions. Pulmonary vasculitis is uncommon but may present precipitously with haemoptysis. The other cause of haemoptysis that requires exclusion is pulmonary emboli, particularly in the setting of the anti-phospholipid antibody syndrome (APLAS). Pulmonary hypertension, usually presenting in patients as dyspnoea, may be the result of recurrent pulmonary emboli or pulmonary vasculitis.

Gastroenterology

Abdominal serositis (peritonitis) may manifest as abdominal pain. One of the most feared gastrointestinal manifestations is vasculitis of the mesenteric blood vessels which may either present subacutely with chronic post-prandial abdominal pain or acutely with mesenteric infarction. Pancreatitis may occur in SLE with or without the co-existent use of corticosteroids. Many SLE patients are treated with non-steroidal anti-inflammatory drugs (NSAIDs) for symptomatic relief and thus may present with peptic ulcer disease or gastrointestinal bleeding. The commonest hepatic abnormality seen in SLE is a non-specific hepatitis with elevation of the transaminases (AST and ALT). This may occur secondary to the use of NSAIDs or other immunosuppressives such as azathioprine or methotrexate. Specific autoimmune liver involvement with characteristic anti-smooth muscle and anti-mitochondrial antibodies are features of autoimmune chronic active hepatitis and primary biliary cirrhosis, respectively. These diseases are organ-specific and are not features of SLE.

Cardiac involvement

The endocardium, myocardium and pericardium can be involved. Clinical features include a murmur, tachycardia, arrhythmia and heart failure. Cardiovascular and coronary artery disease has been reported to be a major cause of premature morbidity and mortality in lupus. The pathogenesis is multifactorial, with contributions from vascular wall inflammation, corticosteroid effects on the lipid profile, renal disease, hypertension and thrombosis in the setting of anti-phospholipid antibodies. With the exception of anti-phospholipid antibody-induced thromboses, the other factors tend to impact after 10–20 years of lupus activity.

Anti-phospholipid antibody syndrome

These are autoantibodies directed against components of the cellular membrane. The APLAS or anti-cardiolipin antibody syndrome has three components: (1) arterial and/or venous thrombosis; (2) thrombocytopenia or a reduced platelet count; and (3) spontaneous abortions associated with persistently positive anticardiolipin antibodies or lupus anticoagulant. It may occur as a primary event with no apparent cause or in association with an

---

Case 9.1 SLE: 3

Clinical case

Recall that Melanie was anaemic when she flared. In SLE this can be due to a number of factors, including the anaemia of chronic disease, renal failure, autoimmune haemolysis and iron deficiency due to poor dietary intake or blood loss induced by NSAIDs. In our patient, the two main factors were an anaemia of chronic disease compounded by poor dietary intake. There was no evidence of autoimmune haemolysis on the blood film, her serum creatinine level was in the normal range and she was not on any NSAIDs. Her ESR was markedly elevated at 112 mm/h and her CRP was also elevated. The ESR and CRP are objective markers of inflammation. Inflammation leads to an increase in serum proteins such as fibrinogen, immunoglobulins, ferritin and alpha-1-antitrypsin, which are known as acute phase reactants. These proteins cause red cells to become adherent to each other and hence sediment faster. An ESR is a sensitive but not particularly specific test for inflammation. The presence of a significantly elevated ESR (>100 mm/h) should raise the suspicion of a connective tissue disorder, chronic infection such as tuberculosis or bacterial endocarditis, malignancy or a paraprotein. In the elderly with headache and an elevated ESR, giant cell (temporal) arteritis should be considered (Ch. 1).

The CRP is a specific acute phase reactant whose hepatic synthesis is upregulated predominantly by interleukin-6 (IL-6), which in turn is upregulated in inflammation. Its half-life is only a few days. As such, the CRP tends to mirror the clinical course of inflammation more closely than an ESR.

Melanie's twin sister becomes symptomatic with fatigue and arthralgia and questions if she could also have lupus. Investigation reveals a positive ANA and the presence of antibodies against dsDNA. The development of lupus in her sister raises questions about aetiology and the role of genetic versus environmental factors in the predisposition to disease. The issues surrounding aetiology, management and clinical outcome are discussed below.

---

underlying connective tissue disease (secondary). About half of all patients with the APLAS have the primary form of the disease. Anti-phospholipid antibodies are found in approximately one-third of all patients with lupus and up to 2% of normal controls. Both primary and secondary APLAS have similar manifestations and the activity of APLAS in SLE is independent of the clinical activity of the lupus. Long-term anticoagulation is generally indicated.

Aetiology

Environmental factors

The aetiology of SLE is unclear but probably results from an interplay between susceptibility genes and environmental stimuli. Potential environmental stimuli that could trigger the process include stress, sunlight, drugs/chemicals (procainamide, hydralazine, sulphonamides), pollutants/toxins, hairsprays, diet (alfalfa sprouts) and infections (viruses, bacterial superantigens). As yet, there is no convincing evidence for involvement of a specific infective agent in the aetiology of SLE. Viral agents possibly implicated in SLE are CMV, EBV and retroviruses.

It has been postulated that an environmental agent, such as a microbe, may produce autoimmune disease in a genetically susceptible host by 'molecular mimicry'. That is, the antigen incites antibodies that cross-react with the host's proteins. Alternatively, the inciting agent may alter the structure of proteins in the host, thus resulting in a breakdown of immune tolerance in the host.

Superantigens are antigens that interact with major histocompatibility complex (MHC) class II molecules on the surface of antigen-presenting cells and with specific elements of the T-cell receptor (TCR). This mode of immune activation can trigger T-cell proliferation and the release of large concentrations of cytokines leading to fever, malaise and, at times, shock. In addition, superantigens may bridge T cells and B cells, allowing rapid polyclonal B-cell activation with autoantibody secretion. Superantigens may originate from bacteria and thus may provide the link between infection and triggering of autoimmunity. As yet there is no clear evidence indicating that superantigens may directly trigger SLE in human beings.

Genetics

Persuasive evidence for a genetic influence on SLE predisposition has arisen from twin studies, familial aggregation, studies of ethnicity and experimental animal models of the disease. In SLE, supporting data for each of these parameters makes the case for genetic predisposition compelling. In twin studies, there is a higher concordance for disease in monozygotic (24–60%) than in dizygotic twins (5%). Similarly, family studies have provided convincing evidence of a genetic basis in SLE by identifying an increased prevalence of disease in siblings from the same family compared with the normal population.

Numerous studies have attempted to find associations between candidate genes and patients with SLE. Of these the major histocompatibility locus (MHC) genes have been the most extensively studied. The B8-DR3 haplotype is associated with SLE in Caucasian individuals. Since these genes are in linkage disequilibrium with other MHC genes, the extended haplotype associated with SLE is A1-B8-C4A0-DR3-DQW2. The DQ genes have been shown to correlate better with autoantibody formation than with clinical phenotype, for example anti-Sm has been associated with DR2, 4, 7 and DQ6; anti-Ro with DR2, 4 and DQbeta; anti-phospholipid antibodies with DR4, 7 and DQ6 and 7.

Much of the genetic information about human lupus has come from experimental studies in murine lupus models. These studies have identified several susceptibility loci

predisposing mice to develop lupus. There is no one single gene defect as the cause of SLE. It appears that a number of genes are required that collectively contribute to the clinical syndrome.

Treatment

The management of SLE is largely dependent on the severity of the disease and the type and extent of organ involvement. Simpler measures such as education and psychosocial intervention can affect morbidity and mortality and should therefore not be underestimated. Infections that can mimic flares should be excluded and/or treated early and aggressively.

General principles (prevention)

Avoid the sun This involves the use of sunscreen cream (at least SPF 15+), a hat, long-sleeved clothing or even a change in occupation.

Avoidance of infections This may require yearly influenza vaccines and prompt treatment of any infection.

Tight control of blood pressure Attention to control of hypertension is important in minimizing damage to the renal vasculature.

Contraception This is important in women with lupus nephritis as pregnancy may cause further deterioration of already tenuous renal function along with increased fetal morbidity and mortality. It is clear from all the published data that as the degree of renal insufficiency increases, the risk that renal function will worsen during pregnancy rises sharply. The issue of contraception is also of strong relevance if cytotoxic therapy is being used as the effects of such therapy on an unborn foetus are of concern.

Regular follow-up Some indicators of disease flares can only be detected by urine or blood tests. Regular follow-up by a physician for potential side-effects from medications or disease flares should be performed regularly.

Drug therapy

Non-steroidal anti-inflammatory drugs (NSAIDs)

These are useful for symptomatic relief and are usually given as first-line treatment, either alone or in combination with the other drugs discussed below, for mild flares of inflammatory symptoms such as serositis and arthritis. The significant side-effects of gastrointestinal bleeding and renal impairment should be looked for closely. Since NSAIDs may affect renal function by decreasing renal perfusion or by causing acute interstitial nephritis, they should be discontinued in patients suspected of having renal involvement. Renal impairment is thought to arise by inhibition of the vasodilatory prostaglandins that mediate renal perfusion and is more prevalent in the elderly and in those with pre-existing renal impairment. NSAIDs may also aggravate hypertension via promoting salt and water retention in the kidney. The newer cyclooxygenase-2 inhibitors appear to require a similar degree of caution in patients with renal failure as conventional NSAIDs.

An unusual feature of ibuprofen (a conventional NSAID) in SLE patients is its propensity to induce an aseptic meningitis syndrome characterized by headache, fever and meningism. The symptoms resolve on cessation of the drug.

Anti-malarials

Hydroxychloroquine is useful for the dermatologic, musculoskeletal and mild constitutional manifestations of lupus. Its mechanism of action is uncertain but it may work by interfering with lysosomal function and thus impairing phagocytic activity. It is a weak immunosuppressant that does not require regular blood monitoring and is usually used in conjunction with sunscreens and topical steroids. Side-effects include corneal deposits and retinal toxicity. These side-effects are less with hydroxychloroquine than with chloroquine. Although the risk of retinal toxicity due to hydroxychloroquine is low, formal ophthalmological review every 12 months to detect any restriction in visual fields is recommended. Anti-malarials are of little value for the 'visceral' manifestations of SLE, such as nephritis or vasculitis.

Corticosteroids

These drugs, already discussed in Chapter 1, form the cornerstone of treatment for the acute active manifestations of lupus. Corticosteroids can be given intravenously for acute life-threatening presentations, intra-articularly, topically, orally and at times intralesionally for discoid lupus. Doses of more than 20 mg/day of prednisone significantly increase the risk of susceptibility to infection.

Immunosuppressive agents

These agents are often used as 'steroid-sparing' agents to provide more potent immunosuppression in those with disease unable to be controlled by the above agents alone.

The commencement of potent immunosuppressive therapy such as azathioprine or cyclophosphamide is never undertaken lightly, especially in a female of reproductive age. Due consideration needs to be given to contraception or even the harvesting of eggs for storage prior to commencement of therapy. The effects of such medication on a foetus are obviously poorly studied and pregnancy should be avoided. This must be clearly explained to the patient.

Cyclophosphamide

This alkylating agent reduces the risk of end-stage renal disease in diffuse proliferative lupus nephritis. Its substantial side-effect profile includes bone marrow toxicity, nausea, infertility, alopecia, bladder cancer and an increased long-term risk of haemoatpoietic malignancy. One of the metabolites of cyclophosphamide (acrolein) is directly toxic to the bladder mucosa and thus the administration of cyclophosphamide should always be followed by a generous fluid intake to flush through the breakdown products of the drug. Mesna (sodium 2-mercaptoethanesulfonate) may be given to further minimize the likelihood of haemorrhagic cystitis. Cyclophosphamide may be administered orally as a daily dose or intravenously on a 'pulse' basis every 4–6 weeks.

Azathioprine

The limiting side-effects of azathioprine are bone marrow toxicity and gastrointestinal intolerance. Long-term usage increases the risk of haemoatpoietic malignancy. While less toxic than cyclophosphamide, it is less effective in severe renal disease. It has a role as a steroid-sparing agent. Co-administration with allopurinol should be undertaken with great caution due to the fact that both drugs inhibit xanthine oxidase and accumulation of high levels of either drug may manifest as profound cytopenias.

Mycophenolate mofetil

This drug is growing in popularity and increasingly used in the treatment of lupus nephritis because of its efficacy and good tolerability. The compound is a potent, selective, uncompetitive and reversible inhibitor of inosine monophosphate dehydrogenase which inhibits the de novo pathway of guanosine nucleotide synthesis necessary for DNA synthesis. Because T and B cells have no other salvage pathways of producing guanosine, mycophenolic acid has a very specific and potent cytostatic effect on these cells.

Cyclosporin

This is another drug which is sometimes used as a steroid-sparing agent, particularly in patients unable to tolerate one of the more 'traditional' drugs mentioned above. Its mode of action is by complexing with an intracellular protein, cyclophilin, to inhibit IL-2 production and suppress T-cell activation. Unfortunately, it has a long list of potential side-effects, including renal impairment, hypertension, hirsutism, tremor and immunosuppression. Renal toxicity is dose-dependent and predictable, occurring especially in those with pre-existing renal impairment. It is not recommended in those with lupus nephritis. Another complicating factor is its potential interaction with other medications metabolized by the cytochrome P450 enzyme pathway. These include macrolide antibiotics (erythromycin) and certain calcium channel blockers which elevate serum cyclosporin levels. Regular monitoring of renal function, blood pressure and urinalysis is mandatory. Unlike its use in transplant medicine, routine monitoring of cyclosporin blood levels is unnecessary as the doses used in rheumatology are significantly lower.

Other agents

The role of methotrexate in the treatment of SLE is uncertain despite it having established itself as the drug of choice in the treatment of rheumatoid arthritis (see Ch. 1). Dapsone is sometimes used in the management of discoid, subacute cutaneous, bullous and profundus skin lesions due to SLE. Haematological side-effects are common and should be monitored. Danazol is useful in the treatment of discoid lupus and lupus thrombocytopenia. There are a number of hormonal side-effects that need monitoring.

Other newer biological modalities, such as Rituximab (anti-CD20 monoclonal antibody) with the ability to deplete B cells alone or in combination with cyclophosphamide shows potential as new therapy in patients with lupus nephritis refractory to the conventional immunosuppressive therapy. Anti-tumour necrosis factor antibodies (anti-TNF) are not indicated for the treatment of SLE.

Variants of SLE

SLE is a heterogeneous disorder that may manifest in a variety of presentations that collectively form a syndrome. These include:

Subacute cutaneous lupus erythematosus

This term refers to a specific group of patients distinct from systemic lupus erythematosus characterized by photosensitive skin lesions which wax and wane without residual scarring. They are usually distributed in the 'V-shaped' area of the chest and extensor surfaces of the arms. The skin lesions are usually papules or plaques with a small amount of scale and may be associated with arthralgia or arthritis and a positive anti-Ro (SS-A) antibody in approximately 70% of cases. They may enlarge into confluent areas which may mimic psoriasis.

Neonatal lupus

Some children born to mothers with SLE may develop a lupus dermatitis that fades over the ensuing months. They may display transiently positive ANA tests. Thrombocytopenia due to maternal antiplatelet antibodies traversing the placenta, haemolytic anaemia or leukopenia may also occur. Less commonly, the infants may develop congenital heart block which requires placement of a permanent pacemaker. Anti-Ro/La (SS-A/SS-B) antibodies are present in approximately 80% of mothers of children with congenital heart block and are thought to play a pathogenic role in this disorder.

Drug-induced lupus

This syndrome is seen in patients without a prior history of SLE that have recently been placed on a drug and develop fever, arthritis and serositis typical of SLE. These clinical features are usually less florid than those with 'idiopathic' lupus. Serology reveals a positive ANA with antibodies to ssDNA (single-stranded DNA) but not to dsDNA. Antibodies to histones occur in 90% of cases. The anti-histone antibodies are non-specific and can be seen in a small percentage of idiopathic SLE. Complement levels are usually normal. Unlike SLE there is no renal or CNS involvement. Drugs implicated include procainamide, hydralazine, sulphonamides, methyldopa and isoniazid. Procainamide is the drug most strongly associated with drug-induced SLE. Clinical symptoms improve when the drug is withdrawn. Of recent interest has been the association between the patient's acetylator status and the propensity to develop drug-induced lupus. Slow acetylators tend to develop ANA and features of drug-induced lupus quicker than rapid acetylators.

Further reading

Harris Jr, E.D., Budd, R.C., Ruddy, S. (Eds.), 2005. Kelley's Textbook of Rheumatology, seventh ed. Elsevier Saunders, Philadelphia.
Hochberg, M.C., 1997. Updating the American College of Rheumatology revised criteria for the classification of systemic lupus erythematosus. Arthritis Rheum. 40 (9), 1725.
Hochberg, M.C., Silman, A.J., Smolen, J.S. et al. (Eds.), 2008. Rheumatology, fourth ed.. Mosby, St Louis.
Klippel, J., Stone, J.H., Crofford, L.J., White, P.H. (Eds.), 2008. Primer on the Rheumatic Diseases, thirteenth ed. Springer, Wien.
Manolios, N., Schrieber, L., 1997. Systemic lupus erythematosus. In: Bradley, J., McCluskey, J. (Eds.), Clinical Immunology. Oxford University Press, Oxford.
Weening, J.J., D'Agati, V.D., Schwartz, M.M., et al., 2004. The classification of glomerulonephritis in systemic lupus erythematosus revisited. Kidney Int. 65 (2), 521–530.

TRAUMA AND THE MUSCULOSKELETAL SYSTEM

10

*Andrew M. Ellis
and Thomas Taylor*

Chapter objectives

After studying this chapter you should be able to:

1. Understand the biological basis of fracture healing.

2. Outline principles of management of fractures and understand how to initially manage injuries of the musculoskeletal system.

3. Recognize broad groupings of complications of fractures.

4. Understand the principles by which life- and limb-threatening injuries are assessed and priorities of management are assigned.

5. Understand the functional anatomy of the knee and recognize and describe the significance of ligamentous injuries of the knee.

Introduction

Musculoskeletal injury frequently occurs in the setting of major trauma. The energy required to produce fractures, especially of diaphysial bone in young people, is considerable. Such energy is often associated with falls from a height, motor vehicle accidents, workplace accident or assault. Blunt trauma is more common but penetrating trauma (from bullets in particular) is not uncommon in some parts of the world. The key factor to appreciate is that musculoskeletal injury may occur in association with life-threatening injury such as tension pneumothorax, for example. Such other injury receives priority of treatment during initial assessment. Recognizing that life-threatening injury has many reversible elements, the American College of Surgeons has developed a programme that is taught worldwide to provide a system of recognition, prioritization and treatment of such injury.

This system, known as advanced trauma life support (ATLS), provides a systematic approach in which life-threatening injury is first identified in a process known as primary survey. Problems with the airway, breathing, circulation and neurological disability are sought and treated (ABCD) while the patient is resuscitated, and then other less important injury is identified by means of secondary survey. It is beyond the scope of this chapter to deal any more with this system, except to say that it forms the backbone of modern trauma management. ATLS is a registered trademark of the American College of Surgeons Committee on Trauma, and medical practitioners working in the field of injury are strongly advised to seek this qualification.

Interesting facts

Injury deaths worldwide are estimated at more than 5 million per year. Motor vehicle crashes (road traffic accidents) cause more than 1 million deaths annually and 20–50 million significant injuries. Trauma remains the leading cause of death between 1 and 44 years of age. By 2020, it is estimated that more than 1 in 10 people will die from injury. Global trauma-related deaths are estimated to exceed US$500 billion annually.

Source: American College of Surgeons Committee on Trauma 2008 ATLS Student Course Manual, 8th edn.

Terminology

Developing a precise but common language is important for both communication and understanding of the mechanisms and patterns of fracture.

- *Fracture*: a structural break in the continuity of bone.

- *Open fracture*: where the overlying skin is breached, allowing communication between the fracture and the outside. Open fractures are often referred to as compound fractures but the former is the preferred and more correct term.

- *Closed fracture*: the overlying skin is intact.

- *Pathological fracture*: a fracture caused by normal force in abnormal bone.

- *Stress fracture*: a fracture caused by repetitive 'normal' forces.

- *Insufficiency fracture*: a type of pathological fracture occurring in osteoporotic bone, e.g. a compression fracture of the thoracic vertebra occurring in a postmenopausal woman (see Ch. 5).

- *Greenstick fracture*: a type of incomplete fracture that occurs in children. Because of the relatively high moisture content and strength of collagen in children, bones tend to bend or fracture incompletely. The fracture looks as the name implies.

- *Growth plate or physis*: consists of cartilage until skeletal maturity.

- *Diaphysis*: shaft of a long bone. Consists of cortical or lamellar bone. Loads well in compression but does not tolerate torque (twisting) force well.

- *Metaphysis*: the flare of a long bone towards the joint. Consists of cancellous or trabecular bone.

- *Epiphysis*: the part beyond the growth plate leading up to the joint surface. Blends with the growth plate scar to form the metaphysis beyond skeletal maturity.

- *Dislocation*: disruption of a joint such that the normally opposing joint surfaces have no contact with each other.

- *Subluxation*: disruption of a joint such that the normally opposing joint surfaces have some contact with each other but are not congruous.

Pathophysiology

Bone has a remarkable capacity to heal, far exceeding that of all other connective tissues. Unfortunately, hyaline articular cartilage has none (see Ch. 6). The inherent determination of fractures to repair is viewed as a highly efficient, primitive response to injury. Moreover, many residual deformities from fractures can remodel with time and leave no trace of the original injury.

The repair process is different in cortical and cancellous bone and this is not at all surprising when one considers the functions and biology of the two tissues (summarized in Table 10.1; return to Ch. 5 to review this in more detail).

In general terms, cancellous or trabecular bone is strong in compression and weak in tension. Most often its honeycomb, sponge-like structure fails in compression, for example a crush fracture of a vertebral body with excessive axial loading as sustained in a fall from a height. The tissue is compacted as the trabecular bone fails. Healing is directly between endosteal surfaces with no significant

Trauma: 1

Case history

Max is a 20-year-old apprentice plumber. He is travelling home from visiting family in the country when he is involved in a high-speed motor vehicle accident. His car hits a tree near the outskirts of a large town. The police report suggests that high speed, alcohol and fatigue have all contributed to the accident. The ambulance report shows that he is conscious (Glasgow Coma Score 14), was restrained and has signs indicative of a right knee injury, an open fracture of the right femur and a fracture of the right ankle. He has no other injuries.

He is brought to the Emergency Department where life-threatening injury is excluded and resuscitation commences along the ATLS guidelines discussed above. The Glasgow Coma Score (GCS) is a uniform system for quantifying the extent of neurological injury. It is particularly important for monitoring change in levels of consciousness and neurological deterioration because of increasing intracranial pressure after head injury. Such a cause of change after injury might be an expanding extradural haematoma, for example. The GCS allows accurate monitoring of this change and, because of standardization, interobserver error and vagaries of description are minimized. Three main areas are assessed and the sums of the sections are combined to give a score. A GCS of 8 or below has become the generally accepted definition of coma. In this case, our patient has a GCS of 14, indicating that he is not in a coma and has a mild head injury only.

Radiographs are taken after the patient has been stabilized. These show a fracture-dislocation of the right femur through the diaphysis (Fig. 10.1), a fracture-dislocation of the right ankle (Fig. 10.2) and a swollen right knee without any obvious bony injury.

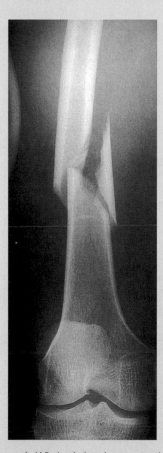

Fig. 10.1 Radiograph (AP view) showing a comminuted fracture of the shaft of the femur with a large butterfly segment.

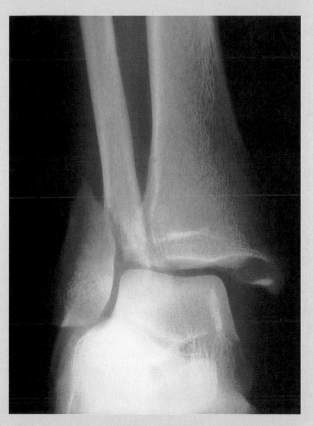

Fig. 10.2 Radiograph (AP view) showing fracture/dislocation of the ankle.

periosteal (indirect) contribution. The process is favoured by immobility (fixation) and the close apposition of the fracture surfaces. Hence, the very mechanism of injury produces circumstances conducive to healing. The rich blood supply is central to the reparative process. Non-union of a vertebral crush fracture is unknown.

According to the mechanism of certain cancellous bone fractures, there may be a gap at the fracture site. A displaced metaphyseal fracture is an example of this. Endosteal bone does not proliferate to fill the defect and delayed or non-union occurs. This is the rationale of open reduction and rigid internal fixation of widely displaced

Table 10.1 Features of cortical and cancellous bone

	Cortical	*Cancellous*
Location	Diaphyseal (shaft) bone	Metaphyseal (marrow) bone (carpal, tarsal, vertebral and flat bones)
Function	Mechanical	Primarily metabolic
Cortex	Thick	Thin
Periosteum	Thick	Thin
Turnover	Slow	Rapid
Blood supply	Slow	Rich

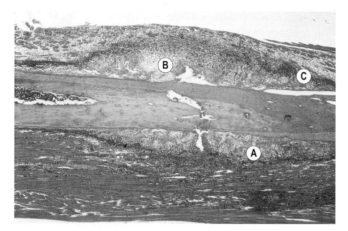

Fig. 10.3 Histology of healing fracture of diaphyseal bone: (A) early woven bone from organization of haematoma, which is well advanced (B); (C) note that the periosteum has been lifted by trauma.

metaphyseal fractures in adults. Fracture fragments are reduced and rigidly internally fixed.

Diaphysial bone is fractured by either direct or indirect (transmitted) violence. Obviously, the forces involved are very variable. So too are the resultant fracture patterns, which vary according to the way in which the forces are applied.

The reparative tissue has two components—one from the periosteum and the other produced by osteoinduction of primitive local mesenchymal stem cells. It is a highly efficient healing mechanism (Fig. 10.3).

The periosteal component When the periosteum is lifted from the underlying cortical bone, whether it be by trauma, tumour or pus, it responds by laying down bone. This is an activation of the normal process of bone formation. This component is always most in evidence in a fracture on the side with the least tissue disruption. It does not entail endochondral ossification and results from activity of osteoblasts in the inner *cambium* (Latin: bark) layer of the periosteum. Periosteal new bone formation is stimulated by movement and is abolished by rigid internal fixation. In osteosarcoma (a primary tumour of bone), the periosteum is lifted by the tumour and new

bone may form under the elevated periosteum giving rise to the radiological sign called Codman's triangle.

Osteoinduction The fracture haematoma provides the tissue scaffold for the transformation into the definitive reparative tissue. This is a complex process that until recently was not well understood. Local, primitive mesenchymal cells are transformed into osteoblasts under the influence of bone morphogenetic proteins (BMPs) of humoral and platelet origins, and other undefined cytokines. This transformation sees a spectrum of cellular events in the resultant callus. The histological picture is far from homogeneous. Areas where an endochondral sequence is proceeding are seen immediately adjacent to foci of ossification without an antecedent cartilage phase as well as areas of intermediate cellular appearance. The overall picture is one of intense cellular activity. A biopsy of callus, viewed out of the context of trauma, could easily be misinterpreted as a neoplastic process.

The haematoma is rapidly invaded by blood vessels (angiogenesis) and the subsequent callus acquires its own circulation. This is essential for normal healing. It has been postulated that the local release of vascular stimulating factors is central to this event, but the control mechanisms have not yet been identified. Further, it follows that successful vascularization will depend upon the integrity of the encompassing soft tissues. Hence, a variable degree of impairment of repair, even to the point of non-union, is not an unexpected sequel in those injuries where the surrounding soft tissues are severely crushed and traumatized.

Fracture callus is best viewed as temporary tissue. It is gradually formed into a three-dimensional mesh of relatively disorganized woven bone, which under the influence of physical forces, and especially muscle activity, is gradually transformed into highly organized lamellar bone with a cortex with central remodelling and re-establishment of the medullary canal.

Ligaments, tendons and joint capsules are designed to transmit tensile forces and are thus extremely strong in tension. They are far stronger in tension than is cancellous bone. When there is a traumatic angular deformation of a joint, the ligament may be injured (partially or completely ruptured) or it may be torn off (avulsed) from its metaphyseal attachment, taking with it a piece of bone which may be small (often erroneously called a 'chip') or quite large, according to varying circumstances. Such injuries are called avulsion fractures and in many instances, the fragment will not unite with its bed because of the displacement and the inability of the underlying cancellous bone to bridge the gap.

Functional anatomy of the knee joint

The key anatomical structures of the knee relevant to osteoarthritis were reviewed in Chapter 6. Here, we will review the anatomy of the knee joint with an emphasis on its functional anatomy relevant to musculoskeletal injury.

Case 10.1 Trauma: 2

Case note: Potential damage to the knee joint

Max's left knee is observed to be swollen with obliteration of the normal contours. The swelling extends above the patella. It is important to examine the knee joint for evidence of ligamentous damage, as it is known that a significant percentage of patients with a fracture of the shaft of the femur have concomitant knee ligament injury. This is not surprising given the forces that must be applied to the limb to produce a diaphysial fracture.

General joint morphology

Inasmuch as major morphological changes were required for hominids to walk upright and to stand erect with minimal effort, these are unique to the human knee and set it apart from the knee joints of all other creatures.

In the erect position, the line of centre of gravity passes behind the hip joint and in front of the knee and ankle joints. In full extension, the hip and knee joints are said to be 'locked'. Extension of the former is restrained by the substantial iliofemoral ligament, the strongest ligament in the body. Stability of the locked knee is dependent upon the femoral condyles, which are flattened in an anteroposterior direction (a human trait), and the collateral ligaments, which become taut in extension, as does the anterior cruciate ligament (ACL). Further, the upper surface of the tibia slopes backwards, resisting hyperextension.

The locking of the hip and knee joints allows humans to stand without activity of the respective extensor mechanisms. The reader can readily confirm this. As the hip and knee flex, as they do when we walk or run, these muscle groups come into action to stabilize the joints. Standing is a very efficient mechanism. On the other hand, the ankle joint cannot be locked and the plantigrade position is maintained by the tonic activity of the calf muscles, which force the foot against the ground. The reader will recall that humans get sore and stiff in the calves on prolonged standing, but not so in the buttocks and thighs. Next, stand with the hips and knees flexed at about 20°. You will soon appreciate that it takes considerable muscle effort to maintain this position. Hence, a flexion contracture of the knee joint constitutes a significant disability, particularly if the joint is painful owing to an arthropathy. A flexion contracture of up to 30° in the hip joint can be accommodated by increasing lumbar lordosis.

Because of the widened human pelvis, the femur makes a coronal plane angle of 6–10° with the tibia in the fully extended position. This is relatively larger in the female because of the wider pelvis. This configuration results in a tendency for the patella to move laterally when the quadriceps muscle contracts (Fig. 10.4). This is resisted by the elevated lateral femoral condyle, which

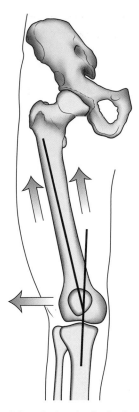

Fig. 10.4 Patella instability. The longitudinal axis of the femur makes an angle of approximately 6–10° with the tibia. The angle is slightly more in females because of the wider pelvis. A strong contraction of the quadriceps muscle will tend to displace the patella laterally. This is resisted by the direct attachment of the vastus and medialis components of the quadriceps to the inner margin of the patella.

is well seen in profile. The upper surfaces of the tibial plateaus are increased in an anteroposterior direction to accommodate the flattened femoral condyles (those of the chimpanzee are much rounder). Lastly, the ACL, which becomes taut in extension, helps guide the femur medially on the tibia in the last 15° of extension—the screw-home movement. This crucial mechanism results in grooving of the anterolateral surface of the intercondylar notch and the smooth depression can be easily seen and felt in well-preserved bones.

Muscle control

The extraordinarily powerful quadriceps group is attached distally to the readily palpable tibial tubercle. It becomes well developed and very strong in athletes, especially weightlifters—you lift with your knees. The vastus medialis controls patellar position by virtue of its fleshy attachment to the medial patella margin and it aids in the 'screw-home' movement required for full extension. It is the most specialized part of the quadriceps mechanism and atrophies quickly with disuse. Moreover, once weakened and atrophic, it is difficult for it to regain full strength and muscle bulk.

Range of motion

The normal range of movement is from 0–150° and approximately 60° of flexion is required for normal gait on flat ground. Because the cruciate and collateral ligaments become taut in full extension, no rotation is possible in this position. When the knee is flexed, there is approximately 15° of internal and external rotation and these movements are produced by the medial and lateral hamstrings, respectively. This is a small degree of freedom in both directions given the enormous stresses that athletes place upon their knees, particularly when the foot is fixed to the ground by cleats or rubber soles. Little wonder then that athletes are plagued by self-induced knee injuries. Natural selection did not take the demands of soccer, basketball and the like into its deliberate, gradual determinations.

Ligaments

Ligaments, like tendons, are composed almost exclusively of type I collagen. The lateral collateral ligament can easily be felt when the knee is flexed to 90° and crossed over the opposite thigh. This structure plays a relatively minor role in stability of the fully extended knee. When the knee is flexed, as it is in all human activities except standing, lateral stability is efficiently and effectively provided by the strong, wide iliotibial band. This is tensed by the action of the gluteus maximus muscle, three-quarters of which is inserted in the fascia lata, of which the band is a specialized part. The reader can verify this by standing on tiptoe with the knee and hips slightly flexed. The band is easily felt and will be noted to become less taut in the fully upright stance.

The medial collateral ligament is fan-shaped and distally has a wide attachment to the upper, inner aspect of the tibia, this strong structure being needed medially to combat the valgus deformity force in weight bearing, secondary to the femorotibial angle. The axis of flexion and extension passes through the condyles.

Joint capsule

This is 'redundant' anteriorly and posteriorly to allow flexion/extension by virtue of a loose criss-cross arrangement of capsular (collagen) fibres. Small amounts of elastin are so placed between bundles to assist in recoil after deformation. When a capsular injury or inflammation occurs, periarticular collagen is laid down (fibrosis) but then it is along the lines of stress and not in the preferential way described. Collagen is a virtually inextensible molecule and so too are ligaments and tendons—they have to be to serve their designated functions. Hence, capsular and periarticular fibrosis is an important cause of joint contractures and the associated disability.

Menisci—the semilunar cartilages

These structures are fibrocartilaginous notwithstanding the loose terminology. They are peculiar to joints where movements on either side of them are in different planes. They are crescentic in shape with tibial attachments at both ends (horns). The outer one-third is made up of distinct circumferential fibrous lamellae and it has a limited blood supply at the periphery. Centrally, the lamellated structure is lost and the avascular, more homogeneous tissue, is distinctly more cartilage-like. This tissue pattern indicates that the outer regions must withstand tensile forces and, more centrally, compression.

By their contour, with the upper surfaces being slightly concave, the menisci enhance joint stability. They also help in the distribution of synovial fluid essential for joint lubrication. They function as 'thrust pads', familiar to engineers. That is, they move in and out of the joint with flexion and extension. The reader can substantiate this as follows. Place the index finger immediately above the sharp anterior tibial margin adjacent to the patella tendon. Here the firm, rubbery meniscus can be palpated. With the knee flexed to 90° there is a shallow depression, which is obliterated as the joint is extended. The flattened inferior surface of the femoral condyle pushes the meniscus in a centrifugal fashion. The articular surface of the femur is grooved anteriorly to articulate with the meniscus and a shallow depression for this contact is seen in lateral radiographs.

Movement in the sagittal plane largely takes place between the femur and the meniscus and rotation between the meniscus and the tibia. As stated earlier, the femur rotates medially on the tibia as the joint is fully extended. If these movements are not synchronized, the meniscus may be trapped between the ends of the two bones and tear. It may occur, for example, if the foot is firmly fixed to the ground in an internally rotated position, and the flexed knee is suddenly extended as in rising quickly from a semi-crouched position. The medial meniscus is more liable to injury than its lateral counterpart, because it is attached to the inner aspect of the medial collateral ligament, which makes it more immobile than its lateral fellow. The popliteus muscle is a flexor of the knee joint and its tendon is attached to the posterior part of the lateral meniscus. Hence, when the joint is flexed, the lateral meniscus is retracted posteriorly out of harms way.

When a meniscus is torn in its mid-substance, the tear will not heal spontaneously (cf. hyaline articular cartilage). Longitudinal tears in the outer vascular lamellae have the capacity to repair, as do peripheral detachments.

Diagnosis of fracture

Diagnosing most fractures is usually easy. When a fracture occurs, a patient can usually give a history of a significant event, immediate and significant pain associated with loss of usefulness of the affected part and certain signs on examination (Box 10.1).

If the fracture is in a weight-bearing bone, a patient will find it very difficult to walk; if it is in the forearm, the patient might have to hold or support it with the opposite arm. To the examining doctor there may be swelling and bruising, and very marked local tenderness along the palpable part of the bone; deformity may be present and the patient will not easily use the affected limb. In some cases, the sign of crepitus will be demonstrated. This is the unique grating feeling of bone against bone and should not be actively sought in the conscious patient because of the amount of pain involved.

Most fractures occur in the way that Max's has; as the result of a single episode by a force powerful enough to fracture normal bone. An abnormal force has been applied to normal bone leaving the fracture. Cortical bone usually fails when a torque or twisting force is applied that exceeds the strength of a bone to resist a fracture. Occasionally, a normal force can be applied to abnormal bone leading to fracture, and in this case, this is known as a *pathological fracture*. Pathological fractures occur in abnormal bone and these might be bones affected by neoplastic disease (primary or secondary) or by metabolic process (e.g. rickets, osteomalacia, osteoporosis or Paget's disease). An accurate history is very important in ascertaining the exact mechanism of the fracture. Often it is the relatively minor nature of the injury that occurs that alerts the treating doctor to the presence of a pathological fracture.

Another type of fracture occurs when a normal stress is applied to normal bone but in an abnormal way. This is known as a stress fracture and occurs often when repetitive stress is applied in such a way as to cause fatigue failure of bone by means of a small crack that propagates under the repeated stress. Such a fracture might occur in athletes who over-train or in army recruits who do an excessive amount of marching.

The examining doctor should be able to localize the area very well and have a high suspicion of the presence of fracture in a conscious patient (Table 10.2) and thus be able to organize specific investigations (usually plain X-rays will suffice).

Management of fractures

After attention to first aid and treatment of associated injuries or haemorrhage, treatment involves reduction of the fracture (if there is displacement) and holding the fracture reduced. Early stability, from the time of injury or first medical assessment, can be provided by means of external temporary splints. Such temporary splints, made of padded boards, temporary plaster half casts (back-slabs) or specially made adjustable tubular frames, are an important part of the first aid of fractures.

Box 10.1 Physical signs of fracture

- Exquisite local tenderness
- Crepitus
- Deformity
- Swelling
- Loss of function

Undisplaced fractures may be well treated by closed means without the need to align or 'reduce' the fracture. A well-moulded cast may be all that is required for many fractures. Use of such a cast usually involves splinting the joint above and below a fracture so that the muscle forces that might lead to further displacement are neutralized. In the first few hours and days, swelling must be looked for, the plaster checked to ensure that it is not too tight and the limb rested and supported. This might be done with a triangular sling in the upper limb or by means of crutches and not bearing weight in the lower limb. Healing would be expected along the lines discussed previously. Generally, a cancellous fracture of the upper limb (e.g. radius) would heal in an adult in about 6 weeks. A diaphysial fracture takes twice as long, and a potentially weight-bearing fracture might need protection for a further period. In children, fractures often heal in about half the time of healing in adults, given their accelerated biological mechanisms.

Fractures that are displaced usually need to be aligned or reduced, to prevent the complication of malunion (healing in a non-anatomical position) and the resultant loss of function, obvious deformity or altered biomechanics that this might produce. Reduction may be closed (skin envelope intact, alignment achieved by manipulation of the limb) or open (the surgeon operates, opens the fracture and directly aligns it). Holding the fracture reduced may be by continuous traction, plaster or internal fixation. Reduction by closed manipulation usually involves traction along the line of the bone and, if further reduction is required, application of a force usually opposite to that which caused the fracture. Reduction must be confirmed by X-ray examination. Operative or open reduction is indicated if closed reduction is not possible or inadequate. Some of the indications for open reduction are listed in Table 10.3. The principles of treatment of an open fracture such as Max sustained are outlined in Box 10.2.

Box 10.2 Priorities of treatment of open fractures

- Identify and treat associated life-threatening injury
- Intravenous fluid resuscitation
- Intravenous antibiotics
- Splint limb and dress wound
- Tetanus prophylaxis, appropriate to immunization status
- Early surgical consultation
- Early surgical debridement and stabilization of fracture

Table 10.2 Decision-making in musculoskeletal injury

Questions	Answers
What was the mechanism of injury?	Does the history fit the fracture pattern?
	Reduction is achieved by reversing the mechanism of injury (dislocation also)
What are the deforming forces?	These must be overcome to achieve reduction. Remember gravity works 24 h a day
What are the neurovascular structures and organs (solid and hollow) at risk?	Always (in your mind's eye) paint the anatomy on the radiographs in three planes
Would further views or another form of imaging be helpful?	Anteroposterior and lateral X-rays are the minimal requirement
Is the bone normal?	Pathological fracture
Is it a fracture through cortical (diaphyseal) or cancellous bone?	Different mechanisms of healing
	Different methods of management
Is the fracture stable or unstable?	Examination under anaesthesia may be required. If deduced to be unstable, it must be made stable, or more so, by closed (plaster cast, etc.) or open means (internal fixation)

Case 10.1 | Trauma: 3

Clinical examination of the knee

The collateral ligaments

The stability of a joint is first examined in full extension. The tip of the index finger is placed over the middle of the joint line laterally and a varus stress is applied distally. If the lateral ligament is intact, there should be no opening of the joint space. The medial collateral integrity is similarly tested with a valgus stress. However, the anterior cruciate ligament (ACL) is taut in full extension, and if the medial collateral ligament (MCL) is ruptured, it may not be possible to open the joint medially. Hence, to test the MCL, the joint should be flexed 15–20°, and in Max's knee the examining finger detects a slight but definite opening at the joint line in its midpart. This indicates a partial tear in the MCL. If the anterior cruciate and medial collateral ligaments are both ruptured, then the joint can be widely opened with a valgus stress when the knee is in full extension.

The cruciate ligaments

Both knees are flexed to approximately 90° with Max supine and the feet placed together and parallel on the table. The joints are then viewed from the side. If the posterior cruciate ligament is ruptured, the tibia on the injured side will sag posteriorly on the femur. If the ACL is disrupted, common in football or skiing injuries, then the tibia can be passively drawn forward on the femur to a much greater degree than on the uninjured side (the anterior drawer sign). Slight anterior movement of the tibia on the femur is observed in normal knees. Further, with an ACL rupture, the knee can be passively hyperextended (into recurvatum). The cruciates are judged to be intact in Max's knee.

Pathology of ligament injuries

The configuration of the bundles of collagen in ligaments, and especially those that are fan-shaped, is such that for any given position of a joint, there is not equal tension on all collagen bundles. Further, the collagen is irregularly dispersed in the attachment to bone (Sharpey's fibres). When an angulatory force is applied to a joint, those bundles under maximum tension absorb the energy first, where it may be dissipated with only a small number of fibres actually rupturing. This is a safety mechanism. It explains why minor sprains are so common, moderate sprains such as Max sustained are rather infrequent and complete ruptures are unusual. In Max's case with slight opening on the medial joint line, the effective functional length of the ligament has been increased. The ligament does not shorten (contract) and some laxity will remain as a legacy to the injury. A complete rupture of the MCL is an indication for surgical repair. Moderate injuries such as Max has are not amenable to surgery. In minor sprains, the functional length of the ligament is not altered and there are no long-term consequences.

Longer-term considerations

The future of Max's knee will depend much upon maintaining the quadriceps mechanism in good condition and, as soon as pain and fracture healing permit, a regular isometric exercise programme will be instituted. Provided good muscle control is regained, Max will be able to function well from the point of view of his knee and even participate in sport. Many professional athletes have persistent laxity of the collateral ligamentous complexes and even cruciate-deficient knees, but still participate at a high level provided they have good muscle control. All sport is conducted with the knees flexed and here muscle control is vital. The player with persistent ligamentous laxity is always apprehensive about being caught off-guard, such as when he is tackled, and this is one reason why recurrent injuries in the ligamentous-deficient knee are so common.

Case 10.1   Trauma: 4

Fracture diagnosis and treatment priorities

In Max's case, physical examination revealed marked swelling in the mid-thigh and ankle associated with quite marked pain and a tendency for abnormal movement to occur as the limb was being examined. Pain limited the examination. Palpation of the bony landmarks around the ankle and the lateral border of the right femur showed that tenderness was particularly localized to the areas of fracture. Max was unable to move his right limb and was in significant pain.

Plain radiographs proved to be all that was required to see the obvious break in cortical bone in Max's femur with significant displacement (Fig. 10.1). The X-ray image of the ankle showed a degree of subluxation of the ankle joint that is obvious (Fig. 10.2).

Question

Look at the X-rays of Max's fractures and attempt to describe them so that another doctor could paint an accurate picture of the fracture without looking at the X-rays.

Fractures might be described in their radiological appearance in terms of the following parameters:

- site
- extent
- configuration
- relationship of the fragments to each other (displaced, angulated, rotated, lengthened, or shortened)
- whether the fractures are open to the skin or not.

Fractures can be associated with significant bleeding, and the priority of initial treatment with Max is to restore the circulatory loss associated with his hypovolaemic state. Loss of blood volume can be associated with quite marked physiological change. Initially, venous return falls leading to a decrease in the diastolic filling pressure and/or volume of the heart. This leads to a fall in cardiac output and may lead to significant failure of perfusion of end-organs, which untreated, might lead to death. The body has a number of protective measures in place to compensate for this, including the ability to sense a decrease in mean arterial pressure (by carotid and aortic baroreceptors, leading to an immediate sympathetic response). The sympathetic response leads to release of adrenaline and noradrenaline, allowing immediate constriction of arterioles, causing a rise in peripheral resistance and also helping to control bleeding. There is a reflex tachycardia in an attempt to improve output and perfusion and there is vasoconstriction of non-essential vascular beds (e.g. in the skin and abdomen). These changes often lead to a measurable alteration in signs and symptoms, including a fall in blood pressure and a rise in the heart rate; the patient may be pale, sweaty and peripherally shut down. The respiratory rate will increase in an attempt to improve oxygenation and the urinary output will fall in response to decreased renal perfusion.

Table 10.3   Fractures that require surgical stabilization

Type of fracture	Reason
Pathological fractures	Unlikely to heal spontaneously
Intra-articular fractures	To optimize joint function and to prevent secondary osteoarthritis
Open fracture	To reduce risk of infection
Unstable fracture (e.g. short oblique tibia and fibula)	Rates of malunion high by closed means
Slow-healing fracture (e.g. fractured neck of femur)	Surgical treatment leads to early mobilization and reduction in complications of prolonged bed rest (pneumonia, pressure sores, thromboembolic complications). Public health benefit from reduced hospitalization costs
Associated high levels of avascular necrosis (e.g. comminuted proximal humerus, subcapital femur)	Joint function likely to be affected. Often require artificial joint replacement (arthroplasty)

Fractures need careful follow-up and monitoring by an experienced practitioner. This is to ensure that the position is maintained, the adjacent joints exercised and that plasters and splints are maintained. Radiographs are used to monitor healing and position (Figs 10.5–10.7). Physiotherapy is an important adjunct to treatment, especially to regain joint motion after a period of immobility.

Interesting facts

Internal fixation of fractures generally does not speed up time to union but will reduce rates of malunion (healing in poor position), improve function, reduce hospitalization time and cost and hasten return to work.

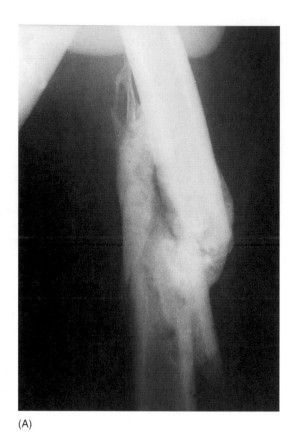

(A)

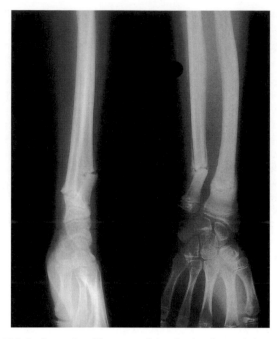

Fig. 10.6 Radiographs of fractures of the distal radius and ulna at 4 weeks post-injury in a child aged 8. In the ulna, periosteal new bone formation is less marked on the radial aspect where it was disrupted. There is metaphyseal osteopenia from immobilization and the open growth plate.

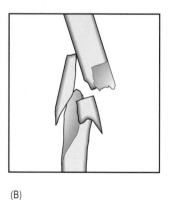

(B)

Fig. 10.5 (A) Radiograph of healing bone. Note the immature callus of early healing: although trabecular patterns are evident, the new cortex is yet to be established. At this stage, the femur would not withstand unprotected weight bearing. (B) Line drawing of original fracture fragments.

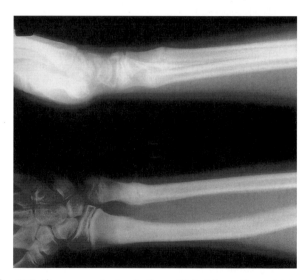

Fig. 10.7 The same patient as in Figure 10.6 at 6 months post-injury. The effect of remodelling has led to an improvement in alignment.

Interesting facts

Fractures of the distal radius are the commonest type of fracture, accounting for one-sixth of all fractures seen in the Emergency Department. After hip fracture treatment, half or more of patients fail to gain their preoperative level of mobility.

Complications of fractures

Fracture complications are best thought of as *early* or *late*. Early complications are those that might be considered to occur within the first few days. Hypovolaemia and infection are the two main examples of early complications.

<table>
<tr><td>Case
10.1</td><td>Trauma: 5</td></tr>
</table>

Management

Max's initial management aims to treat the pathological changes that occur with hypovolaemia and to support the physiological response. He will be given oxygen to improve his oxygen saturation and intravenous fluids to replace loss and to help maintain his cardiac output. Two large-bore intravenous lines might be inserted so that the fluid can be delivered quickly and a urinary catheter might be passed to measure his urinary output. He will be given analgesia to relieve his pain, and the leg will be splinted for this reason as well.

We know from our examination that Max has a fracture of the shaft of his femur, an injury to the medial collateral ligament of the knee and an intra-articular fracture of the ankle. We know from basic principles that his fractures would heal if they were managed by closed (non-operative) means. However, a diaphyseal fracture of the femoral shaft might take some months to heal. A single bone fracture of cortical bone is quite likely to be unstable and there will be a degree of shortening and perhaps rotational deformity unless the fracture is accurately reduced. There are strong pulls of muscles, both quadriceps and hamstrings, which will tend to shorten the limb, and the pull of the adductors distally might lead to a varus or bow deformity of the femur.

The intra-articular fracture of the ankle has some subluxation. Articular cartilage does not bear abnormal force well as you already understand from considering the pathogenesis of osteoarthritis in Chapter 6. An intra-articular fracture, not anatomically reduced, will lead to high contact pressures and the development of premature secondary osteoarthritis within the joint in a high percentage of cases. Without restoring congruity of the ankle joint, the patient is likely to develop a painful secondary osteoarthritis within 10 years (Fig. 10.8).

For these reasons, surgery is indicated in Max. Additionally, you recall that there is an open wound over Max's femoral fracture. This makes it likely that Max's femur has become contaminated with skin organisms, or possibly with debris from the road or his clothing. Without surgical cleaning of this area, he is likely to develop a deep infection, which could lead to the development of osteomyelitis, as will be discussed in Chapter 11. For this reason, surgery is indicated to provide wound toilet (Fig. 10.9). This is the act of debridement and cleaning of a contaminated fracture that much reduces the risk of osteomyelitis. *Debridement* comes from the French—to unbridle, and means to separate the risk of infection from the better outcome expected by the patient. Surgery combined with antibiotics is the only way to do this.

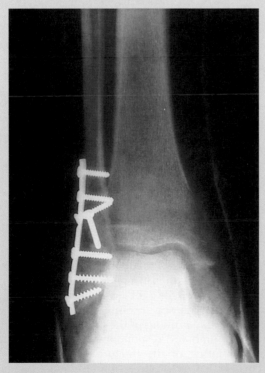

Fig. 10.8 AP radiograph of Max's ankle after internal fixation.

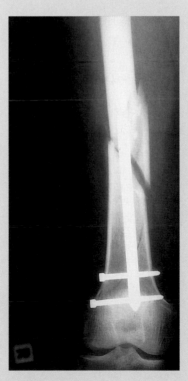

Fig. 10.9 AP radiograph of Max's knee after intramedullary nailing.

Table 10.4 Classification of open fractures after Gustilo: severity of fracture is strongly linked with prognosis

Classification	Description	Deep infection rate (%)
Type I	Clean wound <1 cm	0
Type II	Laceration >1 cm, without extensive soft tissue damage	1–2.5
Type IIIA	Extensive soft tissue damage or resulting from high-energy trauma	
Type IIIB	Extensive soft tissue loss with periosteal stripping and bone exposure	10–25
Type IIIC	As above but with arterial injury requiring repair	

Infection

Continuity of the fracture site with the bacteria-laden outside world is a serious complication. Infection (osteomyelitis) jeopardizes healing as well as bringing with it other complications such as excessive joint stiffness. Uncontrolled or poorly controlled sepsis may lead to limb loss. Open fractures are exposed to the outside and always result in a variable amount of dirty, devitalized and dead tissue around the fracture site, and these favour infection (Table 10.4). This is why wound debridement and lavage should be carried out as soon as possible and, ideally, in less than 6–9 h after the injury. Prophylactic antibiotics should be given to all patients with open fractures.

Infections in open fractures include gas gangrene, which is caused by the organism *Clostridium welchii* and associated with significant mortality and morbidity due to a toxin produced by the organism. Amputation and death are distinct outcomes when a patient contracts this infection. Tetanus, caused by *Clostridium tetani*, has been a significant problem in the past, but now is thankfully very rare (in the first world), because of a programme of immunization and the ready availability of tetanus immunoglobulin. *Clostridium tetani* elaborates a neurotoxin, which causes significant contracted paralysis of muscles that may lead to failure to ventilate and thus death. In the face, the contracted paralysis produces the *risus sardonicus tetani* or violent contraction of muscles, which can be prevented by anaesthesia or by nursing the patient in a darkened quiet room. Infections of the musculoskeletal system are discussed further in Chapter 11.

More commonly, however, deep infection usually occurs with skin commensals and in up to 85% of infections associated with open fractures, *Staphylococcus aureus* from the patient's own skin is implicated.

Fat embolism syndrome

When a diaphyseal bone is fractured, fat embolism syndrome may develop. Whether this occurs through direct release of marrow fat into lacerated venules or by means of precipitation of chylomicrons within the intravascular system is subject to some controversy. The features of this syndrome are often associated with an acute respiratory distress and the presence of petechial haemorrhage (often best seen in the conjunctiva or axilla). The development of adult respiratory distress syndrome is strongly associated with the presence of fat embolism. The fat precipitates in the capillary system of the lung, causing impaired oxygenation and may attenuate confusional states associated with hypovolaemia and decreased cerebral perfusion. The treatment is largely supportive by means of oxygenation of the patient, which may be achieved by simple measures such as oxygen by mask, but might lead to the need to intubate and ventilate the patient by means of an endotracheal tube in an intensive care unit.

Injury to adjacent vessels and nerves

Nerves and vessels are intimately associated with the skeleton, and neurovascular injury must always be excluded when dealing with a fracture of the skeleton. Peripheral pulses must always be palpated and both the sensory and motor functions of individual peripheral nerves formally assessed. There are some fractures that are particularly prone to the development of neurovascular injury because of the particularities of their anatomy. For example, the common peroneal nerve passes very close to the head of the fibula, near the knee, and is often injured in high fibula fractures. The radial nerve is intimately adjacent to the humerus in the radial groove in the mid-posterior portion of the humerus. Fractures of the humeral shaft in this area may cause nerve injury. Nerve injury most commonly occurs by means of stretching, occurring once the stabilizing function of bone has been lost. Such stretching injury (neuropraxia) is not uncommon and resolves for most individuals in less than 6 weeks. If, however, the stretching has been so significant that the nerve has been torn or even lacerated by the sharp bone ends, such recovery is unlikely to occur without formal exploration and nerve repair. If the neural sheath is intact, this condition is known as axonotmesis; if the nerve sheath is torn, it is known as neurotmesis. Return to Chapter 3 for a review of nerve injuries.

Arterial injury is not uncommon. In most, it is simply associated with a kinking of the artery caused by malposition of the limb and responds well to simple measures such as splinting of the fracture. However, the artery may be lacerated or torn in a similar way to the nerve. In dislocations of the knee, there is an up to 70% incidence of injury to the popliteal artery. This is a surgical emergency, as muscle ischaemia cannot last longer than 6 h without unrecoverable damage. Early surgical opinion is warranted and the patient may require an interposition arterial graft.

Compartment syndrome

This is not an uncommon complication of fractures, especially of the tibial diaphysis. It is also occasionally seen in forearm and femoral fractures. Compartment syndrome is associated with bleeding into an area of muscle surrounded by tight fascia; commonly such systems are found in the lower limb and forearm. Bleeding and tissue damage causing swelling within the closed fascial system can lead to pressures being raised within the fascial envelope. Fascia is unyielding and has no ability to stretch. Pressures soon exceed the relatively low venous capillary emptying pressure, allowing further swelling to occur because arterial capillary filling still continues. This compounds the swelling until arterial capillary pressure is exceeded, and the muscle can become ischaemic. Note that it is still possible for a palpable distal pulse to be present as arterial capillary filling pressure is only about 35–40 mm Hg. The signs and symptoms that alert to a compartment syndrome include intense pain (unrelieved by analgesics), pain on stretching the affected muscles and altered sensation (paraesthesia and decreased sensation); motor paralysis is a late sign.

Regional pain syndromes

An occasional but significant complication of fracture is the development of a pain syndrome that occurs even when the fracture is well healed. This syndrome is vague and ill-defined but is associated with significant alteration of sympathetic nervous function of the limb, including altered sweating, swelling and vasomotor change. The limb often develops a severe regional osteoporosis owing to disuse. Early mobilization, physiotherapy and sympathetic blocks have all been used for treatment. The condition has been known as reflex sympathetic dystrophy or Sudeck's atrophy in the past. The treatment is usually multidisciplinary and difficult, and the condition is slow to resolve.

Malunion

This occurs when the fracture heals in a less than anatomical way. Small degrees of malunion may have little functional import but significant malunion can be a major problem. For example, if Max's femur were to heal with a greater than 10° varus malunion, he may develop secondary osteoarthritis of the medial compartment of the knee joint owing to the shifting of his mechanical axis of the knee to the medial side.

Non-union

This occurs when a fracture fails to heal as expected and when radiographs show no progress to union in successive films. Non-union is relatively rare, but Max has had a high-energy fracture of his femur with tissue stripping and loss of some local blood supply, so he has about a 5% risk of non-union of his femur. Of all fractures, the tibia in its distal third is most susceptible to non-union because of its poor blood supply. Surgical intervention by means of bone-grafting or surgical stabilization is often required.

Avascular necrosis

Fractures occurring in bones with a precarious blood supply may lead to this complication. Avascular necrosis is a significant clinical problem in subcapital fractures of the femur, and fractures of the scaphoid and the talus.

Further reading

Apley, A.G., Solomon, L., 2001. A System of Orthopaedics and Fractures, eighth ed. Arnold, London.

Bullough, P.G., 2009. Atlas of Orthopaedic Pathology with Clinical and Radiological Correlations, fourth ed. Mosby, Philadelphia.

McRae, R., 2006. Pocketbook of Orthopaedics and Fractures, second ed. Churchill Livingstone, Edinburgh.

INFECTION AND THE MUSCULOSKELETAL SYSTEM

11

Sydney Nade

Chapter objectives

After studying this chapter you should be able to:

1. Understand how microorganisms reach bones or joints.

2. Understand the possible effects of microorganisms on bones, growth plates, articular cartilage and intervertebral discs.

3. Diagnose infection in musculoskeletal tissues.

4. Understand the principles of management of musculoskeletal infections.

5. Describe the possible outcomes of infection in bones, joints and intervertebral discs.

Introduction

Microorganisms abound in nature, and many find the environment and nutrients needed for growth and reproduction on or within other living organisms. Such microorganisms live in a balanced situation with their host that ensures survival of both host and parasite. Humans have developed a complex immune system that allows such co-existence to continue.

Infection is the process by which a microorganism enters into a damaging relationship with its host. If the microorganism injures the host to a sufficient degree, disturbances result in the host, which manifest as disease. Included among the microorganisms that cause disease in the musculoskeletal system are bacteria, fungi (and fungus-like organisms), protozoa, helminths and viruses. In addition, inflammation in joints (synovitis) can occur without direct invasion by microorganisms, but as a reaction to infection elsewhere in the body, perhaps as a response to circulating breakdown products.

It is the combination of the presence of microorganisms, inflammation and tissue destruction that constitutes 'clinical infection'. The case histories that follow are typical of musculoskeletal infections, and their discussion provides not only a clinical picture, but also knowledge of physiological and pathological mechanisms that are essential for the understanding of principles of management. If those principles are followed, then the outcome should be favourable in restoration of the balance of the host–parasite contest, thereby minimizing the potential adverse effects on the normal function of the host.

General principles of musculoskeletal infection

In the musculoskeletal system there are three types of infection:

- *A primary process,* in which the microorganisms attach to the target tissues, having reached them by the bloodstream (such as acute haematogenous osteomyelitis).

- *A potential process,* in which an alternative portal of entry to the tissues has been made by breach of the integument, either by accidental trauma, or by intentional surgical incision (such as osteomyelitis after an open fracture).

- *An unwelcome process,* occurring after entry to the tissues by one of the above routes, for which the methods used to eradicate the infection are likely to cause greater loss of function than the process for which the original surgical operation was performed (such as chronic osteomyelitis after hip replacement).

Case 11.1 Acute osteomyelitis: 1

Case history

Simon, 4-years-old, complained to his mother that his leg was sore. That night he did not eat his evening meal with his usual enthusiasm. In the early hours of the morning, he awoke crying, and complaining that his leg still hurt. Later in the day his mother saw that he was reluctant to run around. She felt he was warm. In the afternoon, she took him to the doctor, who asked him to point to where his leg hurt and he indicated just below the knee on the inner side of the leg. When the doctor pressed at that spot, Simon said 'Ouch'. The skin was not discoloured. Lymph nodes in his groin were not palpable. Although he was reluctant to walk for the doctor, his knee joint range of movement was normal. His body temperature was elevated at 38.5°C. The doctor did not find any other abnormal clinical signs and made a provisional diagnosis of acute osteomyelitis of the tibia.

Once infection is established, it is the outcome of the host and parasite contest that determines the effect of the infection. Microorganisms may:

- be repelled and eradicated, with restitution of the tissues to their normal state

- cause such tissue damage that the host is unable to survive

- be eradicated by the host but tissue destruction and inflammation lead to the formation of repair tissue that leaves a fibrous scar at the site of invasion (the most common outcome)

- remain dormant in the tissues but there is 'clinical resolution' of the disease.

The 'clinical outcome' is the recovery of function in the host and is determined by the tissue responses. Those responses may be modified by effective treatment, tipping the balance between microorganism and host in favour of the host.

The mere presence of microorganisms is not sufficient to produce disease. They must demonstrate an ability to invade the host tissues, to enter, multiply, spread and produce toxic substances. The body has defences against invasiveness and toxigenicity. The ability to produce a disease is known as *pathogenicity*. The comparative pathogenicity of various organisms is known as *virulence*. Very small numbers of virulent bacteria produce disease, whereas larger numbers are required of less virulent organisms. The invasiveness of microorganisms relates not only to the toxins that they produce, but also to enzymes, which may allow them to spread by tissue dissolution and protect them from host phagocytes.

Portals of entry

In order to produce diseases of the musculoskeletal system in man, organisms must gain access to those tissues. There are several ways in which this may occur:

- haematogenous spread by bacteraemia or septicaemia from a primary site of colonization (skin, mouth, gut) if barriers to spread have been breached

- direct access by puncture of the skin and deeper tissues following injury, with organisms carried in by the penetrating instrument

- direct access at the time of elective surgery or following surgery for open injury

- local spread from infected adjacent tissues.

Interesting associations

Certain clinical observations are useful in trying to understand the basis for musculoskeletal infections. The common sites of infections in infants and children are in the lower limbs, both bones and joints, whereas the spine is the bone site most commonly affected by haematogenous infection in adults. This probably reflects the larger vascular beds or the nature of blood flow in the vessels in those sites. Acute haematogenous osteomyelitis and septic arthritis are more common in boys than girls; however, the reason for this is unclear.

The organisms involved are not randomly distributed. *Staphylococcus aureus* is a common cause of bone and joint infections in all age groups, but in the past 40 years it has been recognized that *Haemophilus influenzae* was a not infrequent cause of septic arthritis in children between the ages of 6 months and 2 years. This may represent a modification of the immune competence of children in that age group. *Salmonella* has a predilection for black-skinned races with sickle cell disease. The site of infection in adults is usually the diaphysis of a long bone, while the common site of infection in children, as in Simon, is metaphyseal.

Host defences against infection

The host, for its part in the host–parasite relationship, has a resistance to invasion by microorganisms and the effects of their toxins that can be assessed in terms of non-specific and specific factors.

Non-specific factors are those acting against a variety of microorganisms:

- physiological, physical and chemical barriers at the portal of entry (skin or mucous membrane)

- phagocytosis (intracellular killing of microorganisms)

- the reticuloendothelial system

- the inflammatory response.

The specific factors are those that confer resistance against a specific infectious agent and come under the heading of immunity. Such immunity may be natural (not acquired through previous contact with the infecting agent), or acquired (passively or actively). Passive acquired immunity is a state of relative temporary insusceptibility to an infectious agent that has been induced by the administration of antibodies that were formed in another host, rather than formed by the individual person. Monoclonal antibodies, or polyvalent antisera, are examples. Tetanus immune globulin is a product of autologous human serum that contains antibodies against tetanus toxin. Active immunity is a state of resistance built up in an individual following effective contact with the foreign antigens; that is the microorganisms or their products. Active immunization against tetanus requires injection of deactivated tetanus toxin. The antibodies are manufactured by the host. Adaptive or acquired resistance to infection requires a specific response by the host to enable it to eradicate a particular infection.

The resistance of acquired immunity is a complex subject, but as reviewed in Chapter 1, there are two major subgroups:

1. *humoral immunity,* or the active production of antibodies; and

2. *cellular immunity*, in which certain lymphoid cells recognize material as foreign and initiate a chain of responses that permit them to destroy intracellular organisms.

Humoral immunity involves the production and secretion of special protein molecules called antibodies by cells of the lymphoid system. The antibodies circulate in the blood and body fluids, having been stimulated to appear by the presence of antigens. Antibodies may induce resistance to infection because they:

- neutralize toxins or cellular enzymes

- have direct bactericidal or lytic effect

- block the infective ability of microorganisms

- agglutinate microorganisms, making them more susceptible to phagocytosis

- opsonize microorganisms and therefore aid phagocytosis.

Cell-mediated immunity depends on the ability of sensitized lymphocytes to kill foreign cells by direct contact. Lymphocytes are found in lymphoid tissue (bone marrow, thymus, spleen, lymph nodes and lymph) and in the blood. In Chapter 1 we described how humoral immunity is mediated by B lymphocytes derived from stem cells in the bone marrow. These are stimulated by antigen to divide and form plasma cells, which then secrete antibodies against the antigen concerned. The other lymphocyte population, the T lymphocytes, are responsible for cellular immunity.

The presence of antibodies, and their amount, can sometimes be used to determine whether or not a person has had contact with an antigen; this is useful in the diagnosis of some infections and in determining a person's response to treatment. Similarly, the ability of T cells to respond to challenge by some antigens can be used as a diagnostic technique.

The tissues that are regularly in contact with the external environment, such as skin, mucous membrane and cornea, have adaptations that resist invasion by microorganisms, and it is usually only at times when the continuity of the tissue surface is breached that infection occurs. The deeper tissues such as bone and joint do not have the same natural barriers to infection. Muscle is also a deeper tissue, but has a lower incidence of primary infection than bones or joints, for unknown reasons.

Also important are alterations in function of one or more organ systems in the host. The normal ecological balance of symbiotic organisms resident on the host may be upset by burns, trauma, surgery, hospitalization or antibiotic therapy. Disrupted anatomical barriers consequent on burns, trauma, bites, other infections, ischaemia or the presence of foreign materials (including implanted prostheses) alter normal relations. If the person has diabetes, renal failure, diseases of the haematopoietic system or is taking immunosuppressive drugs, the normally protective inflammatory response may be altered. Diseases of the lymphoreticular system, cancer, debilitating diseases, malnutrition and cigarette smoking have an effect on the way the body meets challenges from microorganisms.

Blood supply of bone

The clinical patterns of acute osteomyelitis are different in infants, children and adults. The most likely explanation is that the blood supply and structure of bone in the three age groups is different (Fig. 11.1). You will recall from Chapter 5 that children have a well-defined growth plate (physis), while adults do not have a growth plate. In infants, a growth plate is present, but it is less well defined, and has some vessels that penetrate it and thereby connect the epiphysis and metaphysis of the bone. The physis is

cartilaginous, and therefore capable of being 'expanded' by dividing and growing cells, whereas adult bone can only grow by apposition on its surface. At the junction of metaphysis and physis, small blood vessels are open-ended, growing towards the physis. At that point, the contents of the lumen can escape and lie adjacent to physeal cartilage. If an embolus of bacteria (septicaemia or bacteraemia) escapes from such a vessel, and the size of the inoculum is sufficient to cause an infection (a measure of virulence), and there is a tropism (attraction) of the pathogenic bacteria for cartilage, then an infection may be initiated.

Once a metaphyseal infection is initiated, cell death occurs and an inflammatory process follows. Intramedullary (within the marrow cavity) inflammation in the metaphysis of a long bone further impairs the circulation to the bone and ischaemia occurs around the initial septic focus or abscess. Because the direction of flow of blood in bone is dependent on pressure differences in capillaries, the nutrition of the cortical bone of the metaphysis may be secondarily impaired. The ischaemic necrosis of bone allows pus (the consequence of infective inflammation) to spread from the initial focus within the cancellous bone of the metaphysis through the bone cortex, and through the medullary cavity.

Acute infection of bone and joints

Diagnosis of acute bone infection

The absolute diagnosis of infection in bone requires that microorganisms be detected at a site in bone. The simplest

---

Case 11.1 Acute osteomyelitis: 2

Case note: Aetiology

The doctor made a diagnosis of acute haematogenous osteomyelitis. Osteomyelitis is inflammation (-itis) of bone (osteo-) and bone marrow (myel-), and is normally due to infection. Some books call it *osteitis* but it is not possible to distinguish if bone can be infected without the marrow component. The primary infection is usually blood-borne in infants and children and the first site of lodgement of the bacterial embolus is in small blood vessels within the medullary (marrow) cavity of the bone.

Case 11.1 Acute osteomyelitis: 3

Case note: Relating clinical features to pathology

The fact that Simon pointed to the metaphyseal region of his tibia as his site of pain, and the doctor found tenderness at precisely that site links the anatomy of the region to the pathology and observed clinical picture. In adults, metaphyseal osteomyelitis is uncommon, and haematogenous osteomyelitis is less common than direct invasion of bone. When haematogenous in adults, osteomyelitis is most frequent in the vertebrae.

Had Simon been examined when he first complained of his leg being sore, the doctor may not have found tenderness at the tibial metaphysis. However, the pathological sequela of the infectious process in the intervening hours, then untreated, leads to purulent oedema fluid collecting beneath the periosteum of the bone cortex, providing a critical clinical sign—*finger point tenderness at the metaphysis of a long bone in a child*. If this sign is found, acute osteomyelitis should be considered the most likely diagnosis until proven otherwise.

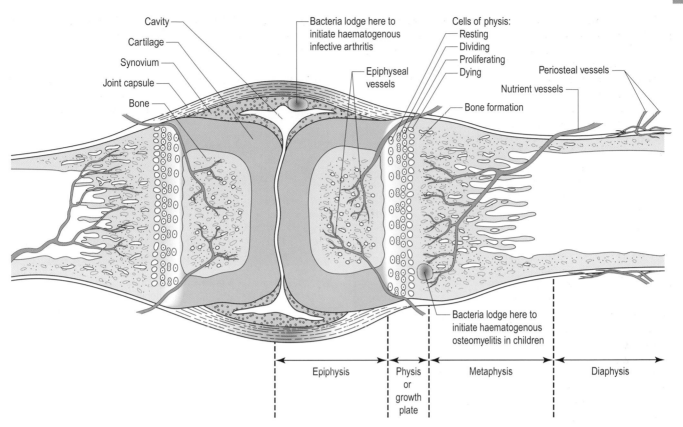

Fig. 11.1 The anatomy of bone and joint in a child. The terms used to describe the parts of the bone are shown. Note the relationship of the site of initiation of a metaphyseal abscess to the blood supply and junction of dead cartilage and forming bone adjacent to the physis.

way to confirm bone infection is to put a needle at the site of tenderness and to aspirate for pus. Any material collected should then be subjected to Gram staining and microbiological culture. However, this is not always possible and other investigations are usually necessary.

Although bone is an easy tissue to image, changes in bone on plain radiographs, characteristic of infection, do not appear for several days after the infection has started. When present, the most typical change is the laying down of thin layers of bone on the periosteal surface (Fig. 11.2). By the time that occurs, the infective process may be well established and difficult to abort by treatment. Nevertheless, plain radiography should always be performed as it may show an alternative diagnosis. The best investigation to perform is ultrasound imaging. It is non-invasive, not painful, and shows an image of the tissues in real time. An anechoic zone adjacent to bone (that is, under the periosteum) means a collection of liquid and in the clinical setting confirms a diagnosis of osteomyelitis (Fig. 11.3). Furthermore, an aspirating needle can be guided by the ultrasound image to enter the liquid for the collection of a sample.

Blood cultures should also be performed, since organisms can be grown in cultures of blood taken from about half the children who have acute osteomyelitis, confirming also the septicaemic nature of the condition.

Haematological examination may show neutrophil leukocytosis or a rise in the erythrocyte sedimentation rate (ESR) or C-reactive protein (CRP) level, but they are not specific for osteomyelitis. The principal reason for such tests is to ensure that the patient does not have any underlying condition that has affected the immune status, thereby permitting the infection to be initiated.

In typical cases of acute osteomyelitis, no other investigations are required for diagnosis. A management scheme for a patient with pain, fever and loss of joint function in which a provisional diagnosis of osteomyelitis is considered is shown in Figure 11.4. Sometimes the condition is *atypical*, affecting an unusual bone (e.g. clavicle, calcaneus), a site that is concealed (e.g. vertebra, pelvis), or due to an uncommon pathogen (fungus, *Salmonella*). Then it may be appropriate to determine whether or not it is bone that harbours the pathology, and which bone. The most sensitive test for determining altered bone metabolism is a radioisotope bone scan. Bone scans usually employ ^{99m}technetium as the γ-emitter and a bisphosphonate as the molecule that binds to bone. Very small increases in bone formation, such as a response to infection (although not specific for infection) can be detected. Bone scans may thus locate a site, but not necessarily the pathological process. If tests locate the bone site, then it may be necessary to biopsy that site by needle or trephine aspiration to confirm an infection and identify the causative organism. Magnetic resonance imaging (MRI), if available, provides valuable information about soft tissues adjacent to bone, including the presence of pus.

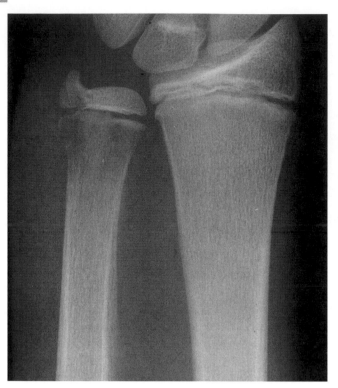

Fig. 11.2 Plain radiograph showing the effects of osteomyelitis involving the distal end of the ulna. Note the thickness of the soft tissue shadow of the skin adjacent to the distal ulna. It indicates the swelling that should be clinically obvious. Note the loss of bone that has occurred in the metaphysis of the ulna, which follows the site of initial abscess formation. Note the layers of bone that have been laid down by periosteal activity just proximal to the focus of the intramedullary osteomyelitis. In this radiograph you have evidence of bone destruction, bone formation and inflammation. These findings would be typical about 10 days after the osteomyelitis started.

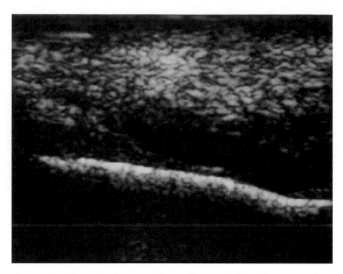

Fig. 11.3 Diagnostic ultrasound image from a child with osteomyelitis of the tibia. The cortex of the tibia is depicted by the continuous white line in the lower part of the figure. Overlying muscle is depicted by the dappled grey and black lines in the upper part. Between the two is an area from which there are no ultrasonic echoes (anechoic), appearing black. It is adjacent to the bone and represents a collection of pus.

Case 11.1 **Acute osteomyelitis: 4**

Case note: Investigations

In Simon's case, the diagnosis of acute haematogenous osteomyelitis of the proximal tibia was almost certain, as he had classical clinical features. Plain radiography was normal. Ultrasound imaging showed that there was a liquid collection adjacent to his proximal tibia on its medial side. His haemoglobin level was 142 g/L, his white blood cell count was 14×10^9 cells/L with 79% neutrophils, and his ESR was 45 mm in 1 h and CRP 100 mg/L.

Treatment of acute bone infections

The appropriate treatment depends on knowledge of the causative microorganism. Treatment demands that the use of antibiotic drugs, surgery, or both, be considered. Most of the infants and children who have acute haematogenous osteomyelitis are infected with *Staphylococcus aureus*. The sooner the treatment commences after making

---

Case 11.1 **Acute osteomyelitis: 5**

Case note: Treatment

Simon was treated with the intravenous administration of flucloxacillin in a dose of 100 mg/kg body weight per day, given 6-hourly, after checking that he did not have an intolerance to penicillins. As his condition improved quickly, assessed by his general wellbeing, loss of pain, decrease in tenderness, and improved appetite, the intravenous line was removed 60 h after his admission to the hospital and the same dose of the antibiotic continued orally. It was given between meals and he was *not* given ice cream 'to help the medicine go down'!.

---

the provisional diagnosis of acute osteomyelitis, the more likely the condition is to be aborted and the amount of tissue destroyed by the infection to be minimized (Fig. 11.5).

In contrast, chronic osteomyelitis, discussed below, requires that the causative organism be determined before treatment starts, as the likely organisms are much more diverse and, therefore, selection of an antibiotic on a 'best-guess' principle is more likely to be wrong. In chronic osteomyelitis, the urgency of intervention is much less, as the level of pain is less, the risk of septicaemia is less, and the structural alteration of the tissues has already occurred.

Interesting facts

It is essential to begin treatment of suspected ACUTE osteomyelitis without delay, but in CHRONIC osteomyelitis it is essential to identify the causative organism before treatment begins.

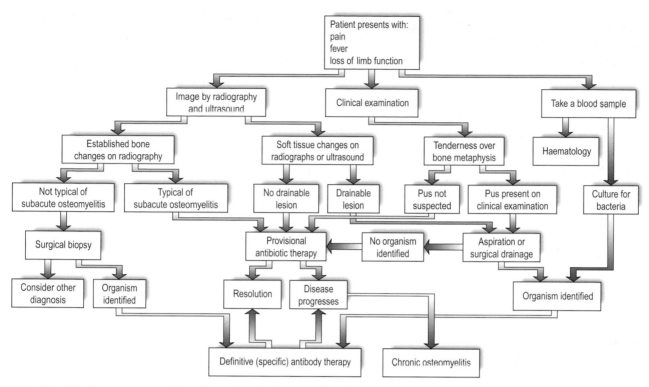

Fig. 11.4 Algorithm for management of a patient with pain, fever and loss of function in a limb when a diagnosis of osteomyelitis is considered. Note that the three important tasks are: (1) take a history; (2) take a blood sample; (3) image by ultrasound and plain radiography.

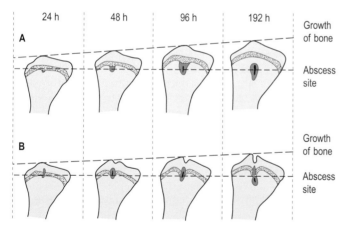

Fig. 11.5 Effects of infection of growing bone. (A) The growing end of a bone at four successive time periods demonstrating how the bone growth moves relative to the initial site of abscess formation. As a consequence of growth, the growth plate (physis) moves away from the site of the abscess, leaving behind a sequestrum of dead unresorbed cartilage (depicted by a vertical line), which harbours masses of bacteria. (B) What may happen to the shape of the articular surface of the joint and the physis, if the site of lodgement of the initial embolus is within a vessel that crosses the growth plate. Growth adjacent to that site is prevented because the dividing cells within the physis are destroyed by the infection.

Diagnosis of acute joint infections

Any non-traumatic acute condition affecting a joint should be assumed as being an infection until proved otherwise.

The best way to confirm the diagnosis is to aspirate the joint and examine its contents by Gram stain, cell count, crystal examination and culture. Infection initiates an inflammatory response and neutrophils enter the joint cavity. A cell count of greater than 10^5 cells/mm^3 is consistent with an infection, while half that value or more is suggestive. The analysis of synovial fluid and the information that can be gained from it was addressed in Chapter 1. It will be the next day before any bacterial colony growth may be seen but treatment should start before then. If the Gram stain demonstrates bacteria, it can also guide the choice of the correct antibiotic, as the organisms that commonly cause septic arthritis are limited in number. *Staphylococcus aureus* and streptococci are Gram-positive cocci, while *Haemophilus influenzae* are Gram-negative rods.

Interesting facts

Since immunization against *Haemophilus influenzae type b* has been introduced, the incidence of that organism as a cause of septic arthritis in children has decreased markedly.

The larger joints of the body are those most commonly infected. If an unusual joint is involved or if the infection has followed an inadvertent joint puncture (e.g. tooth, thorn or fishbone), then it is likely that an unusual organism will be the cause. If the immune state of the patient is impaired (see 11.2: 1—Sylvia has diabetes) or if the portal of entry has been from intravenous recreational drug use, the causative organism might be unusual, so every

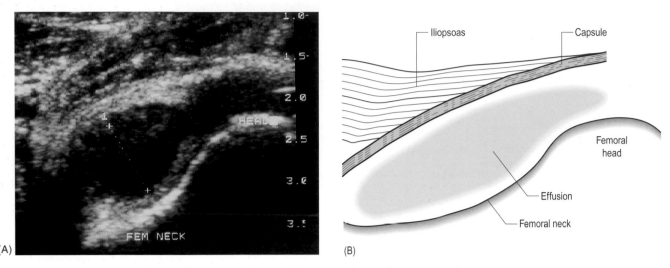

Fig. 11.6 (A) Ultrasound image of joint effusion in the hip joint. (B) Drawing showing key anatomical structures.

attempt should be made to arrive at a definitive identification of the organism and its antibiotic sensitivity.

In neonates and infants 'pseudo-paralysis' of a limb is an important clue that warrants suspicion of infection of bone or joint.

Sometimes it is difficult to determine whether a swollen joint contains liquid (an effusion) or proliferative synovium, or both. Moreover, in deeper joints such as the hip or shoulder, the joint cannot be palpated. If uncertainty exists as to whether a joint contains an effusion, the best tool to confirm it is ultrasound imaging (Fig. 11.6). It is a much cheaper, quicker and easier examination than magnetic resonance imaging, which will also delineate a joint effusion.

Interesting facts

In any joint in which there has been rapid onset of pain, in the absence of trauma, infection must be suspected, and assumed to be present until proved otherwise.

Treatment of acute joint infections

An algorithm for the management of suspected septic arthritis is shown in Figure 11.7. The important principles of management of bone and joint infections are shown in Box 11.1.

Location of the site of infection Locating the site of infection involves clinical examination and usually imaging procedures. Confirmation should be by identifying microorganisms there; however, it is not always necessary to do that before starting treatment.

Identification of the causative organism This should always be pursued, although it may not always be successful, and if an organism is strongly suspected, the administration of antibiotics should not be delayed. As well as identifying the organism, the microbiological laboratory is able to determine susceptibility of the organism to antibiotics.

Case 11.2 Septic arthritis: 1

Case history

Sylvia is an overweight woman aged 67 years who has had mild discomfort from both knees for about 5 years. For about 2 days she had noticed that the pattern of her knee pain had changed from being present on the inner side of each knee on bearing weight to a more severe, constant, pain in her left knee, which did not settle when she went to bed the previous night. She regularly tested her blood glucose, as she was a diabetic who needed oral anti-diabetic agents. She consulted her doctor because her blood sugar level had risen from its previously well-controlled range. Her doctor noted that despite her weight and bow-legged stance, Sylvia had swelling in her left knee region and some mild reddish discolouration of the surrounding skin. When he attempted to put her knee through a range of motion, she resisted the movements and said that it increased the pain. He found that she had a fungal infection between her fourth and fifth toes. He disinfected the skin around the knee and aspirated her knee joint, finding cloudy yellow liquid, not the normal clear straw-coloured appearance of synovial fluid described in Chapter 1. He then telephoned the local hospital to arrange urgent admission.

Acute septic arthritis is commonly due to *Staphylococcus aureus*, but in unimmunized children between the ages of 6 months and 2 years, *Haemophilus influenzae* is a common cause. It is important to note this, because the 'best-guess' antibiotic to choose for initial treatment is different for the two bacteria. In the presence of implanted foreign material, such as internal fixation for fractures or prosthetic joints, unusual pathogens such as *Staphylococcus epidermidis* may be the cause of infection. After traumatic open fractures with destruction of the tissues, organisms such as *Escherichia coli*, *Pseudomonas aeruginosa*, *Bacteroides*, streptococci, and

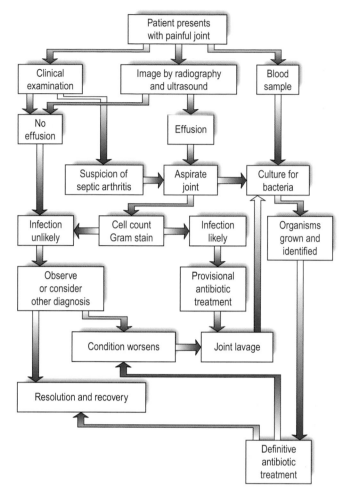

Fig. 11.7 Algorithm for management of a child with septic arthritis. Note that the three important tasks are: (1) take a history; (2) take a blood sample; (3) image by ultrasound and plain radiography.

Box 11.1 Principles of management of infection in bones and joints

- Locate the site of infection
- Identify the causative organism
- Sterilize the infected region
- Remove pus, necrotic tissue and foreign material and restore blood supply
- Monitor progress of the patient

clostridia may be found. In sexually active young people, aged between 15 and 30, it is becoming more and more common to find gonorrhoea as a cause of acute arthritis. Recreational drug takers, and immunosuppressed people may also have bone and joint infections with unusual organisms, including fungi, and therefore every attempt should be made to obtain a tissue specimen for identification early in the diagnostic process. *Kingella kingae* is now recognized as a causative organism, particularly in those cases in which there is no growth on routine microbiological

testing; but if specimens are placed in blood culture bottles it is often found!

In chronic osteomyelitis there is no urgency to commence treatment and in all cases, identification of causative organisms should precede the starting of antibiotics. In spinal infections, aspiration biopsy should be performed, as *Mycobacterium tuberculosis* is a frequent cause, particularly in the patient originating from an area of endemic tuberculosis.

Sterilizing the infected region The effective way to sterilize the infected region is to use antibiotic drugs. In order to be effective, antibiotics must be able to reach the bacteria. This requires patent blood vessels sufficiently close to the periphery of the infective focus for the antibiotic to diffuse in sufficient concentration to inhibit bacterial division. The microbiological laboratory can determine the sensitivity of organisms to various antibiotics and, if necessary, determine blood levels of antibiotics. By their presence in the tissues peripheral to an infected focus (abscess), antibiotics control the spread of invading bacteria to surrounding tissues. Bactericidal antibiotics are more effective than bacteriostatic drugs but antibiotics do not remove pus.

Surgery The principal role of surgery is to remove pus and necrotic tissue. It should be performed in all patients with septic arthritis, unless the likely cause is *Neisseria gonorrhoeae* or *Kingella kingae*, as soon as possible after diagnosis. Thorough and copious lavage is necessary. Lavage of joints can be performed using an arthroscope, being minimally invasive, or by open arthrotomy. In acute osteomyelitis, all patients should be prepared for surgery, although it may not be required in those who have a prompt clinical response to antibiotics alone. The indications for surgery are:

- the presence of pus as assessed on clinical grounds (and probably if detected by ultrasound imaging)

- failure of the patient to improve between two examinations by the clinician, 4–6h apart, after the administration of an adequate dose of provisional antibiotic and rehydration.

Antibiotic therapy

Initially, an appropriate dose of provisional ('best guess') antibiotic is given. In infants and children this should be on a body weight basis. Currently, it is appropriate to give an anti-staphylococcal bactericidal antibiotic in four daily divided doses to all children suspected of having acute osteomyelitis or septic arthritis. The precise selection of antibiotic depends on keeping local records about the causative organisms that have previously been found, and their antibiotic sensitivities. Change to a specific antibiotic, if necessary, will be guided by the results of microbiological cultures. In chronic osteomyelitis a mixed growth is often obtained. If an operative procedure is performed as part of the diagnostic process in chronic osteomyelitis to obtain a specimen for culture, the risk of bacteraemia or septicaemia at the time of surgery should be minimized by giving a single dose of an anti-staphylococcal antibiotic at that time. There is no place for the topical administration of antibiotics or washing of infected sites or wounds with antibiotic solutions.

The route and duration of antibiotics

The route and duration of treatment with antibiotics often excite debate, but current evidence does not support the prolonged use of intravenous administration. When the patient is feeling better and tolerating food, antibiotics can be given by mouth. It is important to ensure that the dose is administered regularly and that it is swallowed. Antibiotic absorption can be inhibited by food in the stomach; therefore it is advisable to administer oral antibiotics between meals. Recall that Simon was given his antibiotics between meals and his mother was told to avoid concomitant ice cream (see 11.1: 4). Oral administration can usually be started within 3 days of the initiation of treatment. The total duration need not be prolonged.

- In the uncomplicated case of acute osteomyelitis or septic arthritis, when clinical recovery is prompt, pain disappears and function returns, a total duration of 3 weeks is probably adequate to minimize the risk of recurrence.

- In chronic osteomyelitis, the duration relates more to the type and number of surgical procedures performed than to any other indicator.

Where antibiotics are used to suppress, but not cure, chronic osteomyelitis the requirement for antibiotics can be tested by suspending the medication after a reasonable period and watching for the clinical effect. Should symptoms recur then antibiotic medication can be recommenced, without deleterious effect on the patient. It is usual to offer such a therapeutic challenge after 6 weeks of initial treatment for chronic osteomyelitis.

Monitoring progress

Clinical examination should be based on the temperature chart, the appearance of the patient, the degree of tenderness, and the restriction of movement. There is no indication for repeated radiological ultrasound or radioisotope imaging to monitor progress, provided the patient makes progressive clinical improvement. CRP monitoring may be a useful guide, especially if not falling promptly.

The ideal outcome is to abort the infection and restore normal function, without structural deformity of the affected skeletal tissue, or other long-term sequel. As acute haematogenous osteomyelitis usually affects infants and children, there is an enormous capacity for repair as the child grows. In normal growth, infants' bones are completely replaced as their size increases by new bone laid down adjacent to the growth plate for length, and circumferentially under the periosteum for width. If acute osteomyelitis, which commences in the metaphysis, involves the growth plate by local spread, future growth in length may be affected, leading to a short, or curved bone (see Fig. 11.5). Once destroyed by infection, growth plates cannot repair or be replaced. Articular cartilage also has a limited capacity for repair and, if completely destroyed by the infective process in septic arthritis, ankylosis of the joint occurs, meaning that it cannot move.

Chronic infections of bones and joints

In contrast to acute infections, in subacute, chronic, or unusual presentations of musculoskeletal sepsis, diagnosis must precede treatment. Little is lost if antibiotics are withheld for a few days, but much is lost if they are administered in an inappropriate dose without a clear diagnosis.

Chronic infection after an open wound

Skin is a remarkably effective barrier against invasion by the parasitic organisms that live on its surface. Once that surface is broken, however, a pathway exists for infection to occur. The natural defence mechanisms of the body, both cellular (phagocytes and macrophages) and

Case 11.2 Septic arthritis: 2

Case note: The causative organism

The liquid aspirated from Sylvia's knee was examined and a Gram stain revealed clumps of Gram-positive cocci consistent with a diagnosis of septic arthritis. The next day there were colonies of bacteria on the culture plate, which were identified as *S. aureus*.

Case 11.2 Septic arthritis: 3

Case note: Treatment

Following her admission to hospital, Sylvia had an intravenous line inserted. Fluid was administered via the line because she was nauseated, has diabetes and had not drunk much that day, and an antistaphylococcal, bactericidal antibiotic was given intravenously by a bolus dose every 6h. Her blood sugar level was measured and found to be 14mmol/L. When Sylvia was rehydrated and her blood sugar level had been reduced to normal by administration of insulin, she had lavage (washout) of her knee joint with sterile water, using an arthroscope to view the inside of the joint under spinal anaesthesia. The surgeon had warned her that if a satisfactory washout of the joint could not be achieved by that technique, the joint would have to be opened (open arthrotomy) to achieve the same result.

humoral (antibodies), are stimulated to act. Where there has been major transfer of energy sufficient to fracture a bone, there is inevitably disruption of other tissues and blood vessels. Tissue that has been devascularized cannot play a role in the defence process. Whether or not an infection follows depends on the size of the inoculum of bacteria that enters the wound, and the ability of the surrounding tissues to combat those microorganisms. Measures that must be employed to reduce the risk of infection after any open wound are:

- surgical toilet, meaning copious lavage with large volumes of water to wash out and dilute the inoculum and any other foreign material, together with excision of any devitalized tissue; and

- inhibition of bacterial cell division by the use of antibiotics. The principle of prophylaxis is to give large doses of appropriate antibiotics as soon after the injury as possible, and to continue them for only a short period.

The organisms that are most likely to cause infection after open wounds are *S. aureus*, *Pseudomonas aeruginosa*, clostridia and anaerobes, such as *Bacteroides*.

Case 11.1 Acute osteomyelitis: 6

Case note: Progress

Simon became free from pain 3 days after treatment commenced. He was discharged from hospital and his mother was told that the antibiotic treatment with flucloxacillin must continue, with regular dosage, between meals, for the next 2 weeks. He has not had any further problems. In view of his good progress, assessed clinically, no further investigations were performed, as they were unlikely to influence any therapeutic or prognostic decisions.

Case 11.2 Septic arthritis: 4

Case note: Progress

Sylvia did not fare as well as Simon. She continued to have some pain in her knee, and the swelling persisted. She had a further arthroscopic lavage, and it was found that there was very little articular cartilage remaining on her medial femoral and tibial condyles (from her osteoarthritis, although more may have been lost because of the infection). The surgeon told her that she could not have total knee replacement surgery as the risk of a prosthesis becoming infected was high, in view of her recent acute septic arthritis. Remember that the presence of a foreign body decreases the local tissue defences against infecting organisms, and a small inoculum of bacteria may then cause an infection, even with organisms of low virulence or pathogenicity.

If fractures are treated by internal fixation, bacteria may adhere to the foreign surface and surround themselves with a slime (called glycocalyx), which can prevent the penetration of antibiotics in to the bacterial colonies. Such colonies may remain dormant for long periods and emerge as acute infections when the general state of the patient, nutritionally or by disease or change in immunity, alters. It is also inevitable that bone death occurs at the site of fracture, because of the disruption of blood supply. Removal of such dead bone in the evolution of fracture healing requires considerable osteoclast activity over a long period. Some of the dead bone (sequestrum) may become incorporated into the fracture repair callus and new living bone, but act as a nidus for infection at a future date.

Joint replacement surgery has been a great advance in treatment for arthritis during the last 30 years. The surgery of joint replacement requires the excision of considerable amounts of bone adjacent to the joint in order to insert a prosthesis. The prostheses used are manufactured from several different materials—metals, high-density polyethylene, ceramics and polymethyl methacrylate as a bone cement. Such foreign material can act as a repository for bacterial colonies inevitably introduced during the surgical operation. Furthermore, wear particles from the articulating surfaces may affect the way phagocytic cells function. Infection may occur in up to 2% of patients who have joint replacement. The effect is chronic osteomyelitis for which the prosthesis may have to be removed (Fig. 11.9). Antibiotic prophylaxis should be given for joint replacement surgery, using the same principles as for open fractures.

Chronic osteomyelitis

Chronic osteomyelitis is a significant health problem with substantial morbidity but low mortality. Whether it arises from acute haematogenous infection, after trauma, or following an implant, the general principles of management are identical. There is no guarantee that cure can ever be achieved, so suppression is probably a better concept. Recurrences can occur a very long time after the initial infection.

Staphylococcus aureus remains the most common isolate, reflecting the acute infection that initiated the process. In many parts of the world, particularly where there is malnutrition, overcrowding or poverty, tuberculosis is endemic. *M. tuberculosis* reaches bones and joints by haematogenous spread, stimulating chronic inflammation, which has a different pathological pattern from that of acute inflammation but a similar association of destruction and repair of tissues. In chronic inflammation, the onset of pain is gradual rather than sudden and its severity is less intense. However, the inflammation has frequently been present for a long period before treatment is sought and irreversible structural changes may have occurred in the bones and joints involved.

The fundamental problem is the persistence of organisms. The pathological anatomy reflects the consequences

Case 11.3 — Chronic infection: 1

Case history

Stewart loved his motorcycle. When he was 18 he crashed it at high speed and sustained a comminuted open fracture of his right tibia. He was taken to the nearest district hospital where he was treated without delay by the administration of an antibiotic, surgical toilet of the open wound and insertion of an intramedullary nail to internally fix the fracture after it had been realigned to an almost anatomical position. Some 10 days after his accident, his temperature rose to 39°C and there was a serous discharge from the wound. A specimen of the discharge was taken for culture, and antibiotic medication was recommenced; 10 days later he was allowed to go home, as he was feeling well. He is now 20 and has not been able to return to work as an apprentice plumber. He has continuing mild discomfort from his right leg, particularly when bearing weight. He had to use crutches for 9 months, as plain radiography did not show healing of the fracture. Every 2 or 3 months he has an acute exacerbation of pain in his tibia, a feeling of being unwell, and discharge of a small amount of pus from his shin. After taking antibiotics for a few days, he generally feels better and the pain decreases. He is now concerned that his orthopaedic surgeon might suggest that his leg be amputated below the knee (Fig. 11.8).

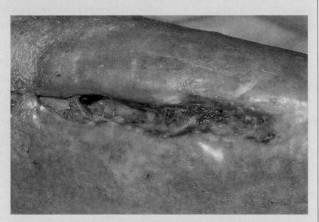

Fig. 11.8 The state of Stewart's leg on one of the occasions when he had an exacerbation of pain and purulent discharge. Note the redness and swelling of acute inflammation of the skin, the ulceration of the skin because of necrosis, and in the base of the ulcer the coagulated slough of dead tissue and pus lying on exposed bone. When bone is allowed to dry like that, it dies and acts as a reservoir for bacteria. Such dead bone is called sequestrum, and it is essential that it be removed before healing can occur. Dead bone cannot contribute to the fracture-healing process.

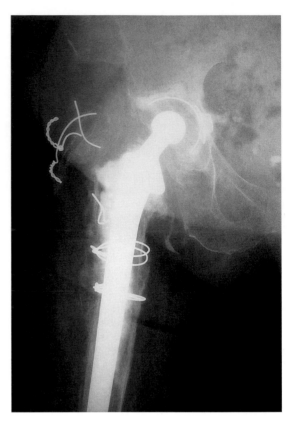

Fig. 11.9 Plain radiograph of infected hip prosthesis.

Case 11.3 — Chronic infection: 2

Case note: Prognosis

Until all dead and foreign tissue has been removed, the risk of such exacerbations of infection always remains in cases of chronic osteomyelitis. This is the most likely reason why Stewart has had a 'flare-up' of infection in his leg. If Stewart is left with an ununited fracture of his tibia and an intermittent or continually discharging sinus, he may never regain normal function of his limb. The potential for chronic infection was caused by his open fracture in the first instance. The severity of disruption of the tissues at the time of the initial trauma is a major determinant of outcome. The incidence of chronic osteomyelitis after open fracture may be as high as 10%.

of continuing necrosis and repair. Dead bone that has become detached from surrounding living bone is called *sequestrum*. The accumulation of pus in the tissues is an abscess, and a sinus is a track from the depths of a tissue to the exterior, usually made by the passage of pus. Reactive new bone is called an *involucrum*. The balance between necrosis and repair determines the outcome; the aim of management is to tip the balance in favour of the host.

Diagnosis of chronic bone and joint infections

If the mouth of a discharging sinus is sampled to obtain a specimen, a diverse mixture of organisms may be cultured. Most of them are likely to be commensals which have

Table 11.1 Relation of radiological signs to pathology in chronic infections

Pathological process	Radiological sign
Oedema	Soft tissue swelling; obliteration of tissue planes
Medullary infection	Osteopenia and lysis of cortical bone
Cortical infection	Cortical lucency and lysis
Subperiosteal abscess	Periosteal new bone, involucrum
Soft tissue abscess	Soft tissue swelling; obliteration of tissue planes
Localized cortical and medullary abscess	Single or multiple radiolucent cortical or medullary lytic lesions with surrounding sclerosis
Cortical necrosis	Sequestration of bone
Fistula	Migration of cortical fragments

colonized the superficial tissue; only tissue specimens from the depths of a sinus, or blood cultures, are useful in identifying the true causative organism in chronic osteomyelitis. Vertebral osteomyelitis is not usually associated with a sinus, so a biopsy, which can be done by a trephine or needle using radiological monitoring, is an important part of the diagnostic process. Plain radiography is usually sufficient to make a diagnosis of chronic osteomyelitis (Table 11.1).

If further detail is required, computerized tomography and sometimes magnetic resonance imaging may be helpful. A sinus can be delineated by injection of a radiological contrast agent along its track, or at the time of surgery by injecting a coloured dye, such as gentian violet. Any tissue sample removed should be subjected to histological examination to seek features of infection. That may be the only direct evidence.

Management of chronic infection

The principles of management of chronic infection of bones and joints, regardless of aetiology or the site of infection, are:

- correct and complete microbiological diagnosis
- assessment and modification of host defence mechanisms
- anatomical definition of the extent of local disease in bone and soft tissues
- correct antibiotic therapy
- surgical removal of necrotic and poorly vascularized tissue and all infected granulation
- obliteration of dead spaces left by the surgical debridement
- restoration of stability of the skeleton to allow function
- rehabilitation.

Case 11.4   Tuberculous osteomyelitis: 1

Case history

Sachin was born in Cambodia and had grown up during the civil war in that country. At the age of 36 she had been granted emigration rights. As part of the immigration process she had undergone a medical examination, and had a chest X-ray examination. She was found to be healthy. Two years after re-establishing her family life in another country she had consulted a medical practitioner who spoke her native language, because of pain in her back. She had not sustained any injury that she could recall. The pain was not related to her menstrual periods. It was a constant dull ache that was progressively becoming more severe. She had not experienced a fever. She had lost a little weight. Examination showed her to stand with a slight scoliosis of her thoracolumbar region and she had lost the normally expected rhythmic pattern of movement of her back when she was asked to bend forwards. She had an area of impaired light touch sensation on the anterior aspect of her left thigh. Her left knee jerk reflex was slightly less prominent than the right. You will recall from Chapter 4 that these neurological abnormalities would constitute a so-called 'red flag'. Moreover, the report of the X-ray examination of her back stated 'infection should be excluded'.

Case 11.4   Tuberculous osteomyelitis: 2

Case note: Diagnosis

The spine is a more frequent site for tuberculous osteomyelitis than acute osteomyelitis. The destructive effects are on intervertebral discs as well as bone, leading to potential impairment of spinal cord function because of structural and mechanical deformity of the spine. In Sachin's case, it was the characteristic loss of the intervertebral disc height between two vertebrae that alerted the radiologist to make the comment about the possibility of infection. Regardless of the infecting organism, the structural changes in bones and joints are similar. It is essential to identify the causative organisms before commencing treatment.

There are limited indications for surgery:

- significant disability for the patient's lifestyle or general health
- appropriate patient expectations and commitment to multiple surgeries and prolonged treatment
- prior stabilization of systemic disease (including cessation of cigarette smoking)
- adequate local conditions (skin, blood supply) in the affected limb
- technical feasibility of any planned reconstruction.

Case 11.4 Tuberculous osteomyelitis: 3

Case note: Pathology

Osteomyelitis of the spine destroys intervertebral discs and parts of the adjacent vertebrae so that an angular deformity, or kyphus, results. The hunchback of Notre Dame probably had tuberculosis. The vertebrae usually fuse together when the infection is controlled. The level of the spine infected determines whether spinal cord dysfunction may follow as a result of the cord being stretched over the kyphus. In the lumbar region, nerve roots occupy the spinal canal and are less vulnerable to stretch. Pus from the infection may, however, enter the spinal canal and produce an extradural abscess with nerve root or spinal cord dysfunction. This may explain the abnormal neurological findings in Sachin's case.

If a vertebral body is affected, the pus may track forwards causing a paravertebral abscess. In the lumbar region such an abscess frequently enters the substance of the psoas muscle(s) and tracks down to the groin within the psoas sheath, leading to a 'cold abscess' in the groin when the sinus breaks through the skin. Chronic osteomyelitis in a long bone may lead to pathological fracture of that bone—if that occurs, the fracture may not unite.

The use of antibiotics may be an alternative to suppress the disease. Usually a prolonged course is not necessary, although short courses (6 weeks) may have to be repeated from time to time. However, in tuberculosis, antituberculous antibiotics, given as multiple drug combinations, are usually effective in controlling, and eradicating the disease after about 9 months' administration.

Further reading

Gillespie, W.J., Nade, S., 1987. Musculoskeletal Infections. Melbourne, Blackwell.

Norden, C., Gillespie, W.J., Nade, S., 1994. Infections in Bones and Joints. Boston, Blackwell.

Parsch, K., Nade, S. Infections in bones and joints. In: Benson, M.K.D., Fixsen, J., Macnicol, M.F., Parsch, K. (Eds.), Children's Orthopaedics and Fractures, third ed. (in press).

alopecia – excessive loss of hair.

ankylosis – when the joint becomes stiff or fused in a particular position.

arthropathy – pathology in a joint, but sometimes used as a generic term for arthritis.

arthroplasty – surgery to a joint to modify its surface or structure including joint replacement.

arthrotomy – surgical incision of a joint capsule.

autoantibody – an antibody directed against self-components.

bursa – a 'cushioning' sac, lined by synovium and normally containing a small amount of synovial fluid, lying between areas of friction to allow opposing surfaces to slide smoothly against each other.

capsulitis – inflammation of the outer lining of the joint, i.e. the joint capsule.

chondrocyte – principal cartilage cell responsible for synthesis of extracellular matrix.

condyle – a rounded protuberance that occurs at the ends of some bones.

crepitus – grating sound elicited on moving a joint.

cyclooxygenase – an enzyme responsible for synthesis of prostaglandins and thromboxanes.

cytokine – polypeptides which act non-enzymatically and regulate host cell function.

denervation – interruption of the nerve supply to muscles or skin.

depolarization – the sudden surge of charged particles across the membrane of a nerve or muscle cell.

dermatome – the skin segment of the body supplied by a given spinal nerve.

diaphysis – the shaft of a long bone.

dislocation – disruption of a joint such that the normally opposing joint surfaces have no contact with each other.

effusion – excessive synovial fluid accumulation within the joint cavity.

enthesopathy – inflammation at site of tendinous insertion into bone.

epicondyle – the protuberance above a condyle.

epiphysis – the end of the long bone beyond the growth plate leading up to the joint surface.

erosion – localized loss of integrity of the articular surface, usually due to invasion by inflamed synovium.

fracture – a structural break in the continuity of bone.

glomerulonephritis – inflammation of the glomerulus of the kidney.

glycosaminoglycan – complex polysaccharides consisting of long chains of sugar molecules attached to an amino group.

haemarthrosis – blood within synovial cavity.

haplotype – the particular combination in any individual of specific HLA gene alleles.

histocompatibility antigen – a white blood cell marker determined by certain genes important in transplant graft acceptance or rejection; sometimes called HLA (human leukocyte antigen).

humoral – refers to the 'fluid' component of blood, as opposed to circulating cells.

immunosuppression – suppression of immune system, usually by drugs.

intima – the inner layer of the wall of a tissue such as the synovium.

labrum – a lip like structure around the margins of joint.

malar – a rash over the facial cheeks typically seen in systemic lupus erythematosus.

meniscus – fibrocartilaginous discs that divide the cavity of certain synovial joints.

mesangium – the part of the glomerulus comprised of phagocytic cells and extracellular matrix.

metalloproteinases – a family of enzymes which contain a metal atom in their structure and can degrade cartilage and other connective tissues.

metaphysis – the flare of a long bone towards the joint.

monarthritis – joint inflammation involving only one joint.

myopathy – a disorder of skeletal muscle.

nociception – the sensation of pain.

oligoarthritis – joint inflammation involving less than six joints.

open fracture – a fracture where the overlying skin is breached, allowing communication between the fracture and the outside.

osteoblast – the cell responsible for bone formation.

osteoclast – the cell responsible for bone resorption.

pathogenicity – ability to cause pathology (disease).

pathological fracture – a fracture caused by normal force in abnormal bone.

periarticular – occurring 'near the joint'.

physis – the growth plate in a long bone.

polyarthritis – joint inflammation involving six or more joints.

proteoglycan – large molecules made up of glycosaminoglycans linked to the proteins.

radiculopathy – pathology involving a spinal nerve root.

serositis – inflammation of the lining surface of the heart (pericarditis), lungs (pleuritis) or abdomen (peritonitis).

spondyloarthritis – inflammation involving spinal joints.

spondylosis – degeneration affecting the intervertebral discs.

stress fracture – a fracture caused by repetitive 'normal' forces.

subluxation – disruption of a joint such that the normally opposing joint surfaces have some partial contact with each other.

synovectomy – removal of synovium either by surgery or by treatment with radioactive isotopes.

synovium – a normal thin layer of tissue within the joint that produces synovial fluid.

tendonitis – inflammation of a tendon.

tophus – collection of sodium urate crystals in tissues.

valgus – a deformity that displaces the distal part of a joint away from midline.

varus – a deformity that displaces the distal part of a joint towards the midline.

vasculitis – inflammation of blood vessels.

Index